A NEW PRESCRIPTION FOR WOMEN'S HEALTH

A NEW PRESCRIPTION FOR WOMEN'S HEALTH

BERNADINE HEALY, M.D.

Getting
the Best Medical Care
in a Man's World

VIKING

VIKING
Published by the Penguin Group
Penguin Books USA Inc., 375 Hudson Street, New York, New York 10014, U.S.A.
Penguin Books Ltd, 27 Wrights Lane, London W8 5TZ, England
Penguin Books Australia Ltd, Ringwood, Victoria, Australia
Penguin Books Canada Ltd, 10 Alcorn Avenue, Toronto, Ontario, Canada M4V 3B2
Penguin Books (N.Z.) Ltd, 182–190 Wairau Road, Auckland 10, New Zealand

Penguin Books Ltd, Registered Offices: Harmondsworth, Middlesex, England

First published in 1995 by Viking Penguin, a division of Penguin Books USA Inc.

10   9   8   7   6   5   4   3   2   1

A NOTE TO THE READER
A New Prescription for Women's Health sets forth current information and opinions on subjects related to women's health. It is not the intent of the author to diagnose or prescribe. Various medications described herein can only be prescribed by a physician. While issues covered in this book have been checked with sources believed to be reliable, some material may be affected by developments and discoveries in the medical field made after the manuscript for this book was completed. This book is not intended as a substitute for medical treatment by a physician; the reader should regularly consult a physician in matters relating to health.

The names and identifying features of the patients discussed in this book have been changed.

Grateful acknowledgment is made for permission to use the following works: Adaptation of an extract from *Good Fat, Bad Fat, How to Lower Your Cholesterol & Beat the Odds of a Heart Attack* by Glen C. Griffin and William P. Castelli, Fisher Books, Tucson, AZ, © 1989. By permission of the publisher. "Sorrow" by Edna St. Vincent Millay, from *Collected Poems*, HarperCollins. "The Courage That My Mother Had" by Edna St. Vincent Millay. From *Collected Poems*, HarperCollins. Copyright © 1954, 1982 by Norma Millay Ellis. Reprinted by permission of Elizabeth Barnett, literary executor. Table on pages 53–54 adapted from *Diet and Health: Implications for Reducing Chronic Disease Risk*, National Research Council. Copyright 1989 by the National Academy of Sciences. By permission of the National Academy Press, Washington, D.C.

LIBRARY OF CONGRESS CATALOGING IN PUBLICATION DATA
Healy, Bernadine, M.D.
A new prescription for women's health : Getting the best
medical care in a man's world / Bernadine Healy, M.D.
    p.   cm.
    Includes index.
    ISBN 0-670-85550-2
1. Women—Health and hygiene.   I. Title.
RA778.H4445   1995
613'.04244—dc20   95-10719

This book is printed on acid-free paper.

Printed in the United States of America
Set in Sabon
Designed by Katy Riegel

To my husband, Dr. Floyd D. Loop,
my love, my limerence, and my haven

ACKNOWLEDGMENTS

The many women who came before me, the energetic women who are now my contemporaries, and the new generation of young women who are just now coming along all share a fate on matters of health and quality of life. Together we all yearn to know more about our health. I acknowledge all of these women for being the inspiration for this book, and for many of the better things I have accomplished in my first fifty years.

There is no doubt that the concrete idea for this book came out of my time as director of the National Institutes of Health, that glorious federal institution established more than one hundred years ago with the sole purpose of improving and safeguarding the health of every American. There I found friends and colleagues who helped me focus daily on the many and vital priorities for medical research, and who informed me and prepared me for endless hearings and meetings in a wide range of science and medical arenas. This daily work included our several initiatives on women's health and making women's health research a national priority.

I am honored to officially thank those who were the backbone of the NIH with me at the time, in particular Jay Moskowitz, my "strategic" and creative deputy, and the enthusiastic and energetic John

Diggs and Lance Liotta; and the many others who do so much for so many, including William Harlan, Vivian Pinn, Darla Danford, John Ruffin, Mary Chunko, and Kendra Dimond; Jack Mahoney, Leslie Platt, Diane Armstrong, Linda McCleaf, Dixie Kanagy, Kim Kurilla-Gray, Charlette Bronson, and Shirley Everest; two physicians and women's health advocates of the Department of Health and Human Services, Secretary Louis Sullivan and Assistant Secretary James Mason; the institute directors, including Sam Broder, Anthony Fauci, Claude Lenfant, Carl Kupfer, Don Lindberg, Kenneth Olden, Francis Collins, Ada Sue Hinshaw, Duane Alexander, and the many others who worked so well together when it really mattered. My heartfelt thanks to Johanna Schneider, who taught me that you need to communicate well if you are ever to have an impact. Although this book was written after I left the NIH, the spark that lit the fire ignited in Bethesda.

In this book I hold a conversation with women as I would with an individual patient, trying to convey what I think they need to know, sometimes straying into the technical, but only because it is so important or the information so powerful and elegant. I thank all my patients through the years, men and women alike, who gave me an understanding of what we are all looking for as we enter a doctor's office.

As a specialist in heart disease but a generalist in medicine, I also am most appreciative of the detailed review of individual chapters by a distinguished array of Cleveland Clinic Foundation specialty physicians and other experts, including Drs. Jerome Belinson, Elliot Philipson, Susan Rehm, Gita Gidwani, Beth Ann Overmoyer, Ronald Bukowski, Maurie Markman, George Tesar, Eric Topol, Fetnat Fouad, Fredric Pashkow, Vinod Sahgal, Jeffrey Frank, Anthony Furlan, Angelo Licata, Martin Gorbien, and Cynthia Moore. Also thanks to Susan Finn of Ross Laboratories and president of the American Dietetic Association. I valued and relied on their reviews and re-reviews of selected chapters, and I thank them for their comments and their time.

I warmly appreciate those who read all or parts of the proposal or manuscript from a woman's perspective, with a reader's eye, including my mother, Violet; my husband's mother, Marie; my teenage daughter, Bartlett; my sweet twenty-something friend and baby-sitter, Stacie Kreisher; my ever-present distant supporters, Mary Foy and Isabelle MacGregor; and my dear, all too generous, local critics, Sehan Soylu, Pat Modell, Maria Miller, Norma Lerner, and Suzanne Timken. And, with a man's eye, my special advisor, Floyd Loop.

Gail Ross has been a continuous source of encouragement and

advice, the book agent who is always there and in touch with each page and each thought, and prodding with good cheer. Nan Graham, a graceful force and my first editor at Viking, introduced me to the impressive and enthusiastic Viking team, including Courtney Hodell, who faithfully read every word and queried endlessly and wonderfully; Mindy Werner, my strong yet gentle editor; the warm and witty Cathy Hemming; and Viking's new publisher, Barbara Grossman. Early in the effort, Carol Cohan and Robert (Mac) Overmyer assisted me in background research and thinking for several chapters. Jody Rein became my literary coach, advisor, and pal, nurturing this project chapter by chapter, while at the same time nurturing her firstborn, Peter Tobias, trimester by trimester. Peter and I were both fortunate to have her in on our early development.

On the Cleveland front I was helped by the enthusiasms and hard work of Kathy Vaughn and Valerie Stump, by Lynn Berner's scholarly commentary, and by the sharp research and editorial eye of my indispensable Christine Kassuba.

Although he is not here now, I must thank my late father, Michael Healy, for always being there to push me on to do what seemed too hard to do, to inspire and to encourage, and never to lose faith in me or his three other daughters, Suellen, Michelle, and Catherine. Mom, always his soul mate, has carried on his sturdy involvement and always manages to be there. I thank both my parents from the depths of my heart.

And in the nest, I thank my ever-supportive family, who tolerated a house full of reprints, journals, books, papers, archive boxes, computers, faxes, and phone calls with such love and kindness. Sometimes it was not easy for them, as my eight-year old, Marie, recently made clear to me when she said, "Mom, I don't mind if you run for the Senate again, but please don't write another book!" Marie, Bartlett, Floyd, thanks for being there with me in all my adventures.

CONTENTS

A NEW PRESCRIPTION FOR WOMEN'S HEALTH

ONE

TURNING POINTS

*Throughout the ages, the problem of women
has puzzled people of every kind.*

— SIGMUND FREUD,
IN A LETTER TO HIS STUDENT
MARIE BONAPARTE, 1933

I'm a woman and a cardiologist. Generally, when someone with heart trouble finds his or her way into my office and sees that I'm a woman, nothing happens. There is no reaction. With rare exceptions my patients, who are far more concerned with their own health than they are with my sex, treat me with the same deference and respect they would, I imagine, afford any other professional caretaker.

I, on the other hand, place a great deal of emphasis on the sex of my patients, as do most physicians today. I do so because the reactions of a woman's body to both illnesses and remedies are often vastly different from those of a man's, and gender is therefore a critical consideration in any responsible analysis of a patient's condition and in the choice of recommended treatment.

Does this seem like common sense? To me, such thinking borders on the miraculous; I do not for a moment take for granted either the medical world's recognition of the biological differences between the sexes or my patients' easy acceptance of being treated by a woman doctor. These understandings are the flip sides of a freshly minted coin—the coin of the unequivocal acceptance of women in society, each woman valued according to her worth without prejudice. The attitudes underlying the seemingly mundane interactions I experience as a woman physician are critical to the health and well-being of all women. These attitudes are also new to our culture; for many reasons they are quite tenuous and in urgent need of attention and nurturing in order to become permanent personal and societal visions. It is for this reason I have written this book.

We are in a time of transition. Today's quiet battle for accurate and responsible health care for women marks the third phase in our campaign for equal rights and opportunities. Less than a hundred years ago, thousands of women—Republican and Democrat, rich and poor, accomplished and uneducated, professional and unskilled—joined together to demand the right to vote. With the achievement of that right, women won a voice—but not admittance. The second phase of this women's campaign has lasted for about thirty years. With the new goal of personal advancement, women swelled the ranks of universities and professional schools—whether they were wanted or not—and then claimed their economic rights, becoming scientists and engineers, bankers and corporate executives, lawyers and judges, senators and governors. Women sought equality—perhaps at the expense of personal identity, as many felt the need to deny the value of gender differences in order to achieve our overall goals in the workforce.

Regaining that identity is the goal of this perhaps final stage in women's struggle for true equality. Thanks to the monumental efforts of women over the last one hundred years, we can vote, as men can, and we can work, as men can. Now our cause is more subtle. We must be seen clearly both as women and as individuals of value who deserve attention not only for our differences from men but also for those qualities that we share with men. And we must see ourselves in this same light, treating our mental, emotional, and physical selves with attentiveness and respect. Nowhere are these attitudes more critical than in the care of our health.

A woman's sense of herself, her degree of personal power, her ability to use her talents in society are all tightly linked to her overall health and well-being. When women demand equal care, we declare our equal capacity to contribute fully to society. A woman who sees herself as only a child bearer and child-rearer sometimes minimizes her own value when her nest empties. A woman who aims for success in the working world by attempting to be the same as a man diminishes her power by denying her own substance.

But when we learn about and value our bodies, we become truly powerful. If a woman envisions herself living well into her tenth decade, as all women should, and being a continuing force in the lives of her family and community, she will be concerned about her long-term mental and physical health. A woman who says with conviction, "My health is worth fighting for" is saying "*I* am worth fighting for."

THE CAUTION OF HISTORY

> *Women are already the equals of men in the whole realm of thought, in art, science, literature and government. The poetry and novels of the century are theirs, and they have touched the keynote of reform, in religion, politics, and social life. They fill the editor's and professor's chair, plead at the bar of justice, walk the wards of the hospital, speak from the pulpit and the platform. Such is the type of womanhood that an enlightened public sentiment welcomes today, and such the triumph of the facts of life over the false theories of the past.*

> —*ELIZABETH CADY STANTON, 1892*

Elizabeth Cady Stanton was a brilliant speaker and writer. However, her optimistic interpretation of the position of women in her society was clearly premature, although the first admittance of women into a few professional schools and the first blooming of the feminist movement convinced her otherwise. In our own times we've seen a tremendous awakening to the importance of women's health, and as a result we've made enormous advances. Now life is easier for us, woman patient and woman physician alike. Nonetheless, I'm concerned that we won't be able to make the advances of the present stick without an awareness of the past. As a New York cabbie said to me recently, "Hey, doc, don't ever forget where ya come from."

OUR NOT SO DISTANT MEDICAL PAST

The Victorians of nineteenth-century America placed woman on a pedestal and situated that pedestal firmly within the home. The uterus was the holy of holies in the Victorian cult of motherhood; childbearing and -rearing were considered a woman's ultimate—and only—worthwhile contributions to society. For physicians of the time, "women's health" meant one thing: maternal health. In fact, one esteemed physician writing in 1882 expressed the opinion that the "Almighty, in creating the female sex, [has] taken the uterus and built up a woman around it."

This kind of thinking led to the passage of the so-called Comstock laws, meant to stamp out obscenity. In 1873 Congress explicitly banned the transport of every article, written material, or "thing" that would prevent conception, induce abortions, or be used for "immoral purpose." Ironically, the twentieth century's crusade for women's rights began in response to the dismal state of women's health resulting from these laws and out of the recognition that women's health problems were tied to the political disenfranchisement of women. It was not a coincidence that early feminist Margaret Sanger was an obstetrical nurse working in poor areas of New York City at the turn of the century. She saw women and their children suffering in poverty, mothers and their infants dying in a plague of unhealthy and unwanted maternity, desperate women suffering the consequences of botched illegal abortions and the ravages of sexually transmitted diseases (about which most women knew little or nothing and, in fact, whose very existence was often kept secret from women).

Threads of the kind of thinking that outraged the suffragettes have wound their way around medical research and thought throughout much of this century. We'll see in specific instances throughout this book that the Victorians, followed by the Freudians, and much of the modern medical profession for too many years, believed that women are naturally hysterical and hypochondriacal. Because of this misconception, women have often been deprived of definitive diagnosis and treatment. Just as harmful was the overzealous Victorian-bred consensus that women and their unborn must be protected from harm, resulting in the banishment of women from many medical studies. Until very recently, research on diseases, drugs, even human growth and development, continued to use men as the standard from which we can extrapolate what is normal. This was not done with malice, but reflexively, without a thought that there could be another way. Women's health concerns—menopause, female cancers, osteoporosis, for example—got short shrift. All these factors resulted in a deficit of information about women's health and about important gender differences in health as well as disease.

Women themselves were in no position to remedy this situation. It was not until the end of the nineteenth century that they were grudgingly allowed to enter the medical profession, and then they were restricted in their areas of practice, and were seen as unwelcome oddities by both men and women patients.

Dr. Helen Taussig brought home to me rather vividly the difficulties women faced only a generation or so ago. When as a young woman she had applied to medical school, she was turned down by Harvard; they were unwilling to accept female applicants. Later she wanted to intern in medicine at Harvard but was again refused. Her father, a prominent Harvard economist, advised her to continue at Hopkins; "Stay where you are wanted," he said. Johns Hopkins allowed her to stay, but only to study pediatrics. On the assumption that as a woman she'd make an ideal baby-sitter, she was given responsibility for the most difficult and hopeless of patients, the "blue babies."

After years of caring for these previously incurable babies, she designed a blood vessel operation to create a "shunt" that would redirect blood into the lungs and turn these little infants instantly from blue to pink. She was not a surgeon, however, so she needed a collaborator who had the training and experience. She visited the famous vascular surgeon Robert Gross of Harvard Medical School, who dismissed her ideas in no uncertain terms; he closed shunts and was not going to help her make them. With great persistence, she convinced Dr. Alfred Blalock of Johns Hopkins to try her innovation in 1944, and the Blalock-Taussig operation was born. Her work not only ushered in congenital heart surgery but paved the way for all open-heart surgery.

By the time I met her in the mid-1970s she was a physician world renowned for devising the "blue-baby" operation and for other accomplishments.

Helen was a gracious and grandmotherly woman, but it was with a still-wounded conviction that she told me this story. Her anger welled into amusement as she remembered the day Harvard finally called, to award her an honorary degree—after she had been heaped with awards and feted worldwide and was named the first woman president of the American Heart Association. When she accepted this highest of Harvard honors, she told all that she viewed this as a degree issued through the back door. She let none present forget she had been turned down by Harvard three times earlier when she knocked on the front door.

A PERSONAL AND MORE RECENT PAST

I was born in 1944. I remember when women, especially widows, were seen as helpless dependents or as unwelcome outsiders. I remember the schools and clubs and scholarships that were open to men only—including Yale, Harvard, Princeton, virtually every downtown business club, and of course the Rhodes scholarship.

In 1964 I applied to medical school and was invited to my first interview—the beginning of my medical career and my introduction to the world of coeducation. It's hard to express the meaning this encounter held for me and the strangeness of it. I had attended all-girl schools and a women's college up to that point, and I was raised in a family of four sisters. I had encountered only encouragement for my dreams and plans for my future career.

In this interview I ran head-on into the way the world of the sixties operated. The man interviewing me held a powerful position—he helped determine who would be admitted into one of the top medical schools in the country. At the time, while colleges were filled with women who wanted to train as physicians, the medical schools maintained an unofficial "quota"—they admitted as few women as possible, and those women who did get in had to be much more qualified than any male candidate. My interviewer obviously felt that even this unspoken quota was too high. He asked me little about my scholastic interests or future plans, but he did want to know more about my mother: Was she menopausal and therefore frustrated? Had she inspired my clearly deviant life choice? Was my neurosis caused by the fact that my parents hadn't graduated from high school?

I rebelled against these attitudes by withdrawing my application from that interviewer's school, but only *after* I was accepted to other medical schools. At Harvard I was to face similar attitudes from some faculty members and fellow students. The standard of the time, continuing throughout my internship at Johns Hopkins, can be summed up in the words of a resident who—after frantically working with me for more than an hour to save a desperately ill patient—studied my blood-soaked clothes, face, and hair and said: "You shouldn't be here doing this. You should be at home with a husband and children. This job is not for a woman. What's wrong with you?"

We women ignored the jabs, the lecturers who showed slides of naked women in distinctly nonmedical positions to lighten up a discussion, and the comments that disparaged female patients. We didn't take issue with the attitude that we were oddities and outsiders, invading a world that inalienably belonged to men, because we were grateful to be there.

By the time I became a full professor at Johns Hopkins in the early eighties, I felt neither wounded nor grateful—I felt quite secure in my knowledge and in the correctness of being exactly where I was. In fact, I felt like stirring up some trouble. The school at the time had been running its age-old, males-only medical school rite of spring, the Pithotomy show, staged by the all-male Pithotomy Club. This collection of comedy skits, fully condoned by many devoted faculty advisors, was supposedly about life at Hopkins and life in medicine. But unlike many mildly ribald comedy skits, which roast people with good humor, the celebration of Pithotomy was a mean-spirited, X-rated orgy. As one commentator, Malcolm Gladwell of the *Washington Post*, analyzed it several years later: "The show . . . was a bonding ritual for male students and faculty, a chance for the once and future elite of American medicine to gather for obscene songs and skits, get drunk, and then—because the club had only one toilet—urinate together in the alleyway next door. F. Scott Fitzgerald immortalized the 'Pit' in a short story. H. L. Mencken said the only time he had seen something cruder was in a show put on by sailors in London."

Originally, the skits were by and about men. Over time, however, the show began to target women medical students and physicians, who were not off-limits the way a mother, sister, or wife would have been. I never liked the idea of this juvenile rite, and I was plenty vocal about my feelings. Finally, perhaps in retaliation for my well-known disapproval of the all-male club and its activities, I was made a "star" of the show, with no apparent limits on the sexual fantasies acted out at my expense by a student in drag. I couldn't see where pornography fit into a med school curriculum, particularly when made so medical and so personal.

I decided to give the club a scare. I wrote a legal-seeming letter asking for the names of all club members and put my lawyer sister's name on the bottom of the page. The boys ended up quite contrite and apologetic, but to my surprise, many faculty members, including several of the deans, implored me to recognize how important the club was to student life and student-faculty rapport—male student, that is. I was supposed to be consoled by the fact that students were afraid to wear their Pithotomy ties for fear that I would recognize them as members of the exclusive club. This was in 1984.

The issue, of course, got resolved; I would not sue their club, and the show would be canceled until it was cleaned up. It was later reopened, and the club and the show now admit women. What I took away from this experience (besides a bit of embarrassment about the show and my perhaps overblown reaction to it) was a deep understanding of the impact of the attitude of the teacher on the student, the society on the individual, the parent on the child, and the mentor on the protégé.

While those future doctors were being rewarded by their teachers for expressing their interesting attitudes toward women, the actual medical training of both male and female students wasn't doing much to enhance their understanding of a woman's physiological and psychological needs. Although some change from the medical viewpoint inherited from the Victorians was certainly under way in the sixties and the seventies, the profession's inadequate attention to the broader issues of women's health nonetheless pervaded my medical training and the bulk of the early years of my practice. You'll find many allusions throughout this text to what we were and weren't taught. Yes, there were distinctly sexist practices: women patients were typically addressed by their first name and men by their last; we were taught that women should bear their children before the age of twenty-five to maximize the health of both mother and child. If they delayed, they were selfish, and as a punishment would develop a painful and scarring disease of the pelvis called endometriosis, which brought the additional penalty of decreased fertility. But mostly the teachings were couched in the cultural truism of the time: a man's body is the normative standard; a woman's is the deviant. *Women's health* still meant *maternal health* only.

This thinking lies behind the men-only studies with which you may already be familiar: studies of estrogen and heart attacks conducted only in men, of aspirin and mortality only in men, of vitamins and cancer only in men, of cholesterol only in men, and so forth. The results of these studies have been released to the media as if the findings applied to both men and women and have been taught as gospel in medical schools. Some pharmaceutical companies marketed mainly to men; women were viewed as a "niche" market.

AND TODAY?

It's sometimes hard for me to absorb how far we've come in so little time. The very meaning of the term *women's health* has been transformed as much as women's roles; no longer does it imply only a Pap smear and a breast check.

At long last, the "problem of women," as Sigmund Freud put it, has become a national priority. September has been designated Women's Health Month, and President Clinton mentioned women's health research as a national priority in his 1994 State of the Union address; numerous governors made women's health issues major parts of their reelection platforms in 1994. As if responding to a clarion call, major medical centers are now establishing special programs in women's health that include the wide array of medical concerns confronting women of all ages, not just reproductive health. Women themselves are becoming more assertive in their expectations of their personal physicians and the health care system. The number of women in medicine is growing exponentially, and the sight of a female doctor no longer causes a double take—or even a blink.

The cause of today's sudden shift has everything to do with the women's movement begun in the sixties. Women are now in positions of power—in the media, in government, throughout the workforce and even in the medical profession itself. I believe it was outrage that caused this critical mass to explode into action. When it became known that the medical studies mentioned above were in fact tested only in men, women's collective and forceful outcry prompted a national awakening. The passion was present from the ground up!

Further, in 1988, as president of the American Heart Association, I was able to initiate a nationwide campaign against heart disease in women—not because I had the support of the skeptical, mostly male board of directors, but because AHA volunteers (90 percent women) ran with the concept by the thousands. The mainstream media, with their large population of women writers and producers, would not let the issues disappear, and women in Congress took up the cause. Perhaps the ultimate sign: I now hear men ask, "But what about men's health?"

SHAKING UP THE TOP

By the early 1990s, the pressure was on at the nation's most powerful medical research organization, the National Institutes of Health. The NIH is a national treasure with an eleven-billion-dollar annual budget, a federal establishment that funds 90 percent of basic biomedical research in the United States—both in its own laboratories in Bethesda and through a network of universities and research institutes across the country. NIH-supported research generates the basic information needed for most new drugs and treatments. When NIH neglects a field, it is usually neglected everywhere. Such was the case, until the early 1990s, for women's health.

Everything shifted beginning in the fall of 1990: I was named the NIH's first woman director and the Office of Women's Health was established in response to concerns expressed by the Congressional

Women's Caucus. As director, I was able to institute a nationwide re-search effort called the Women's Health Initiative. The NIH itself fi-nally began to enforce its long-ignored policy that a study or trial inappropriately excluding women would not be funded.

WE'VE COME SO FAR, SO FAST . . . SO FAR

This is all clearly more than encouraging—it is breathtaking. It is not a reason to stop fighting, however, but an inspiration to start. We have far to go before we can breathe easily, assured that the programs and atti-tudes so recently evolved are here to stay. At the time I write this book, I am greatly concerned about the critical issues, both health and other-wise, now confronting women, and I invite you to work with me to re-solve them, helping women concentrate on getting and staying well.

THE WOMEN'S HEALTH INITIATIVE

Throughout this text, I'll be suggesting you keep an eye out for research findings released from a study called the Women's Health Initiative. This fifteen-year, $625-million NIH study is the largest clinical re-search study of women and their health ever undertaken in the United States or elsewhere. Initiated in 1991, it now encompasses forty clinical research centers spread throughout the country and will involve more than 150,000 women. The WHI will narrow the health knowledge gap for women in crucial areas. This initiative is the first major study to look broadly at the chronic diseases that threaten women most—heart dis-ease, stroke, cancer, osteoporosis, and depression—in relation to each other and in the context of women's overall health. It is also the first ma-jor study to recognize that cultural, ethnic, racial, and socioeconomic characteristics affect the kinds of illness people develop and the way they respond to treatment. Through its diverse nationwide participant recruit-ment base and its holistic approach to integrating physical and mental

THE REMAINING DEFICIT IN RESEARCH

In her autobiography, *My Life*, Golda Meir described how David Ben-Gurion, then the prime minister of Israel, referred to her as "the only man" in his cabinet. Ben-Gurion saw this as the greatest possible compliment that he could give Meir; not surprisingly, she did not agree. As she aptly noted, "I very much doubt that any man would have been flattered if [it had been] said about him that he was the only woman in the government!"

The mind-set is still with us. In 1991, the *New York Times* ran a story saying, in essence, that women reporters who do not choose the "mommy track" are tough "iron ladies," virtually "honorary men." This attitude leads to women's continued exclusion from many clinical research studies. According to this mind-set, a man is the true model for the way the human body should behave, and any woman who can't live "up" to such a standard in a scientific study is not worth the

health, the Women's Health Initiative departs from the path of most clinical research, which typically focuses on one disease or bodily organ.

The overall goal of the Women's Health Initiative is to promote a woman's total health. To this end, it should lead to a series of needed recommendations concerning practical issues such as diet, hormone replacement therapy, vitamin and mineral supplements, exercise, and a range of biological and behavioral factors that impact women's health. It will also examine the ways various interventions may interact; for example, hormone replacement therapy may be good for the heart and the bones but may introduce a slightly increased risk of breast cancer when taken long-term. If this intervention is combined with a low-fat diet, can the benefit of estrogen be enhanced and the risk be diminished? Blood samples from participants will be stored so that as new molecular markers for disease become available (such as genes for osteoporosis, breast or ovarian cancer, stroke, or Alzheimer's) we will be able to ask whether women with different genetic and biological makeup should get different advice about diet, weight, prevention, or treatment. The results of the WHI will tell us.

complications that her inclusion would cause. A woman can either re-act physiologically like an honorary man, or she can lump it.

With the large and notable exception of the WHI, men remain the normative standard in far too many research studies. Even today, weekly issues of the *New England Journal of Medicine* or the *Journal of the American Medical Association* often carry reports of major clinical trials on subjects as important as heart disease, cancer, or vitamin supplements, conducted only in men.

To be fair, many of these studies began ten years ago, but they nonetheless contribute to a knowledge gap that will take many years—and a continued national commitment—to correct. Redoing these studies to reflect women's physiology is expensive, and resources allocated through politicians is never a sure thing. The NIH ban on funding in-appropriately exclusionary studies could easily backslide; further, studies that "have already been done," however inapplicable the results of those studies may be for women, could remain the standard if funds are not forthcoming for gender-corrected trials and basic research directed at closing the gender knowledge-gap.

IS THERE A WOMAN DOCTOR IN YOUR SCHOOL?

Although women now comprise 70 percent of the health care work-force, they are still poorly represented in leadership positions in academic centers, medical research, hospitals, and medical-related industries. Close to 40 percent of all medical students are now women whose academic performance is virtually indistinguishable from men's, but they rarely achieve top faculty positions in those same schools. The women who *are* on staff occupy what might be called an academic ghetto: half are clustered at the assistant professor level or lower; under 10 percent are full professors; less than 3 percent are medical school deans. These trends for women in medicine are also reflected in virtually all other scientific disciplines.

As I write this, I ask myself whether I'm being a reverse sexist, im-plying that any woman should be on a staff simply because she's a woman. I guess the charge holds some water; I believe that patients should have equal access to male and female doctors and other health care professionals and that women do bring to the professions an in-sight, intuition, and ability to nurture that is different from a man's. I don't believe, however, that any unqualified woman should be given a position of authority; it's the glass ceiling for the woman of equal talent with which I take issue. If Salk or Sabin had been women, I often wonder, would we have a polio vaccine?

SEXISM GOES SUBTLE

I've shared with you my Pithotomy saga and the story of the resident who so unshakably felt that a woman's place was in the home. I know we all change and grow, and I'm a fervent believer in judging the individual, not the group. Nonetheless I cannot entirely forget that the students of yesterday, the elite of the standard-setting schools, are the leaders of medicine today. With this in mind, it is not so hard to believe the many current reports that women are frequently treated with less respect than men in the medical care system. Far too often, I hear from my own patients that they are "not taken seriously" by their doctors.

Sexism in health care, subtle or not, can do more than emotional damage. The following example may surprise you: I believe the FDA's actions in dramatically taking silicone breast implants off the market to be a sad story in the annals of women's health, involving the manipulation of women in the guise of protecting them from themselves and their silly vanities.

Silicone implants have been shown to be free from any major health risks in study after study for thirty years—and most recently in studies from the NIH, the Mayo Clinic, Harvard, the University of Maryland, and the University of California. On January 6, 1992, the FDA commissioner, against the advice of the FDA's own advisory board, very publicly (in fact, in a mass media frenzy) pulled implants off the market, banning them outright if used for cosmetic reasons, allowing them exclusively on a research-only and limited basis for post-cancer reconstructive surgery—removing them from the control of women and their physicians. The FDA suggested, without any good scientific evidence, that the implants were related to connective tissue diseases such as systemic lupus, scleroderma, and rheumatoid arthritis. (One of many questions remains: if the implants were so dangerous, why give them to cancer patients?!)

This arbitrary and seemingly capricious act frightened millions of women, causing many to have existing implants removed through needless surgery and others to be deprived forever of personal choice in the matter. Implant makers have stopped making them; instead the inferior saline implants are now used.

Removing the implants from the market provided no benefit to women. Rather, the FDA should have alerted women and physicians to the concern and immediately called for a study to determine the truth of the health concerns, as was recommended by the NIH, which, with the cooperation of the National Cancer Institute, was prepared to provide the studies lacking within two years. Women could have made wise choices during the study period, but those choices were taken away.

Here is the kicker: silicone implants had always been and continued to be available to men (until the supply ran out). With all the hoopla at the FDA, no one thought to "protect" men from silicone testicular implants when needed after cancer surgeries or for correcting other testicular problems. Men, it seems, don't need a regulatory agency to pull a product off the market and out of their hands just in case a suspicion of a very rare danger may be found valid. Why were women singled out for this regulatory zeal? What were the motives? I can't speak to that; I only know that women suffered the results.

CHOICE: EVER CONTENTIOUS

The issue of abortion is obviously a very complex one, involving politics, religion, law, philosophy, and women's rights. Unfortunately, politics has seized the abortion issue with a vengeance: "pro-choice" or "pro-life" can form the core of many political agendas and can be the defining position of a political candidate. I question whether the right answer can be found on either extreme of this contentious debate; it would seem to deny the tragic collision between a woman's right to control her own body and the respect that should be given to fetal life.

As a doctor, I can't help but view abortion as an issue of women's health, first and foremost. I will not use this book to persuade any individual woman to have or not to have an abortion on moral grounds: that is a matter for her to decide. (Beware of those who try to make that decision for you, particularly if they speak for political gain, not in the interest of your health and well-being.) Instead, I will give you important information about the implications of abortion for a woman's overall health.

THE DANGERS OF FEMALE APARTHEID

I am also concerned about a well-intentioned solution to the remaining inequities in women's health that I see as no solution at all: the segregation of these issues into a "women's only" track. At the NIH I've attended discussions about whether we need a new Institute of Women's Health to add to our many other institutes or a new medical specialty for research and training called women's health. Separate but equal can be as harmful in health as it has proved to be in education and social settings, both to women as individual patients and as a group. The NIH has close to twenty institutes, most of which were created by Congress to focus attention and resources on a specific disease—such as cancer, heart and lung disease, dental problems, and arthritis—in response to the lobbying of special interest groups. The creation of a female research institute or a new specialty of women's health separated out from disease-oriented institutes or specialty practices would inadvertently condone the continuing omission of women from the mainstream. Meanwhile, treating women's health as the equal of any one specific disease, not as a blanket under which all research must be conducted, would inevitably cause it to be seen as "woman's work" only. The effect would be to close women out of the mainstream of medical research and practice. Far better is to integrate women's health issues and biologically based questions about gender into the fabric of existing research and practice, part and parcel of every research agenda on cancer, heart disease, stroke, aging, the eyes, human genetics, aging, and so forth.

What we need is more emphasis on women's health throughout the medical school curricula and the integration of women's health concerns into all specialties of medicine and surgery. It may be that some internists or primary care physicians choose to focus their practice on women, but that in itself would not justify the creation of a new specialty. In brief, we must take care that women's health be a priority for *all physicians,* not only for a few specialists. Similarly, although women should have the option of choosing a woman doctor, I believe it is wrong for a woman to insist on women physicians exclusively for her care. Rather, she must seek out those physicians who have a reputation for being good listeners and responsive to the needs of their patients, as well as excellence in their field, be they male or female.

Finally, I fear the campaign for attentiveness to women's health could be seriously set back if it becomes part of any polarizing political agenda. It is not "politically correct," nor is it radically feminist, to suggest that disease prevention is critical to the public health of all Americans; it is common sense. One Washington columnist described NIH's efforts in women's health as being part of a "radical feminist agenda"; such commentary serves only to marginalize women's health issues, creating an artificial polarity that can lead to a backlash.

THE TIME IS NOW

There has never been a more opportune moment to take action for women's health. Our society is increasingly educated and receptive, and we've taken remarkable strides forward. But we'll lose the advantages we've won if we now become complacent and allow our momentum to slow. Moreover, the following outside forces render these health issues crucial to us, here and now, and crucial to men as well as women.

WOMEN LIVE LONGER

A relentless fact of life is that women in our society are getting older. Both men and women are living longer, but women now outlive men by seven to eight years.

We may be living longer, but we're not living better. Some five million women in America over the age of sixty-five have disabilities, and more than one million are living in institutions. (That is roughly the same number of men that are in prison because of crime. We hear the former statistic a lot less often than the latter.) Arthritis, multiple sclerosis, urinary incontinence, chronic depression, and even Alzheimer's are more common in women. Women also see more physicians, require more medication, and have surgery more often.

Much of medical research and practice thus far has emphasized *quantity* of life. Clinical trials have tended to focus on dramatic, serious diseases, with the end point of the trial being the life or death of the participant. Judging the comfort level of survival is far more slippery. Some researchers have attempted to measure quality of life by the ability to return to work—this in a time when many women didn't work to begin with; in any case, such a measurement is useless for the population in question—the older women who constitute the majority of the elderly in need of care. If we want to ensure a satisfactory and rewarding life for ourselves as we age, we must lobby now to target research at the diseases that stand to rob us of our peace of mind and wholeness of body, such as stroke, osteoporosis, depression, and poor nutrition.

WE HAVE THE SCIENCE AND THE MONEY

This awakening also has arrived at a point in the history of science when we have unrivaled power to respond to unsolved medical problems of the mind and the body. Few limits hamper our growing ability to understand and intercede in matters of human health and disease. As a nation we are committing the largest resources in the history of the world to medical research, more than twenty-five to thirty billion dollars of private and public money.

These add up to a potent mix of risk and opportunity. We hold tremendous scientific power that must be wielded with self-control and awareness and, of course, concern for women's health. Power can be misused, and money can be manipulated. Decisions about science research money lie in the hands of politicians, who are obviously subject to the influence of both their constituencies and special interest groups. Our existing approach to allocating funding forces us to steal from one disease in order to pay for another. For example, breast cancer has captured attention today; consequently, breast cancer funding was doubled for the 1994 budget. Meanwhile, funding for most other areas of women's health research, including Alzheimer's, osteoporosis, and most other forms of cancer (including lung cancer, which alone kills more women than breast cancer), was effectively *cut*. Seeing across-the-board decreases that are virtually unprecedented in the more than one-hundred-year history of the NIH, we must worry that this philosophy of allocation represents tossing women a metaphorical bone and freeing lawmakers from their larger obligations to women's health.

Additionally, controversial issues in science require broad debate among men and women together—which doesn't always happen in a field so dominated by men. I know that compromise is possible among fair-minded and decent people who disagree on such complex matters as patenting DNA, recombining genes in the laboratory, engineering different forms of plants and animals, or even retrieving tissue from fetuses after abortion. On some issues, however, concession is not a choice; these issues often involve, primarily, the rights and needs—or simply the understanding—of women.

One such issue is the September 1994 NIH recommendation that scientists be allowed to produce human embryos in the laboratory solely for the purpose of scientific research. The embryo would have to be destroyed when its nervous system started to develop visibly.

For many decades there was a strict ban on this kind of work, and, I believe, with good reason. While some of my colleagues may scoff, I feel both intellectually and intuitively that doing experimentation on live human embryos separated from any maternal bond far oversteps the common-sense ethical boundaries on research that have enabled science to flourish for virtually the entire century. Such matters of scientific research will demand women's as well as men's close attention now and in the foreseeable future.

THE HEALTH CARE DEBATE NEEDS OUR INPUT

The debate on national health care is a good example of just how personal and urgent politics can become. I say beware of any program engineered by an election-driven, male-dominated White House, Senate, and Congress. If a special interest group determines that you should get a Pap smear only every three years if you're under the age of fifty, that's what you'll get. But that might not be what you need.

Women are the biggest consumers of health care—and women are the primary health care providers and caretakers of their families. We get the prescriptions filled and take the prescriptions; we fill our nursing homes; we deliver home care, well-baby care, and self-care. Any major change in the health care system will affect women first and foremost; therefore we must play a major role in the decision making behind such changes. We have a great opportunity here—the chance to spotlight the critical position of women in the health care system just when that very system is under close political scrutiny.

THE STRENGTH OF THE INDIVIDUAL WOMAN

Athena is ready to sew a fine seam or become a general, she can play the flute and teach men a thing or two about plowing a field, and she has wit, wisdom, and a sharp moral sense. She is a tender protector of growing children and an effective fighter when the cause is just. She can make an olive tree grow and make a city a better place to live. She is at home in a helmet or flowing gown.

—DR. CAROLYN ELLIOTT

It's one thing to understand the need to continue pressing for change and equity in the health care system; it's another to determine how to do it. When it comes to our health care, I believe that our energy must come from within as much as it does from the force of external events. We must believe we deserve the best life we can possibly have, on all fronts.

I have always felt that the proper zeitgeist of woman is the one captured by the Greek goddess Athena. This is the image of woman as a heroine in an adventure of her own making, but also as a tender protector of children and an effective fighter for a just cause. A woman who will make a city a better place to live while being comfortable in both a helmet and a flowing gown—that is the image of an individual woman empowered—and an image that in no way gathers its strength from diminishing men.

ATHENA THE SOLDIER

The metaphor of battle is often used in medicine: doctors fight wars against specific diseases, we fight the grim reaper, we fight suffering, we fight to recover. Traditionally, these terms are rather macho and masculine; with the symbol of Athena as a model, perhaps we can incorporate both the male aggressor and the female protector.

Women have to be strong to fight this battle for their health; the expression *strong womanhood* is no oxymoron. We have been healers for thousands of years; our exclusion in this century from traditional medicine is no more than a blip on a time continuum that has seen women as herb gatherers, as caregivers and nurturers, as "witches." All too often I've seen women shy away from their own strength, from their grit and brainpower that can make any place a better place to live. I'd like to see this Athena-like image emblazoned in the minds of our young girls and boys—and in the minds of all physicians—replacing forever whatever residual stereotypes remain of woman as passive, lesser, or weak.

ATHENA THE LEADER

The historian/political scientist James MacGregor Burns analyzed leadership in America and in most developed countries and concluded that there is a clear-cut bias against women as leaders in our society, especially at the highest levels of power. It is hard to dispute Burns's conclusion. Femininity in our Western world has been stereotyped as dependent, submissive, and conforming; hence, women have been seen as lacking in intrinsic leadership qualities.

Burns found that women rarely imagine themselves as "leaders and heroes, healers and teachers, producers and presidents" and shy away from having dreams and visions for themselves. In another recent study, researchers found that with few exceptions successful women saw themselves as "lucky," whereas men generally believed they created their own success.

It's time to rethink our vision of ourselves. This perspective is catching on—especially with our daughters. Any prescription for women's health must include an emphasis on women reclaiming the role of leader within and outside of the medical community. One cannot be healthy as chattel, and certainly not as victim.

ATHENA THE MENTOR

Women taking the initiative to become leaders can provide the inspiration this movement will need, but it isn't enough. We must reach inside to find the incentive to share what we've learned with the next generation.

All too often the stereotype of women is that we don't help each other, that petty jealousies keep the few women who have made it from helping those coming along. To me, this directly contradicts an obviously innate characteristic of most women, who are preprogramed at the least to teach their children how to fend for themselves, how to be safe, and how to be healthy. (Of note, in Greek mythology, Mentor, the teacher and guide, was actually Athena disguised as an old man.) Nutrition, reproductive health, hygiene, and outlook are already passed along from mother to daughter; we must add to the lesson plan our expanding knowledge of diseases and disease prevention, and even more importantly, the sense that our bodies and selves deserve the best treatment we and our physicians can give us. We must be role models of confidence, unafraid to ask questions and make demands of the medical community as it evolves, seeking a new paradigm through which to view women's health needs and women as patients.

KNOWLEDGE IS POWER: ABOUT THIS BOOK

Athena is a lovely image; I hope an inspiration. But the clearest path to empowerment is knowledge. If you know about your own health; if you know where your doctor has come from; if you understand the historical context of the health care you receive; if you have a sense of the fundamental causes, treatments, and preventions for the illnesses you're most likely to face as a woman; if you know what questions to ask, you will be able to make change, within and without.

Educated women are healthy women, women with significantly lower maternal, infant, and child mortality rates. Educated teenagers have fewer unwanted babies. And, as has been documented in many studies, the more a woman knows, the longer she lives. Educated women improve the health of entire nations: recent reports of health care priorities in developing countries show that improving the health of a country involves educating the women—it's far more effective than increasing the earnings of men.

I have written this book with a deep commitment to the idea that the empowerment of the individual woman is possible only through knowledge and that the informed, confident woman can find the strength and competence to demand the health care she deserves. Some readers may use the text as a guide to personal health care; for others it may be an incentive to make a political difference. As do many women, I believe the issue of health care goes far beyond which pill to take for which illness. Women themselves cannot be pigeonholed, and a woman's health means far more than the care of her womb. Now I'll give an overview of what you'll find herein, and why.

THE BIG TEN: HEALTH ISSUES MOST LIKELY TO CHANGE WOMEN'S LIVES

Each chapter that follows in this book highlights one of what I believe to be the most important health issues in every woman's life today and for the future. Each cries out for exploration, and all must be a high priority in our federal medical research budget.

I've chosen these topics—nutrition, reproductive health, sexually transmitted diseases, menopause, cancer, depression, heart disease, stroke, osteoporosis, and Alzheimer's—not because you will personally experience every illness named in these chapters but because I guarantee each will make an impact on your life. I hope this text will enable you to limit the impact of illness by showing you how to reduce your risks for any disease that as a woman you're more likely to encounter and by encouraging you to stay aware and involved, continuing to seek answers and information.

Although the text is written so that you don't have to read each chapter and can refer directly to a topic that most concerns you, it is not my ultimate intent that you pick and choose. The book is a whole, just as you are a whole. Your understanding of proper nutrition will have a direct effect on whether you must endure osteoporosis, which also has a connection to your decision about hormone replacement therapy after menopause. Depression can strike at any time, perhaps in relation to other illnesses; heart disease is connected to stroke, which is connected to nutrition—and everything is tied to your second X chromosome.

The order of the chapters pretty much matches the temporal sequence in which you may confront these issues, but you should still be concerned about many of them throughout your life. For example, you won't struggle with osteoporosis until the last third of your life, but you can start preventing it as a teenager.

YOU WON'T FIND . . .

This book is not intended to be an all-inclusive reference manual, or a dry and crusty medical textbook. It is intended to facilitate your leadership in your own health and to inspire you to influence the health of your mothers, sisters, and daughters. Women today are bombarded by the media with sound bites on one new study after another—many directly contradicting previous studies—on subjects ranging from deadly high-sodium Chinese food to killer electromagnetic waves in cellular telephones. I hope in this text to provide you with a framework through which to judge this information for yourself, to know when something sounds out of proportion to reality or clearly raises plenty of questions.

So you won't find information here on the scary disease of the month. I have, however, reluctantly chosen to omit some very important illnesses such as lupus and multiple sclerosis and the less common cancers, and some topics such as plastic surgery or substance abuse. I do believe these are areas in which you must be informed, but they are not likely to affect or threaten every reader, and their inclusion would imply that this book is the encyclopedia it is not meant to be. Should one of these areas concern you directly, I hope this book will help you learn the type of questions to ask and give you the courage to ask them.

Finally, you won't find an introductory section on a woman's physiological makeup. Because I've always found it easier to absorb new information when it's set in a familiar context, I've placed within each chapter all the background information you'll need to understand any of the health concerns discussed. I hope you come away from each chapter with a fresh admiration of your own mechanics and a deep sense that a woman can very much determine her own physiology. Our bodies are dynamic; while we may have certain inherited tendencies, our power to control our own physical destinies is awesome.

BUT YOU SHOULD FIND . . .

Every woman needs her own medical mentor. It might be your primary care doctor, a nurse or doctor associate, or a well-informed friend; someone to guide you to the right place, to encourage you to seek another opinion if need be, or to be a sounding board if you are not sure what you just heard. And you, too, can be a medical mentor—by learning, listening, and keeping informed. There are no "secrets of the temple." When your health is on the altar you must find the resources to demystify and, thereby, gain comfort and confidence. I hope this book serves some of that purpose—a kind of written medical mentor.

HISTORY, POLITICS, AND OTHER SOAPBOXES

You may get weary of my harping on "when I was in medical school." I attempt to place every discussion in its historical context for several reasons.

First, as is probably already quite plain, I firmly believe that the threads of history stretch into the future. Much of our thinking today is built on the beliefs of yesterday, which means that medicine, and particularly medical research involving women's health, is as much about the past as it is about the future. The thinking of the past is a caution to be heeded, and you must be alert to today's advice that appears to be based on yesterday's attitudes and misconceptions.

Second, I mark with intentional frequency how new many of today's attitudes and scientific findings really are. Not only do we have to be vigilant in detecting subtle sexism and insufficient research, we must also be ever questioning and keep in mind the constantly changing nature of the scientific beast. For example, you'll find I strongly recommend hormone replacement therapy based on all available research and would not hesitate to use it myself. For tomorrow? New findings may be released that will change my current convictions.

Third, and perhaps most important, you must be able to put any information or advice you receive in its proper current perspective. Medicine and medical research do not ever and cannot proceed in a vacuum; they intertwine with the events of their times. Through lessons from the past, I hope to encourage and teach you to separate vigilantly any treatment from its surrounding politics. Remember too that physicians bring with them the lens of their own personalities, training, and experience, through which they cannot help but filter any medical opinion.

I hope that an understanding of history prevents feelings of bitterness from emerging about the past or the present. For example, I do not necessarily see malice in the customary relegation of women to the category of "exception" when it came to medical research. This was simply the way people thought until they were educated to think differently.

Let me also add that throughout the book I have more often used the female pronoun for doctor. That is only to remind us of certain historical biases. These frequent "hers" are not meant to be a slight to my thousands of wonderful male colleagues, or to imply that you should see only women doctors!

MY AGENDA

I hold some strong views that influence the tone and content of this text. I'd like to share with you some of my own perspectives here, in the spirit of full disclosure (and in keeping with my advice to you to be wary of the context—not only historical, but personal—of all advice you hear or read).

• You won't find me advocating many government-run policies "protecting" women. I'm on the side of women taking care of themselves, freely controlling their own lives and choices. I fear the seductive entitlement programs passed down by those who cannot possibly have each individual woman's interests at heart. Government should be responsive to women; women should not be dependent on government.

This perspective carries over into the way I view my patients and their illnesses. I judge each case on its own merits and would never deny, or advocate denying, treatment on the sole basis of age, income, or sex. This may seem on its surface to be common sense, but remember that it can turn into a quite controversial point of view in an era when we are considering government rationing of health care by permitting a national board of advisors to dictate priorities and determine who gets what treatment—or doesn't—and where such rationing is commonplace elsewhere.

• You won't find me suggesting you storm your doctor's offices. Any change, I believe, is best made through strong alliances and non-adversarial partnerships with as much respect, tact, and understanding as possible on both sides. Man and woman are partners in life; doctor and patient, partners in health. When I advocate your asking informed and provocative questions of your physician, I suggest you do so in the spirit of mutual education and of furthering the interests of both doctor and patient.

• At the same time, I say be politically active, take chances, and speak out when the cause is important. This can be a risk; I've made plenty of public mistakes. The only way I can live with myself, though, is to know I haven't sat silent while I saw damage being done around me. In my estimation, there is probably no progress without some defeat. And without courage none of your other principles have much meaning.

• I have great faith in the extraordinary power of molecular biology, human genetics, and medical technology to understand disease and to come up with treatments and cures. Medical research is as much about the patient of tomorrow as it is about our needs today, and we have an obligation to that future patient—just as we do to our children—to continue to invest in more and better scientific research.

• As science becomes more powerful in the way it touches our lives, however, we have to be sure that it is used in the right way—both for the integrity of science and the betterment of human life. Science must bow to the legal, ethical, and moral constraints determined both by personal conscience and by the values of the larger community. This view of mine represents a core philosophical division between me and some of my colleagues, who believe that science conducted for science's sake can still lead ultimately to knowledge that benefits humanity. I, nonetheless, don't believe you can take either the goal of human health or the sensitivities of the public out of the science that is being funded and executed.

• In that context medicine is a timeless art with a spiritual dimension and humanitarian purpose. Patients are not clients; doctors are not adversaries. Whatever the ups and downs of health care reform, legal liability, economic pressures, changing forms of practice, and new science, doctors and patients alike must see this art as reality.

ALL THOSE MEDICAL TERMS!
(EXCEPT THE ONE MY DOCTOR PRESCRIBED)

In keeping with my goal of providing you with just enough information to inform and inspire, not to overwhelm, I list only those medications most often prescribed for each specific illness, along with common brand names. In some cases, such as Prozac, I'll call the drug by the brand name, since that's the name with which you're likely to be most familiar; again, this book is not supposed to be a complete and regimented pharmacopoeia.

I don't list all side effects or make any value judgment in choosing which medications I include. You may well find that your doctor prescribes something different; the same drug can have many different names. My goal is to give you a sense of what's out there and a keen understanding of the evolving story of medications. Any medication should be taken with caution, and no medication should be taken without constant scrutiny and review. Always ask these questions: Is there anything new on the horizon? Is this medication still the best for me?

ALTERNATIVE MEDICATIONS

While I don't give much credence to people pushing potions like apricot pits to treat cancer, I do have a certain respect for the secrets that may be locked up in mythology and folk medicine. As a woman I know the value of teachings passed from mother to daughter far outside the sometimes myopic view of the medical establishment. I wouldn't dismiss any alternative treatment out of hand. However, while I believe in the potential of alternative medications, I don't believe they should be given alternative scrutiny. Any outside-the-norm treatments I mention in this book should be subjected to the same scientific and mainstream tests as any standard therapy.

STUDIES TO WATCH FOR

You'll find, scattered throughout the book, references to ongoing research, either within the text or separated in boxes called "Studies to Watch For." As I've said, sometimes what we fervently believe today is derived from the dogma of yesterday and will be contradicted tomorrow. I hope through this device to provide you with a vocabulary for beginning your own investigations.

I also hope you take from this part of the book the understanding that your health ultimately lies in your hands; even a good doctor gets behind in her reading. You must care enough about yourself to question, to probe, to make sure you have the whole story, to get into the habit of asking "What's new?" "What's next?" It is my wish that this book's philosophies stay with you as you continue to get the information you need on your own long after much of the advice in this book becomes obsolete.

ACTIONS TO TAKE PERSONALLY, POLITICALLY, SOCIETALLY

I don't want to mislead you; in this book I won't very often provide you with a step-by-step blueprint to instigating change. In such a rapidly changing world, most specific steps I could recommend would quickly become outdated. And anyway, ultimately it's your choice. What I can do is help you put yourself in a position of such personal, political, and societal power that you can be prepared to take action when the opportunity arises. I didn't go to the NIH to develop a preset plan for the Women's Health Initiative, but I had a framework for what I thought had to be done. I grabbed the chance when I saw it, and I saw the chance because I was prepared, had a commitment, and knew where we had to go.

There are two time-proven methods for being effective in making change: gaining knowledge and speaking up. Women must embrace the existing health care establishment as well as influence it. To this end, I conclude each chapter with a general section on "What Women Can Do Personally and Politically."

Taking charge of your health, though, becomes far more real and crucial when you are sitting in a doctor's office. Advice such as "Be a partner with your doctor" or "Be informed about your disease" can feel pretty empty when you're faced with a health crisis of your own, you're scared, and you need help. For this reason, I list many questions for you to discuss with your doctor regarding each health issue raised, and where appropriate, give you the means to evaluate whether the physician you've chosen is the right one for you. I want all of us to become assertive, informed, and empowered—but most of all I want you to feel good about your own health care.

In my own life, making choices and taking actions, I find guidance and inspiration from the epitaph of a lady I know nothing about. Emily Morrison lived in Colonial Virginia. Almost twenty years ago I stumbled upon her gravestone—a small gray stone tucked away almost imperceptibly among the large, grand monuments with flowery inscriptions marking families and dynasties of her day. Her epitaph: SHE HATH DONE WHAT SHE COULD.

TWO

NUTRITION

Women's Work Becomes Women's Health

Don't dig your grave with a knife and fork.

— ENGLISH PROVERB

When I was five or so, I stumbled upon my dad in our basement as he was hoarding some food in unlabeled brown glass jars. The Korean War was going on, and my father's memories of the recent World War II wartime shortages were still fresh, including the food rationing stamps administered to families during the war; from time to time he would show me and my sisters the stamps that had our names inscribed on them.

Food and nutrition were a high priority for my mom and dad. Both my parents had seen hunger in their own kitchens, growing up in the Depression, each with a widowed mother. My father believed in the science of food—he argued that everyone must eat, that the world was facing a food crunch, and that our knowledge of food technology and food productivity was woefully inadequate. My mother emphasized food in her own way, through formal family rituals around meals. For her, food was about nurturing and healthy living.

As a result, I've always taken nutrition seriously, and so should you. As a living being, and particularly as a woman, what and how you eat has an enormous impact on your overall health—an impact that, as we'll see later in this chapter, has been systematically overlooked in this century by the American medical and research communities. Six of the ten principal causes of death pertain directly to diet, yet, as of 1992, only 25 percent of medical schools offered a basic course in nutrition. We'll explore the reason for this ridiculous discrepancy later; for now, suffice it to say that food and nutrition have long been viewed as "woman's work" and therefore as unworthy of formal study.

Why is nutrition so crucial? On the surface, eating is such an integral and simple part of our lives that, unless you're on a diet (a tremendously unhealthy and counterproductive twentieth-century obsession), paying too much attention to food can feel contrived, even to conscientious folks. It's much easier to understand the impact of a pill that can cure a disease in a week or so than to identify with the long-term impact on your body of a spinach salad or a doughnut. Also, even the best-intentioned doctors and nutritionists can get confused by the constantly changing studies released these days about what's "good for you" and what's not. When I was a child growing up in an extremely food-aware home, cholesterol- and fat-laden calves' liver was thought to be very good for you; meat every day, if you could afford it, was ideal; fish was a religious requirement; and eggs and bacon made up the standard breakfast. Whole milk, potatoes, and white bread were staples. Lard made the best pie crust, and that funny white margarine that you had to color yellow yourself by breaking an orange dye capsule was bought only because it was cheaper. Cod-liver oil was used as a tonic for cold weather; vitamins were just not considered.

Except for "an apple a day . . . ," almost everything that was "right" then is "wrong" now, but people then seemed to be healthy. So why does it matter?

Because our lives depend on it.

We now know that most debilitating diseases affecting our adult population and affecting women's health in particular have some link to diet. Heart disease, stroke, breast cancer, colon cancer, other cancers, osteoporosis, diabetes, arthritis, obesity, and anorexia nervosa can be to some degree prevented or in some cases treated through foods and vitamins. Nutrition has a clear impact on non-life-threatening issues as well. It can influence our state of mind, our ability to learn and concentrate, our level of alertness, the health and development of our brains, the severity of syndromes such as attention deficits and hyperactivity, the overall physical and mental development of infants and children, the duration and intensity of common colds, and even the length of time we keep our teeth.

There is so much in our frantic lives we feel powerless to change or even affect. I urge you to experience that wonderful sense of empowerment you can feel when you take charge of your health through your diet. You will improve the quality of your life—and, in all likelihood, the length of it as well.

WOMEN'S WORK

We can be sure of two things in the uncertain and insufficiently studied world of nutrition: (1) nutrition is probably the single biggest factor in the health and general well-being of a woman at any stage of her life; and (2) historically, nutrition has been labeled a woman's field and therefore has been long undervalued, starved of research resources, and forced to the fringe of medicine.

Nutrition as a modern science incorporating chemistry and physiology was born about a hundred years ago, when scientists discovered that food contained specific vital nutrients—such as carbohydrates, proteins, fatty acids, vitamins, and minerals. At about the same time, the NIH came into being as a small laboratory devoted to the study of disease prevention and health maintenance. Among the early triumphs of the NIH was the groundbreaking discovery that the disease of pellagra—a then common and frightening deadly disease involving deterioration of the skin, the gut, and the brain—was not a communicable disease or a hopeless mental condition, but rather a dietary deficiency. This discovery made it possible to wipe out the disease. So the NIH actually made its early name in the neglected field of nutrition.

While these fundamental discoveries were being made, talented women, such as MIT's Ellen Swallow Richards (the first woman to study for a Ph.D. there and founder of the nutrition and home economics movement in the United States), were time and time again denied positions in the biomedical research laboratories of NIH and elsewhere. While some women scientists were able to obtain jobs, their career opportunities were limited to positions that dealt with the needs of the home. Through this accident of history, women got a foothold in the field of nutrition. Female chemists took their Ph.D.s to college home economics departments, where they were welcome and where they trained other women in "women's concerns": children and food. Ultimately, Lulu Graves and Lenna Cooper, two leaders of the home economics field, founded the American Dietetic Association (ADA) in response to the nutritional needs of soldiers in World War I; the ADA later expanded its mission to promote health and elevate the nutritional status of the population at large. (Today the ADA is an organization of registered dietitians that play a key role in providing reliable and accurate nutritional information and translating the science of nutrition into practical application.)

Despite the accomplishments of these women, the ADA, and the 50,000 or more registered dietitians at work in our hospitals and clinics, the *science* of nutrition has been a stepchild. Inadequately funded by congressional and university budget committees—composed mostly of men—for decades, the research base of nutrition has been starved. Despite its critical importance to health, nutrition in the form of home economics persisted for too long as a female ghetto, either marginalized or ignored by mainstream scientific researchers—also mostly men. Even the NIH, oblivious to its own history, has generally neglected the field of nutrition sciences except as it relates to selected diseases. Resources for the nutritional sciences are scarce, making both male and female research scientists wary about devoting a lifetime to the field. The science has suffered as a result, and so has our general medical view of the importance of nutrition in daily practice.

The inadequacy of our cultural commitment to nutrition came home to me some time ago when I was talking to a friend, the distraught mother of a fifteen-year-old anorectic daughter. The daughter underwent several rounds of in-hospital treatment, and I saw the anguish and frustration that her mother endured as she took her daughter from physician to psychotherapist in the hopes of seeing her child get well. I asked my friend if her daughter was taking supplemental calcium and a multivitamin, since anorexia can take quite some time to conquer, but the nutritional impact is immediate and dire: it undermines healthy bone growth and can put us at risk for osteoporosis later in life. The answer was "no." None of these highly educated specialists had thought to take care of this young girl's most basic needs.

WHAT WE KNOW ABOUT
THE NUTRITIONAL NEEDS OF WOMEN

Given the sad state of nutritional research today, I almost hesitate to make any blanket dietary recommendations for women. Although nutrition has been a field in which women figure prominently as practitioners, no research agenda has seriously focused on the unique nutritional needs of women, except for differences during pregnancy and lactation. The relationship of fat in the diet and cholesterol intake to heart disease has not been studied specifically in women, yet we know that there are major gender differences between men and women with regard to their cholesterol profiles and their risk for heart disease. We do not even adequately understand whether hormonal status at different stages in a woman's life, including the changes brought on by taking oral contraceptives and then hormone replacement therapy after menopause, might affect dietary requirements.

And we certainly can't count on the U.S. government for guidance in this area. The government's national dietary standards, the recommended daily allowances (RDA) that you see on nutritional labels of packaged foods—from cereal boxes to soups to vitamins—were originally based on studies of one rather homogeneous population: young, healthy male World War II military recruits. Although the RDAs are periodically revised, they aren't now and were never intended to be interpreted as ideal amounts of each nutrient. Instead, they list what is safe and "adequate" to meet the needs of most healthy people. If you're not young, healthy, or male, the RDAs will often confuse and mislead you, not help you.

And yet we must live in the world, eating our three meals a day, making nutritional choices constantly. So, with these caveats—that the field of nutrition is primitive; that new studies can directly contradict old ones; and that even an informed physician's advice can swing wildly with each new discovery—I make the following recommendations and explanations, which I hope will clarify some of your nutritional decision making.

A PRIMER OF BASIC NUTRITIONAL FACTS

A woman's nutritional needs vary with her state of life: a pregnant woman has different considerations from a postmenopausal woman, and so forth. We'll take a look at those special needs later in this chapter. First, though, every woman should have a basic understanding of what her healthy body needs (and doesn't need) to operate efficiently.

Much of the information that drives our present knowledge and recommendations for nutrition comes from international population studies. In recent years nutrition news from other parts of the world has bolstered the American push toward a diet lower in total fats and animal protein, higher in fruits, grains, and other vegetables. The Chinese, for example, eat 20 percent more than we do but weigh less. Their diets—composed almost exclusively of vegetables and, depending on the region, rice or noodles—contain 77 percent complex carbohydrates and 15 percent fat, most of which comes from vegetable sources. They eat one-third the animal protein and three to seven times the fiber we do. The Chinese encounter certain cancers, particularly of the stomach and esophagus, more often than we do, but they do not develop breast and colon cancers at nearly the same rate. They don't eat a great deal of dairy products, but they don't get much osteoporosis; they don't eat much red meat, but they don't suffer anemia; they eat much more than we do, but they don't have much obesity. And they have surprisingly low rates of high blood pressure, heart disease, and diabetes. Are the Chinese simply blessed with good health genes? Probably not, because when they emigrate to the West and adopt our eating habits, they also develop our diseases. Of course, these people and similar cultures lead far less sedentary lifestyles than Americans, but by and large the clearest causal link for this difference in health lies in the food that is eaten.

With this in mind, let's take a closer look at the basic elements of our diet, the five essential nutrients: proteins, fats, carbohydrates, water, vitamins and minerals.

PROTEIN

Our bodies are made mostly of protein and water; the proteins in our bodies are in turn comprised of *amino acids*. When we eat protein in any form, our bodies break the protein down into these amino acid building blocks, which then re-form themselves into a multitude of human proteins, personally tailored for us by our genes.

The body can manufacture only a little over half of the twenty amino acid building blocks that we need to make protein; those that our bodies cannot make are called the essential amino acids. (They include histidine, tryptophan, lysine, valine, leucine, isoleucine, threonine, phenylalanine, and methionine.) We can't live without protein, and we can't manufacture it from nothing; we must ingest it.

But the American diet is enormously protein-heavy, for men and for women. Women need only about 44 to 46 grams of protein a day. That's as much as you'll find in a 5-ounce steak, one chicken breast, 6 ounces of tuna, even 5 cups of skim milk. Even a bowl of cereal gives you more than 5 grams of protein. So the odds are that most of us are consuming much more protein than we need.

Too much protein is not a major danger in itself to health, but it doesn't do us any good either. Since fat tags along with protein in meat, we pick up the fat-laden diseases by association. (You can get protein without fat, through plants: peas or beans, tofu, and cereals have little or no fats and no cholesterol.) In any case, if we fill up on protein, we don't leave room for the carbohydrates our bodies need more of. (There is a small health risk associated with consuming excess protein, which we excrete. Protein excretion can put a strain on our kidneys, and some studies have shown that calcium excretion increases with protein excretion, which gives me concern about osteoporosis.)

While I'm not convinced that excess protein poses any serious health risk to women, I strongly recommend that you consume it in moderation, as no more than 15 percent of your daily calories. I'll explain later how to calculate that. Remember, most protein travels in bad company—animal fat (although many red meats have been modified to be leaner with less marbling, and that makes a huge difference. See table on pages 39–40).

FAT AND CHOLESTEROL

By now we've all heard that too much fat is the culprit in many health problems. Fats do some good, though; a certain (small!) amount of fat is essential to our physical and mental health. Fats are an energy source and are key to both the structure and day-to-day functioning of our cells.

When we ingest fat in any form, it is broken down by our digestive system into fatty acids, or *lipids,* which are in turn absorbed into our bloodstream. Fatty acids are the building blocks of fats just as amino acids are the building blocks of proteins. As with amino acids, we can make only some of the fatty acids we need. Those we can't manufacture, called *essential fatty acids,* perform functions critical to our health and well-being. For example, the fatty acid called *arachidonic acid* is converted by the body into *prostaglandins,* fatty acid derivatives that cause contraction and relaxation of blood vessels, clumping of blood platelets to make blood clots, inflammatory responses, and uterine contractions during labor and delivery. Linolenic fatty acids, a subgroup of the *omega-3 fatty acids,* now the subject of extensive research, are found in certain fish oils (like cod-liver oil); they have been shown to improve the function of blood vessels and may benefit the cardiovascular, nervous, and immune systems.

Fatty acids come in two forms in our diets: *saturated* and *unsaturated*, depending upon how they are chemically bonded to hydrogen. The more hydrogen bonds per molecule of fat, the more they are "saturated" and the more they are likely to be solid in texture. (If you want to get technical, saturated fats have no "double bonds"; each hydrogen atom bonds individually to the fat molecule.) Saturated fats are found mostly in meats and in dairy products. (Exceptions are coconut oil and palm oil, saturated fats made by vegetables.)

Most fats found in vegetables are unsaturated and tend to be liquid at room temperature. Unsaturated fat (with one or more double bonds per molecule) comes in two forms: *monounsaturated* fats (with the fewest number of hydrogen bonds, and only one double bond per molecule), including canola oil and olive oil; and *polyunsaturated* fats

A MARGARINAL NOTE

You've probably heard the controversy lately—suddenly studies claim that margarine is no better than butter, after all. The truth is that margarine is a bit better for you than butter, but not much. I don't use much margarine (or generally butter, either) because the chemical process used to create margarine has always worried me. Margarine is created when an unsaturated fat is treated chemically so that it partially hydrogenates: it turns into a somewhat saturated fat in order to harden, although it is never as saturated as butter. As soon as any fat becomes hydrogenated at all, it will raise your cholesterol. When an unsaturated fat is chemically caused to become saturated, another chemical change occurs. Fatty acids called trans fatty acids are created, and recently a few scientists have expressed worries that these "trans" fatty acids could also raise your cholesterol. I'm not surprised—in my book, the more you mess with the chemical content of food, the more likely you are to create something unhealthy.

A healthy alternative to the margarine dilemma is to use extra virgin olive oil in place of margarine or butter when added fat is necessary.

(more complex chemically, with more than one double bond), including corn oil, sunflower oil, and also fish oil. Fatty acids linked together, traveling through the bloodstream, are called *triglycerides.*

CHOLESTEROL

Cholesterol is a fat, made from saturated fat by our livers. It is critical to the membranes encasing all our cells and tissues, to the formation of our brains, central nervous systems, and sex hormones. About one-quarter of our cholesterol comes from our food—in eggs, dairy products, and meats. Egg yolks and organ meats like liver and brain are especially high in cholesterol.

Since oil (fat) and water don't mix, cholesterol has to be attached to carrier proteins to be able to circulate in our blood. The cholesterol-protein complexes in our blood are called *lipoproteins,* which come in two forms: *high-density lipoproteins* (HDL) and *low-density lipoproteins* (LDL). Here is a simple way to think of fats and cholesterol; there are good and bad fats, and good and bad cholesterol—bad meaning when they occur in excess.

Good Fat = Unsaturated Fat. You'll find good fat—not solid at room temperature—in vegetables, vegetable oils such as olive and canola oils, and fish oils.

Bad Fat = Saturated Fat. It is generally solid at room temperature and easy to see in meats and dairy products such as beef and butter; it is also found in oils made from trees such as palm and coconut oils.

Good Cholesterol = HDL. High-density lipoprotein is a scavenger in the blood for bad cholesterol, picking it up and carrying it to the liver, where it is excreted into the bile and eliminated. Women have higher HDL levels than men.

Bad Cholesterol = LDL. Low-density lipoprotein deposits cholesterol in blood vessel walls and clogs arteries with fatty plaque, leading to heart attacks and strokes. Men usually have higher levels of LDL than do women.

Too much fat in any form does great damage. Dietary fat and its resulting cholesterol has been linked to heart disease and colon and breast cancer in women. The association with colon cancer, supported by research dating back to 1975, was staunchly reinforced by a 1990 report of the Nurses' Health Study, a major observational study of female nurses from the Brigham and Women's Hospital (see page 46). Similarly, breast cancer has been convincingly, albeit inconsistently,

STUDY TO WATCH FOR

While I'm convinced by preliminary studies that there is a link between breast, ovarian, and colon cancer and a high-fat diet, these connections have not been definitively proven; nor can we be certain, if there is a link, of how much fat in the diet is too much. Where does the danger start? The only way we can get a sure answer is through a clinical controlled trial, which the Women's Health Initiative (see page 10) is conducting as of this writing. Watch for the results—it is sure to be reported in the popular press within three to four years. If you haven't heard, ask your doctor.

associated with diets high in calories and fats, especially from milk and meat. There are also studies in research laboratories that have shown a link between a variety of cancers and both saturated and unsaturated fat, suggesting that fat acts as a promoting agent early in the development of a cancer, in essence helping an early tumor become established.

Guidelines for Fat and Cholesterol in a Woman's Diet

It's clear that no healthy adult woman should consume large amounts of fat and cholesterol. Keeping track of dietary cholesterol gets pretty cumbersome, but if you keep your fat content low enough, your cholesterol consumption will fall into a reasonable range automatically. After lengthy debate about what scientific evidence actually shows and what the American public might be expected to accept, in the late 1980s the National Cholesterol Education Program hit upon recommending an intake of no more than 30 percent of your daily calories from fat, with no more than 10 percent from saturated fat, and 300 mg of cholesterol. The recommended percentage was ultimately set arbitrarily because it seemed to be realistic and was a target below the 40 percent or so that most Americans were consuming at the time.

On the other hand, there are some who recommend even more stringent diets (as low as 10 percent total fat), particularly for those who have known heart disease. It is by no means clear, however, that such a severe reduction of fat and cholesterol intake is healthy; in fact, such a low-fat, low-cholesterol diet concerns me greatly, and I would not recommend it. Even if a virtually zero-fat diet benefits the heart, some studies have suggested that such a diet may be associated with a higher risk of cancer, depression, suicide, and even violent behaviors.

Aim for 20 percent (and try not to exceed 25 percent) total fat in your diet—that's my recommendation. In fact, if you keep your intake of *saturated* fat between 7 and 10 percent of the total calories in your diet, you needn't worry about other fat sources. If you consider a diet with a total calorie intake of 2,000 calories, this means about 40 grams of total fat and less than 20 grams saturated.

I'm not expecting any woman reading this book to monitor all her meals with a scale and a calculator. I believe most women instinctively feel, like me, that food is meant to be relished, not harshly regulated. Instead, target these goals:

• First, eat more complex carbohydrates, like bread, rice, potatoes, noodles, dried beans, vegetables, and fruit. A gram of any fat, good or bad, has more than twice the calories of a gram of pure carbohydrate (9 compared to 4) and appears to be easier to metabolize. So if you eat a given amount of carbohydrate, compared to the identical amount of fat, you'll ingest fewer calories in the first place and then burn more calories during digestion.

• Limit your consumption of foods notoriously high in cholesterol such as egg yolks, liver, or heavily marbled steak to only a rare indulgence, perhaps once a month or less.

• Be aware that animal protein is inherently high in fat and keep your protein intake to about 6 ounces per day—that is, one small portion. Eat fish and plant proteins (beans, low-fat tofu, etc.) whenever possible.

• Limit your use of visible fats, such as butter or margarine for bread or on vegetables, oil for cooking, mayonnaise and salad dressings. These are all "extras" and with some attention can be markedly reduced if you just think about them. Healthy alternatives include fat-free sour cream or yogurt, and other condiments such as horseradish, garlic, and other flavor enhancers to replace fat.

• When you're reading labels, compute the percentage of fat as follows: multiply the grams of fat by 9 and compare that number to the total calories. (A can of chowder that has 200 calories a serving, with 8 grams of fat per serving, has 72 calories [8 grams × 9 calories] from fat. That's 72 out of 200, or 36 percent of calories from fat—far too much if it reflects your whole diet.) More labels are starting to show the percentage of fat calories automatically; look for that figure and purchase foods accordingly.

• Gradually reduce your fat intake—don't try to go cold turkey (or cold beef, I guess). Start easy: use less butter and no sour cream on your baked potatoes or only jelly on your toast, then continue to cut down over time in your cooking and flavoring. Think, also, of the benefit of what you are doing—increasing your length of time on this planet and decreasing the likelihood that you'll spend that time in a hospital or nursing home.

The following chart illustrates the huge impact your "minor" nutritional choices can make. Look at the difference between whole and skim milk, or ice cream and ice milk, or halibut vs. a marbled steak!

FAT ESTIMATES IN PORTIONS OF FOOD

FOOD—IN SERVING PORTIONS	SATURATED FAT—GM	(CHOLESTEROL—MG)
Whole milk—one cup	5	33
2% milk—one cup	3	18
Skim milk—one cup	trace	0
Regular yogurt—one cup	5	30
Nonfat yogurt—one cup	trace	0
Ice cream—one cup	9	50
Ice milk—one cup	4	15
Cheeses—one oz.	6	30
Mozzarella (part-skim)—one oz.	3	15
Egg	2	275
Egg white	0	0
Marbled steak—6 oz.	22	180
Lean steak—6 oz.	8	100
Chicken with skin—6 oz.	4–6	100–150
Chicken without skin—6 oz.	2–4	90–100
Hot dog with mustard	5–6	25
Bacon—3 slices	3–4	16

FOOD—IN SERVING PORTIONS	SATURATED FAT—GM	(CHOLESTEROL—MG)
Tuna or salmon—6 oz.	1–2	70–90
Flounder or halibut—6 oz.	0.8	100–120
Baked potato	0	0
French fries	6	trace
Most vegetables	0	0
Pasta—one cup with tomato sauce	trace	0
Avocado	5	0
Beans	trace	0
Butter—one tbsp.	7	30
Margarine—one tbsp.	2	0
Palm or coconut oil	7–12	0
Olive oil	1.8	0
Peanut oil	2.3	0
Canola oil	1.0	0
Nuts—¹/₂ oz. peanuts, almonds, pecans	0.8–1.0	0
Peanut butter—one tbsp.	1.5	0

Source: USDA, Human Nutrition Information Service; also Glen C. Griffin and William P. Castelli, *Good Fat, Bad Fat* (Tucson, Arizona: Fisher Books, 1989).

CARBOHYDRATES

Carbohydrates are a crucial source of energy for all women. They can be *simple,* like the carbohydrates found in table sugar, or *complex,* like those found in fruits, vegetables, whole grains, breads, and pastas. Complex carbohydrates include starches and dietary fiber.

SIMPLE CARBOHYDRATES

Sugar is the prototypical "empty calorie" in that it provides pure energy but little else of nutritional value. *Glucose* is the form of sugar our body uses for energy. In fact, glucose is the only energy source the human brain can use (most other organs can burn fat as well). Other simple sugars that occur in nature, fructose and galactose, must be converted to glucose through enzymes in our digestive system to be absorbed. When glucose is absorbed into the bloodstream, it is used immediately for energy or converted by the liver, fat cells, or muscle into a complex carbohydrate—a starch—called *glycogen,* for storage.

Because of the critical importance of a constant level of blood glucose, especially for brain function, the pancreas secretes two hormones that carefully regulate our glucose levels. When glucose levels start to fall, the hormone *glucagon* pours out from the pancreas to signal the storage sites to release sugar by breaking down the body's stored starch, glycogen, back into glucose for immediate use. When glucose rises after a meal, the pancreas secretes *insulin,* which signals the storage sites to take up glucose and convert it into glycogen, thereby lowering our glucose level, and also into fat. If sugar levels fall too low—as with too much insulin—a person becomes unconscious, since the brain has lost its sustenance.

Is sugar too common in our Western diet? Yes, we eat too much sugar—through candy, soda, ice cream, and other desserts—but in reality, sugar poses a far milder health risk than does fat. If you eat much more than 10 percent of your daily calories from sugar, you risk tooth decay and weight gain. But don't worry about a few teaspoons of sugar in your tea; sugar is not the enemy we once thought it was. When it's glued to fat—as it often is in pastries, cookies, doughnuts, and frostings—you should pay attention.

COMPLEX CARBOHYDRATES

Complex carbohydrates are large constructions of sugar molecules that take on the form of either starches or fiber. About 55 percent of your daily calories should come from complex carbohydrates.

Starches

Complex carbohydrates in the form of starch—such as potatoes, pastas, beans, rice, breads, and cereals—are broken down by your digestive system into simple sugars and converted into glucose, to be absorbed into the bloodstream. In the bloodstream glucose is used for energy and the leftover sugar is converted into body fat. As recently as the early eighties, starches carried with them a bad reputation, perhaps because they are readily available, inexpensive, and most heavily consumed by people in lower socioeconomic groups. Also, since when eaten in excess they are fattening, there was a sense that they were therefore not healthy. We have learned this is far from the truth. Diets rich in starches are associated with less diabetes and heart disease. Starch-centered diets are a way of life among healthy Japanese, Chinese, Italian, or Turkish families; in these cultures, animal fat and protein are used more as condiments or flavoring rather than the centerpiece that they have become in the northern European and North American diets.

For some people whose bodies pour out an overabundance of insulin in response to starch and sugar, too much starch leads to weight gain and possibly an increase in circulating triglycerides. This has led some to bash pasta. To me, this information reinforces the need to develop nutritional guidance tailored to the individual's body type and metabolism, as opposed to a one-size-fits-all diet. Nevertheless, I'm still a supporter of pasta and good breads!

Virtually all the starch we get in our diet comes from plants; consequently, diets high in starch are almost always high in fiber. Let's take a quick closer look at this related carbohydrate—fiber—which received so much attention in the late 1980s.

Fiber

Fiber, found in the structural parts of plants, is made mostly of *indigestible* complex carbohydrates (as opposed to starches, which are totally *digestible*).

Fiber can be either *water-soluble,* like that found in fruits, peas, beans, and oats, or *insoluble,* like that found in vegetables, bran, rice, and whole grains. Both insoluble and soluble fiber provide our diets with bulk—a nearly inert mass that serves as a carrier of other foods and nutrients as it courses through the many yards of our intestines. This function may seem small, but it is critical. Not only does the increased bulk decrease constipation and the risk of *diverticulosis* (a disease of the colon in which fingerlike outpouches of the bowel wall form and can become infected), but it also protects against development of colon cancer.

Soluble fiber has a dual role. In addition to providing bulk, it can slow down the upper bowel absorption of carbohydrates and stimulate fecal excretion of cholesterol-rich bile acids. With these two actions, soluble fiber has been shown to help regulate diabetes and improve cholesterol profiles. (A few years ago there was a flurry of interest around the announcement that these water-soluble fibers could lower LDL cholesterol by 50 percent or more and raise HDL choles-terol by as much as 80 percent. The truth is, to get these results, you'd have to eat an impossibly large amount of fiber each day.)

Although fiber is mostly nondigestible and gives us neither ab-sorbable nutrients nor calories, it virtually always comes in good com-pany. A high-fiber diet inevitably means increased consumption of fruits, vegetables, grains, and cereals—a combination that provides starch and plenty of vitamins and minerals. Low-fiber diets, on the other hand, are invariably high in refined sugars and fats. Take a look at the fiber in your diet. Fiber is a good marker of the kind of dietary pattern you have developed and the kind of palate you have cultivated.

WATER

While water itself is not a nutrient, I include it because it is vital to our health. We are made up mostly of water; about 60 percent of our body mass is good old H_2O. It is the medium through which virtually all of our life functions are carried out.

Many sources recommend you take in six to eight glasses of water a day. While I firmly believe a woman must get plenty of water, some people go overboard (it can't hurt you, but it can keep you busy uri-nating!). Our bodies tell us when we need water—we get thirsty. If you pay attention to your body and heed its cues, you'll get sufficient replenishment without having to count cups. You might, however, consider substituting water for soda or coffee.

VITAMINS AND MINERALS

Vitamins and minerals are among the most provocative and contro-versial elements in nutrition today, prompting heated discussions both in the medical community and within the general population.

For all women, at any age, getting adequate and appropriate amounts of vitamins and minerals in the diet is, I feel, crucial to good preventive health care. If necessary, women should supplement their diet with these nutrients in pill form. This philosophy runs counter to conventional American medical wisdom.

We understand what is important about vitamins and minerals mainly because we know what happens when we don't get them. We work backwards from investigating diseases caused by deficiencies, in-stead of forward from a scientific model of study. So our knowledge is obviously limited when it comes to hard documentation of the positive impact of higher than just adequate levels of vitamins and minerals. And scientists today don't really know much about day-to-day positive functions of vitamins and minerals. As far as the conventional (governmental!) wisdom goes, the National Research Council of the National Academy of Sciences still warns against taking daily vitamin and mineral supplements in excess of the RDAs because "no research exists to support the practice."

Such warnings serve only to endanger the health of American women. While certainly vitamins and minerals can do damage in excess, the RDA requirements do not reflect the higher amounts in which some vitamins can provide real health benefits. It's true that vitamin and mineral deficiency is no longer an issue in the health of most Americans. With the few exceptions we'll discuss below, you get the small amounts of the vitamins and minerals you need at a sustenance level from the food you eat; even a McDonald's hamburger is going to be served to you on a vitamin-enriched bun.

What's important for you to know is that some vitamins and minerals might actually *prevent* serious diseases: for example, scattered studies show connections between certain vitamins and cancer prevention. In this section, we'll focus on those that have received the most attention in terms of prevention.

VITAMINS

Vitamins are complex chemicals that are critical to metabolic reactions in virtually all of our cells. They serve as catalysts in biochemical reactions that range from cell division to cell growth, from development to energy production in our bodies. Most vitamins have a very broad range of action, but a few vitamins have a more targeted role. For example, Vitamin D serves mainly to regulate the calcium and phosphate in our bodies; and Vitamin K is critical to the liver's synthesis of factors crucial in blood clotting. But the B vitamins—and, specifically, the antioxidants—have been getting the most attention lately.

The B Vitamins

Within the B vitamin family are a wide range of compounds including thiamine (B_1), riboflavin (B_2), niacin, pyridoxine, biotin, choline, folic acid, and vitamin B_{12}. Some fifty years ago we discovered the B vitamins and their role in disease, and we still are learning surprising new things about them. For example, there seems to be a connection between low levels of folic acid and cancer. According to research at the University of Alabama, women with precancerous Pap smears and smokers with precancerous cells in their lungs also had folic acid levels that were below normal, perhaps due to the fact that folic acid helps certain normal body cells to mature. In addition, adequate folic acid levels are important for development and maturing of the fetal central nervous system. Niacin, in large doses, is currently used as a treatment for people with a high cholesterol level in their blood. Additionally, the B vitamins—particularly B_{12} and folic acid—might protect against blood vessel damage caused by higher than healthy blood levels of the amino acid homocysteine (see page 362). Choline improves muscular function, particularly with excessive muscular effort (as in marathon runners), and might even enhance memory. The B vitamin riboflavin may help protect against certain cancers, particularly of the esophagus.

The B vitamins are water-soluble, which means they are excreted in the urine and must be replenished regularly. These vitamins can be found in a wide range of foods, including dairy products, most vegetables and fruits, and whole grain or enriched cereals and breads. If you eat any kind of a balanced diet, it is hard to escape them. The only possible exception is Vitamin B_{12}, which is found predominantly in meats, fish, eggs, and dairy products—foods that are excluded from some strict vegetarian diets.

Vitamins A (Beta-Carotene), E, and C: The Antioxidants

These vitamins are called *antioxidants* because they neutralize dangerous oxidants in the bloodstream. Oxidants, also called *free radicals,* are the toxic waste left in the blood when our bodies convert food to energy. These oxidants encourage the buildup of atherosclerotic plaque in the coronary arteries, stimulate the genetic mutations that provoke cancer, and play a role in aging.

The antioxidant vitamins—beta-carotene (which is transformed by our livers into vitamin A), vitamin A, vitamin C, and vitamin E— chemically "trap" the free radicals before they do their damage. One study of groups of women consuming large amounts of vitamin C, folic acid, and beta-carotene showed a lower chance of their getting cancers of the cervix or endometrium. Other studies claim that antioxidants seem to prevent heart disease, other forms of cancer, and protect against certain degenerative diseases of the eyes. (Although many studies have given strong support to these benefits, some contradictory findings have emerged, suggesting lesser value when the vitamins are given alone, away from the foods in which they naturally appear. There is substantial value, however, in any form.)

Although there has been a lot of emphasis on the antioxidant value of these vitamins, we should not forget their other benefits. Vitamin A is important to development of strong teeth and bones and for healthy vision; it helps to strengthen the immune system, and to keep the lining cells of the lungs and intestines healthy. Vitamin E contributes to the formation of our body's red blood cells and has been promoted (without substantiation) as a kind of folk medicine for treating hot flashes during menopause. Vitamin C is critical to healthy teeth, gums, and bones and to the functioning of the body's immune system. Its preventive and possible curative properties may not have been well documented, but taking vitamin C to fight a cold is now as common as last generation's chicken soup.

You can find vitamins A, E, and C in fruits and vegetables: A is

STUDIES TO WATCH FOR

We're poised to learn more about the benefits and proper dosages of antioxidants. An NIH-supported project called the Nurses' Health Study, being conducted at the Brigham and Women's Hospital at Harvard, is currently assessing the effect of beta-carotene and vitamin E on heart disease and cancer in forty-four thousand women over age fifty. Another project called CARET (Carotene and Retinol Efficacy Trial), being conducted at the Fred Hutchinson Cancer Research Center in Seattle, is studying whether components of vitamin A, beta-carotene, and retinoic acid can prevent lung cancer and cardiovascular disease in eighteen thousand heavy cigarette smokers and asbestos workers. Other current studies are investigating the effect of vitamins A, E, and C on lung and stomach cancer and the effect of vitamin A derivatives on severe acne and other skin conditions.

found in dairy products and the orange vegetables and fruits such as carrots, squash, cantaloupes, peaches, and apricots. Vitamin E is found in vegetable oils, nuts, brown rice, whole wheat, and green leafy vegetables; and we all know we can find vitamin C in citrus fruits, strawberries, cantaloupes, and of course those green leafy vegetables. Spinach and broccoli have A, E, C, and more. Eating a wide variety of fruits and vegetables and eating them in abundance is undoubtedly the best way to get an ample array of all these beneficial substances. You can also get your antioxidant vitamins in supplement form, but that is more controversial (see page 51).

MINERALS

Minerals are single-chemical elements found in various levels in our bodies—some in abundance, like calcium and phosphorus; others in mere traces, such as iron or copper. Minerals are essential body components, yet our bodies don't manufacture them; we must obtain them through what we eat.

MINERALS FOUND IN LARGE QUANTITIES IN OUR BODIES

Salt

A healthy diet means cutting back on table salt, or does it? More than a decade ago, salt swept the headlines as a major health hazard—a rumor born from valid studies that show low blood pressure levels throughout life in cultures where salt intake is very low. Scores of corporations responded by introducing new products to the American supermarket shelves, and soon it was common knowledge that sprinkling your food with salt at the table would surely lead to high blood pressure and a quick heart attack.

As much as this idea might have benefited some patients who need salt substitutes and low-salt pretzels, most experts now agree that consuming sodium will not cause high blood pressure in otherwise healthy people. (Those people who suffer from heart failure, kidney or liver dysfunction, salt-sensitive hypertension, or any other condition that inhibits the body's ability to excrete salt and maintain a normal fluid-electrolyte balance *are* at risk.)

In 1989, a large epidemiological study conducted by the London School of Hygiene and Tropical Medicine deflated the already tenuous salt–high blood pressure theory. After assessing exact sodium intake on the basis of urinalysis among more than ten thousand people in fifty-two countries, the London researchers found that, with rare exception, sodium intake had nothing to do with high blood pressure. In fact, in China, where sodium intake is greater than anywhere else in the world, average blood pressure is a normal 119/71. In the United States, sodium intake is about average compared to other countries in the world, but our average blood pressure is a somewhat higher normal of 123/74 (see page 387). The truth is, the human body is a miraculous regulatory machine and generally does an excellent job of maintaining a healthy salt-to-water balance.

The National Research Council advocates holding salt consumption to less than 6 grams a day; the American Heart Association says 4 grams. (The average American probably consumes in the range of 6 to 7 grams per day, but there is a wide variation from individual to individual.)

I believe, nonetheless, that stringent limits on salt are unnecessary for women whose blood pressure is normal and who are otherwise healthy. While I don't recommend a jar full of pickles for an afternoon snack, I say, within the boundaries of common sense, don't sweat the salt.

Sodium Nitrites. No discussion of salt is complete without mention of *sodium nitrites,* which are preservatives found in smoked fish and cured meats—like bacon, hot dogs, luncheon meats, and smoked salmon. International studies from countries like China and Japan as well as Hawaii have shown that high levels of nitrites either in the diet or drinking water are associated with an increased risk of stomach and esophageal cancer. Although these preservatives exist in minute amounts in our foods and are safe (within reason), most of those foods that contain sodium nitrites happen to be unhealthy in other ways, such as high fat content.

When it comes to foods containing sodium nitrites, I suggest erring on the side of caution. Not that you can never have a good hot dog with mustard and sauerkraut at a ball game or never eat smoked fish—just avoid them as a staple in your diet.

Calcium

Calcium is not only a building block for our bones, nails, and teeth, but also a major player in muscle contraction and relaxation—even for the muscles of our heart, and the muscles in the walls of our blood vessels and intestinal tract. It is no news that consuming sufficient calcium can help women stave off *osteoporosis*, the brittle bone condition. What might be news, though, is that adequate calcium is as important for young girls as it is for older women, since young girls are building the bone structure that has to get them through life (even though bone mass is continually replaced). And bone mass plummets after menopause unless women take estrogen replacement to slow the process. Supplemental calcium also slows this decline (see chapter 10).

In addition, calcium may well protect women against colorectal cancer, heart disease, and high blood pressure. The Women's Health Initiative (see page 10) will be investigating these possible benefits among women age fifty and over.

The ideal way to get calcium in your diet is through food: skim milk, low-fat yogurt, and green leafy vegetables like broccoli and kale. An 8-ounce glass of low-fat milk gives you almost 350 mg of calcium; 8 ounces of low-fat yogurt, over 400 mg; an ounce of cheese, between 100 and 200 mg; and a 6-ounce glass of calcium-enriched orange juice, 225 mg. A cup of spinach has almost 300 mg of calcium; 3 ounces of sardines with bones, about 350 mg. But few people get sufficient quantities on a daily basis this way, especially if they are lactose intolerant.

We'll discuss the concept of supplements at length on page 51; for now I strongly suggest you consider with your doctor the merits of calcium supplements, since it is difficult to consume the necessary 1,200 mg to 1,500 mg of calcium per day some women need depending on their age. Calcium supplementation of up to 2,500 mg a day will not cause unhealthy calcium buildup in the body or kidney stones, as once was thought, except possibly during pregnancy. There are three common forms of calcium supplements: calcium carbonate, calcium citrate, and calcium lactate. Calcium carbonate is the preferred form of supplement because it is absorbed well and is least expensive. Choose a tablet fortified with vitamin D, since this vitamin helps your body absorb calcium. Finally, check the absorptive potential of the tablets you choose by dropping one into a glass of water and making sure it dissolves within thirty minutes.

TRACE MINERALS

Trace minerals are needed only in small to minute quantities in the body. I don't recommend you take extra supplements of any of these minerals (other than what might appear in your multivitamin), but you should be aware of their potential benefits.

Iron

Iron is an important element in any woman's diet because it's an essential part of the molecules of our blood and muscles. But, unless you're anemic or pregnant, you get plenty of iron through foods, and there is no need for you to take iron pills. Our healthy bodies regulate iron so that we always have just enough in storage. Too much iron can damage the liver and has been associated with heart disease and cancer.

You can get iron from red meat (but don't stock up on red meat for the iron because the fat isn't worth the trade-off), fish, poultry, green leafy vegetables, and grain products—cereal, bread, and pasta—that have been fortified with iron. Meats and vitamin C enhance iron absorption, by the way, so if you have any concerns, eat a bit of chicken or a glass of orange juice with your iron-fortified pasta to get your quota easily.

Potassium

Potassium and sodium act together to regulate the water going in and out of our cells. Some research suggests that increasing potassium might decrease blood pressure and protect against stroke in healthy adults. Virtually all foods have some potassium; foods especially high in potassium include bananas, oranges, and green leafy vegetables.

Magnesium and Zinc

The possibility that magnesium might lower blood pressure bears further investigation. A 1987 epidemiological study showed that in areas where water is "hard" (that is, where water is laden with minerals including calcium and magnesium) heart disease rates are unusually low. Zinc is necessary for the functioning of many of the body's enzymes and is needed for normal growth and for development of our reproductive organs. Inadequate amounts of zinc might stimulate osteoporosis. Zinc deficiency also weakens the immune system. It's hard to become zinc deficient, since you need so little of it and it is present in a wide range of foods, including meats, fish, breads, and cereals. Too much zinc, however, can interfere with iron absorption, and disproportionately high amounts of zinc relative to copper might contribute to heart disease; I don't advise you take zinc supplements.

Selenium

Selenium is another mineral we need only in very tiny amounts, but its positive potential is intriguing. It's an antioxidant and may inhibit skin and lung cancer and slow the aging process. It is found in many foods (including meats, fish, grains, and dairy products) and in many vegetables if grown in selenium-rich soil. Many multivitamin and mineral tablets on the market contain selenium. We certainly don't have enough information to make recommendations, so stay tuned.

Fluoride

We know fluorides are critical to the growth and development of the skeleton, and, as almost everyone knows, tiny amounts of fluoride in water (one part per million) prevent tooth decay. It's possible that fluoride may have a role in preventing osteoporosis, although the jury's still out. Since fluoride is present in most water supplies, we generally do not have to be concerned about it in our diet; however, if you have well water—as I do—you have to decide in particular whether to give your children fluoride supplements with their pediatric multivitamins—which I did. (Having grown up in the New York City borough of Queens at a time when water was not fluoridated, I now have amalgam-filled teeth that bear no likeness to those of my children, who have been entirely cavity free.)

SUPPLEMENTING YOUR DIET WITH VITAMIN AND MINERAL PILLS

According to conventional medical teaching, if you eat a well-rounded diet, you don't need dietary supplements in pill form. For laypeople and professionals alike, the truth about supplements has been conflicting and confusing. One day, you can cure cancer by taking supplements of beta-carotene, which is converted to vitamin A in the body; the next day, you find out that too much vitamin A can kill you. The RDAs don't help at all; any supplements instantly put you over the RDA "limit" if you abide strictly by these government-recommended dietary allowances.

The medical community does endorse the use of supplements in special circumstances. Doctors regularly recommend over-the-counter daily multivitamins to individuals who for any reason are on a low-calorie diet (that is, taking in fewer than 1,200 calories a day). Pregnant women, women who are breast-feeding, and chronically ill people are advised to take specific supplements; smokers are often told to increase their intake of vitamin C.

I firmly believe that supplements are a valid and important means for getting protective levels of vitamins and minerals in a woman's diet. We know we don't have to worry about deficiencies, but I've also seen a sufficient number of studies to believe that women may derive great value from higher levels of many vitamins and minerals, particularly certain B vitamins (like folic acid), the antioxidant vitamins, calcium, and fluoride. I'm not suggesting massive doses of any vitamin. I am advising that you take a safe and established over-the-counter multivitamin.

Of course, the key danger in supplements is that they are concentrated. It is possible to cause harm by taking too much of certain vitamins or minerals. The vitamins that could be risky are the four fat-soluble vitamins—vitamins A, D, E, and K—which get stored in the body, as opposed to being excreted in the urine, when ingested in excessive amounts. Among even the stored vitamins, only Vitamin A has been shown thus far to be dangerous in excess. Stored in the liver, it can cause liver damage; excessive amounts may be associated with birth defects if taken early in pregnancy. Beta-carotene, which is converted to vitamin A by the liver, is less toxic than vitamin A itself, possibly because only partial conversion to vitamin A occurs; if a supplement is used, beta-carotene is preferable to vitamin A.

For most other vitamins there is little information about serious toxic side effects. But, remember, they have not been well studied; therefore, I suggest you only take fat-soluble vitamin supplements (other than what you'll find in a multivitamin) with your doctor's recommendation.

SUPPLEMENTAL THOUGHTS AND RECOMMENDATIONS

Vitamins and minerals are essential to a woman's health. For a healthy woman, the downside of eating vitamin- and mineral-rich food and even supplements is practically nonexistent, as long as you stay well within dosages that have been shown to be safe.

And whatever the RDA or the medical community may recommend officially, I will tell you that increasing numbers of medical professionals are themselves taking supplements of these vitamins. I take supplements of calcium, the antioxidant vitamins, and a multivitamin. My husband and children also take vitamins.

The National Research Council of the National Academy of Sciences has summarized in detail the range for supplements: the recommended RDA levels at the low end and the probable toxic levels for vitamins and minerals at the high end. When taking any vitamin or mineral supplement, check the minimum daily toxic dose and be sure it is not exceeded. Make sure to add together the amounts if you take, for example, a multivitamin plus a calcium supplement. Most food labels generally tell you the vitamin and mineral content of a serving and what percentage of an RDA that serving supplies, but food labels do not tell you what the minimum toxic dose might be.

The following chart should guide you as you make your specific vitamin and mineral choices. Remember, the chart is for healthy adults—if you have any health problems, or are pregnant, menopausal, or elderly, consult your physician.

SAFE AND TOXIC DIETARY SUPPLEMENTS FOR ADULTS
VITAMINS AND MINERALS

NUTRIENT	HIGHEST RECOMMENDED DAILY INTAKE FOR ADULTS BASED ON RDAs	ESTIMATED DAILY ADULT TOXIC DOSE (IU = INTERNATIONAL UNITS MG = MILLIGRAMS)
Vitamin A	5,000 IU	25,000–50,000 IU
Beta-Carotene	3 mg	15–30 mg
Vitamin D	400 IU	50,000 IU
Vitamin E	30 IU	1,200 IU
Vitamin C	60 mg	1,000–5,000 mg
Thiamin	1.5 mg	300 mg
Riboflavin	1.7 mg	1,000 mg
Niacin	20 mg	1,000 mg
Pyridoxine	2.2 mg	2,000 mg
Biotin	0.3 mg	50 mg
Pantothenic Acid	10 mg	1,000 mg
Folic Acid	0.4 mg	400 mg
Calcium	1,200 mg	12,000 mg
Phosphorus	1,200 mg	12,000 mg
Magnesium	400 mg	6,000 mg

Iron	18 mg	100 mg
Zinc	15 mg	500 mg
Copper	3 mg	100 mg
Fluoride	4 mg	4–20 mg
Iodine	0.15 mg	2 mg
Selenium	0.2 mg	1 mg

Source: Adapted by J. N. Hathcock from National Research Council, *Diet and Health* (Washington, D.C.: National Academy Press, 1989), 518.

PECULIARITIES OF THE AMERICAN DIET

SUGAR SUBSTITUTES

Sugar substitutes, to me, are the snake oil of the twentieth century. They have become almost a routine part of the diets of children and adults out of some fear of sugar. Sugar substitutes are chemicals, with dubious effects on the human body. They've not been proven empirically to endanger women at normal consumption levels, but I know,

WATCH OUT

I was distressed, as were many others, by the threat that the Food and Drug Administration (FDA) might take all megavitamins and other supplements off the shelves. Since dietary supplements like vitamins are regulated by the FDA as a food product and not as a drug, these products must meet safety requirements but are not required to have demonstrated efficacy for health or disease treatment. The FDA has stated its intention to increase its regulation of vitamins and other food supplements—in essence, to start treating them as drugs—and some fear it may impede ready public access to vitamins and other nutrients that exceed the federal guidelines as defined by the RDAs. Like my father more than forty years ago, I've started hoarding nutrients; only for me, they are vitamins! (Of course, I'll be in trouble after their expiration date.)

regardless of what actresses or models may tell you, that some women feel bad physically when they ingest sugar substitutes, and that's enough to consider. A Coke won't kill you; neither will a piece of hard candy. Simple sugar in large amounts is obviously ill advised, but high-fat foods that are chemically sweetened and lower in calories are riskier than the real sweet stuff on your low-fat, high-fiber cereal in the morning. Sugar substitutes have been invaluable, however, for those suffering with diseases of sugar metabolism such as diabetes.

FOODS AS ALTERNATIVE MEDICINE

There is no doubt that we should beware of food fads, like bee pollen as a remedy for allergies or ginseng as a source of virility or mental sharpness. Even if the basic claims ultimately prove to be true, the benefits are generally apt to be overstated until we know the proper dosages, and it's possible that huge quantities of any substance can be dangerous (and certainly expensive).

However, although food fads can be food frauds, I in no way suggest we dismiss them entirely. I think the scientific community should heed them and study them, and laypeople should keep a cautiously open mind. We should not forget that digitalis, used for heart failure, is a medicinal plant that has been used as an herbal remedy for hundreds of years, or that Taxol, a new and highly promising anticancer drug, was discovered in the bark of a yew tree. Garlic lowers cholesterol and blood pressure; it decreases blood clotting and may block the tissue effects of cancer-inducing pollutants, limit tumor growth, and boost the immune system. Garlic's wonders have been so widely experienced that many medical researchers are now actively studying it in the laboratory. Onions, scallions, and chives may also share some of garlic's health-giving properties. And the late Linus Pauling turned out to be no quack—his ideas about vitamin C's boosts to the immune system have now been widely accepted.

Looking deeper into these "old wives' tales" about foods, you will find that plants are filled with many chemical substances (traveling along with other good plant components like vitamins and fiber) that do not have defined nutritional value but may well provide benefits to health not yet fully understood. Plant steroids naturally occurring in vegetables may lower cholesterol. Phytoestrogens (isoflavonoids) present in high levels in soy products may actually *reduce* hormone-related cancers such as breast (unlike the estrogens in HRT, which may increase the risk of breast cancer (see pages 208 and 244) and prostate; indoles in broccoli and brussels sprouts may have a similar anticancer effect. Saponins, plant chemicals that are abundant in soybeans, bind cholesterol in bile and may decrease heart disease and colon cancer. Allium compounds are the chemicals in onions and garlic that have health benefits. Mothers for ages have said that vegetables are very good for you; the future may tell us *how* good.

A WORD ABOUT WINE

As is the case with just about everything in this chapter, we don't know enough about the risks and benefits of alcohol consumption. Several well-documented studies have recently shown that mild to moderate alcohol consumption of up to two drinks a day (one drink meaning about a 4-ounce glass of wine, a 12-ounce bottle of beer, or a 1-ounce shot of liquor—in whatever form, a total of less than one-half ounce of alcohol) can increase HDL levels and thereby lower by half your risk for heart attack. Dr. Walter Willett, a Harvard nutritionist, was quoted in the *New York Times:* "Alcohol is astonishing—related to almost every health issue we look at and it's almost never neutral. . . . It's a very potent pharmacologic agent that can be part of a healthy diet and can also be essentially fatal if consumed in excess." Of course, the benefits of alcohol quickly disappear when the amount consumed exceeds two drinks daily—and two drinks is not, for thousands of people, an easy place to stop. There is a very real concern that positive health findings about alcohol consumption could ultimately have a negative effect among those who use such findings as an excuse to overindulge, thereby endangering themselves and others.

Women need to be especially cautious. Because of the distribution of fat and water in a woman's body, she becomes intoxicated more easily than a man and is more quickly exposed to the health dangers of alcohol. We all know that liver damage is a potential and toxic side effect of alcohol; alcohol consumption in women has also been linked to greater loss of calcium and therefore osteoporosis, and (at least in some studies) to breast cancer. In all these concerns, the greater the amount of alcohol consumed, the greater the risk. This is also true for pregnancy (see page 63).

A glass of wine a day with dinner can't hurt and may indeed help. But use your head; drink alcohol in moderation, be sure you can enjoy yourself without it, and never drink if you plan to drive.

THOUGHTS ABOUT CAFFEINE

There's no such thing as a guilt-free cup of coffee anymore. Yet most of us wake up to the pungent aroma of a good cup of coffee and have spent our lives using caffeine as a quick pick-me-up. Coffee bars are the rage in Seattle—no wonder it's sleepless—and the concessions are spreading with the speed of McDonald's from coast to coast. Is this bad? Is it an addiction? Will coffee damage our hearts, breasts, ovaries, and bones? Having reviewed most of the studies to date, I see only that research results are chaotic, unclear, and highly contradictory. A cup of coffee or two has been shown definitively to improve memory, endurance, and certainly mental alertness. Drink four or five cups, and the resulting overstimulation is just as obvious. I say, as with any good thing, enjoy it in moderation.

TIPS FOR A HEALTHY DIET

With all of this sometimes confusing information, can we come up with a notion of the healthy diet? I think so. Just try to keep the following in mind:

• Think of food not in terms of dieting or fads, but in terms of patterns of living. You should start to think about what you eat as an extension of who you are and how you take care of yourself—the way you brush your teeth or shower in the morning or at night. Yes, the information that will be released about specific nutrients will change over time, but if you care about what you eat and establish a consistent healthy pattern of eating many foods in moderation, the changes won't throw you.

• Think peasant thoughts, keeping your diet reminiscent of a more simple life. Eat lots of whole grains, fruits, and vegetables, and less animal fat and protein. Build your meals on a foundation of complex carbohydrates—cereals for breakfast; a baked potato, rice and beans, or corn on the cob for lunch; pasta and vegetables for dinner. We are talking about black beans and rice, pasta primavera, and spaghetti, macaroni, and whole wheat breads. Try to abandon the notion that dinner is incomplete without meat; when you do have meat, try to reduce the size of the portion. Sure, in excess, starches are fattening, but "in excess" is the key phrase here, as it is in all nutrition.

• Consume at least five servings of fruits and vegetables in any combination in the course of a day. This could include orange juice in the morning and a snack of raisins or an apple mid-morning. Consider carrot sticks, salad, fruit cup, banana on your cereal, a potato topped with chili beans for lunch, and melon or strawberries for dessert.

• Limit the amount of animal protein that you eat to 5 or 6 ounces a day, and try to get most of that protein from chicken, fish, and low-fat dairy products.

• With the help of your physician, seriously explore the use of vitamin and mineral supplements.

• Keep the fat down, paying attention to what you already know. Avoid regular servings of fried foods; lighten up on the butter, margarine, and dressings; stay away from heavily marbled red meat; and drink skim milk.

WOMEN AND WEIGHT

The American woman's obsession with weight is, to me, nothing short of a sickness in itself. I find it particularly ironic that women I've seen in different parts of the world—from Japan to France to England to Canada—who don't appear to have this diet obsession also appear to have reasonable body weights. Yet here, where so many magazine covers scream DIET, I see obesity everywhere. I'll leave it to contemporary

THE DIET WITHOUT A DIET

Who has time to keep track of every bite? A lifetime of healthy eating is for me as simple as one-two-three. If you pay attention to nothing else nutritionally each day but these three components, you'll be in excellent health, maintain an appropriate weight, and feel wonderful.

1. Keep saturated fats down to 10 percent of your daily caloric intake and aim for 20 percent for total fat. How? Load up on complex carbohydrates and skip all the fat you can see.

2. Eat five servings of fruits and vegetables a day.

3. Take a multivitamin and a calcium supplement.

authors such as Susan Faludi *(Backlash)* or Naomi Wolf *(The Beauty Myth)* to reveal the societal causes of this sickness (and I heartily encourage you to peruse these excellent books). I'll take a look at the emotional relationship women have with food later in this chapter (see page 65); now, though, let's examine the issue from the physiological side.

No woman should carry around so many extra pounds that her weight poses a threat to her health. But what is that number? You can easily find charts of ideal weight ranges: the tables of Metropolitan Life and the National Center for Health Statistics are the most reliable. But those charts can be confusing by giving wide ranges and often lumping men and women together. So I suggest that if you find you've picked up more than fifteen extra pounds or weigh more than 15 percent of your top ideal body weight according to those charts, talk with your doctor. Is the weight a new gain, or have you maintained it for years? Are you currently eating well? Do you have high blood pressure or diabetes? If your doctor tells you she feels it would be in your best interest to shed a few pounds, pay attention. Otherwise, most simply, if you're eating a healthy diet as described in this chapter and exercising regularly, your weight is probably just fine.

Forget the TV commercials and the bikini-clad next-door neighbor. Weight is a health matter and an individual, not a societal, issue. Ideal weight varies with your body structure, your heredity, your exercise level, the amount of muscle in your body, your age, the time of the month, your height, and the ratio of body fat to lean body mass. If you are watching your fat intake and getting exercise, you are in all likelihood maintaining a weight that is healthy and appropriate for your body. Don't worry, either, if your weight creeps up over the years—in the range of about 10 percent of where you were at "twenty-something." Women gain some weight naturally with age, and epidemiologists observe that women seem to have less trouble with menopause and even osteoporosis in cultures where they are slightly heavier.

If your doctor doesn't tell you to, don't diet. Most women who diet will gain the weight back—and diet again and gain the weight back, and on and on. This "yo-yo syndrome," some believe, is more dangerous than a few extra pounds. According to data from the Framingham Study (a health study that has followed a community of people in New England for more than four decades), this syndrome is more likely to cause heart disease, cancer, and early death than obesity itself. However, a 1994 report in the *Journal of the American Medical Association* challenged this risk of weight cycling. While this medical question is being resolved, one cannot deny that yo-yo weight is hard on your psyche, your wardrobe, and your pocketbook.

If you feel you might face a medical reason for dieting, look at your body. All extra pounds do not carry the same risk for disease. Diseases associated with obesity appear to be tied more to where the fat is carried than how much fat is present. Women with thick waistlines, big tummies, and love handles—the apple shape—are more susceptible to diabetes, hypertension, and heart disease than women shaped like pears. Obesity in general, though, is also associated with gallstones and cancer of the colon, breast, uterus, and ovaries. For all obese people, too, there is considerable evidence that being on the lean end of those weight charts and voluntary weight loss are associated with greater longevity.

If you are obese, first and foremost I hope you recognize that genetics determines a good deal of your predicament. Obesity is a health condition, not a character flaw. Next, see your doctor. You may find help through medication, although be sure to ask plenty of questions. Several studies in recent years have documented that a new generation of drugs can stimulate weight loss, but the jury is still out on how safe they actually are.

For most American women, my strongest advice is to throw out the liquid diets and any magazine with an unachievable body on the cover. As a rule, I say abandon the concept of "dieting," that is, drastically changing the pattern of what you eat for a short time, with a specific goal in mind; replace it with an ongoing commitment to a low-fat diet and regular exercise. With a stable, conscious, and sane point of view, most of us can keep our weight in check, our psyches healthy, and our lives long.

NUTRITION FOR THE STAGES OF A WOMAN'S LIFE

At different times in your life—or in your daughter's life—nutritional needs will vary. I don't attempt to be exhaustive here but instead want to give you a sense of your body's key nutritional needs as it goes through inevitable changes.

THE GROWING GIRL

What mother is not worried that her little ones are not eating properly—or just not enough? Stop worrying. Numerous studies show that children—boys and girls, whose nutritional needs are not yet significantly different—generally eat better until adolescence than their parents. Their protein intake is comparable to that of adults, and their consumption of vitamins, minerals, and carbohydrates is higher. Studies of children repeatedly show that kids will take care of their daily nutritional needs if you offer a variety of healthy foods and don't make an issue of what or how much they eat. Even obese children (of nonobese parents) generally outgrow their baby fat.

Moreover, although children consume excessively high amounts of sugar (up to 14 percent of their diet), little evidence suggests that these empty calories compromise their nutritional status or cause hyperactivity. Surprisingly, even refined sugar isn't the culprit in dental decay that we once thought it was; in fact, caramels wash out of the mouth faster than breakfast cereals and dried fruit.

My only concern when it comes to a girl's diet (up to eleven years of age) is that she get adequate calcium, generally advised to be at least 800 mg per day. (Two glasses of milk a day will give your daughter 700 mg; add a bite of spinach, calcium-enriched orange juice, or some cheese, and she is heading toward 1,000 mg.) A child's vitamin recommended by your pediatrician will easily fill any nutritional gaps.

Overall, though, simply make nutritional foods available to your young children, permit them to eat when they are hungry and stop eating when they feel full, and don't use food as punishment or reward. They will develop healthy eating habits for life.

ADOLESCENTS

Nutritional needs do differ greatly in *adolescent girls* and boys, and a teen girl's needs are different from those of an adult woman. Teenagers grow almost as fast as infants and thus have extraordinary nutritional needs. But in teens, you face two difficult roadblocks.

First, for many kids, junk food rules. Their social life revolves around it, and it's priced just right for a teenager's budget. Even more disturbing, though, is the fact that this critical period of growth in a girl's life coincides with tremendous peer and media pressure to be skinny and popular, to try all the irresponsible diet fads her friends are trying, and to wear the smallest size possible, despite her body's healthy teen tendency to put on fat as she goes through puberty.

A teenage girl's diet can wreak havoc on her body, either from high-fat, low-nutrient junk or what amounts to periodic self-starvation.

(Anorexia and bulimia are always concerns for the modern parent of a teenage girl—but not quite as common as most have come to believe; see page 66 if you have any worries at all.) As an eternal optimist I believe that you can influence your healthy teenage girl's diet *somewhat,* and in any event you should never give up trying. I suggest that you

• Tell your daughter about nutrition. Show her this chapter. Remind her that her current nutritional choices will have an impact on her body for the rest of her life—she can start now to prevent osteoporosis, heart disease, and cancer.

• Make family dinners a rule. When you ritualize eating, everyone pays more attention. Whoever prepares the food does it with forethought; what gets eaten gets seen and tasted by all; and, of course, you can observe your child's eating behavior firsthand. I also believe the mind and soul, as well as the body, get nourished through this regular gathering of the family members.

• Give your daughter a multivitamin at breakfast (after checking with your doctor). Encourage her to drink calcium-fortified orange juice and skim milk. We now recommend that teens and young women increase their daily calcium intake to 1,200 mg. Teenage girls need more iron, zinc, and calcium than boys, and numerous studies have shown that increased calcium in adolescence increases bone mass and can prevent osteoporosis later in life.

• Grin and bear it. Sometimes she will actually listen!

PREGNANT WOMEN

Fortunately, pregnancy is one area of women's nutrition in which considerable research has been done. If you are pregnant, work with your doctor or midwife to set up your best nutrition plan. You'll also find scores of books devoted entirely to the subject. Be sure to learn about the following food and drink issues; if your doctor doesn't tell you, ask.

Folic Acid. We know that supplements of folic acid (one of the B vitamins), taken before becoming pregnant and through the early part of the pregnancy, can prevent some of the worst kinds of birth defects. The Centers for Disease Control and Prevention (CDC) recommends that all women trying to conceive should take 4 mg of folic acid daily.

Calcium. Sufficient calcium—in the range of at least 1,200 mg daily—is essential for a pregnant woman. A growing fetus requires a considerable amount of calcium to develop; the source of this calcium is the mother's body. Pregnant women must replenish the lost calcium in order to prevent their own bones from weakening. Again, talk with your doctor about the proper calcium supplement during your pregnancy, and be sure to obtain additional calcium through calcium-rich foods such as milk, yogurt, cheese, broccoli, spinach, and canned sardines with bones.

Other Nutrients. Make certain you're getting the right amount of iron (during pregnancy your total blood volume increases, and so will your need for iron); zinc (some inconclusive animal studies do show a relationship between birth defects and zinc deficiencies, but you should easily get enough zinc, even when pregnant, from the foods you eat and your multivitamin); vitamin A (early in your pregnancy, avoid supplements in excess of what is found in your prenatal multivitamins because of possible fetal birth defects); protein (your pregnant body needs a bit more, but with our high-protein American diets, you probably won't have to worry about getting enough).

General Supplements. Most doctors recommend, or even prescribe, multivitamins to their pregnant patients. This is an important and valuable practice.

Alcohol. Drinking 2 to 4 alcoholic beverages every day during pregnancy can harm the developing baby, causing mental retardation and other neurologic deficits. However, many studies done here and abroad have failed to find evidence that fetal alcohol syndrome or impaired fetal development is linked to drinking in the range of 1 drink or less per day (which is less than a half ounce of alcohol). To be safe, many women are deciding to abstain from any alcohol from the time they determine that they are pregnant. I concur. My feeling is it's better to be safe, but a woman should not agonize over an occasional glass of wine during pregnancy and especially not torture herself if she happened to have a few drinks before learning she was pregnant. Again, common sense should rule.

General Diet. Listen to your body. If you have a craving, indulge. If you're into food fads, whether bee pollen or ginseng, take a sabbatical. And, as your doctor will tell you, don't take any medication—over-the-counter or prescription—unless she clears it. (An occasional aspirin, however, is okay.)

Weight Gain. Doctors themselves have been giving pregnant women contradictory recommendations over the years about what is an ideal amount of weight to gain. Many years ago you were "eating for two" and could gain almost any amount of weight; when I was in medical school the ideal weight gain was about twenty to twenty-five pounds;

a decade or so later, any more than ten to fifteen pounds was considered excessive. Now the pendulum seems to have hit the middle again: you can gain about twenty-five to thirty-five pounds and need consume no more than an extra 300 or so calories per day during the second and third trimesters.

MENOPAUSE AND BEYOND

The most nutritionally relevant change that takes place during and after menopause is that your body considerably reduces its production of the important hormone estrogen. (We'll take a close look at hormone replacement therapy in chapter 5.) You should be aware of the following nutritional ramifications of reduced estrogen:

Calcium. Bone mass melts away during and after menopause unless you take estrogen replacement to slow the process. Supplemental calcium can slow this decline. Based on the 1984 NIH Consensus Conference on Osteoporosis, I suggest a supplement of at least 1,500 mg of calcium per day if you do not take estrogen or 1,000 mg a day if you do (with your doctor's approval).

Fat. Recent studies have shown a significant correlation between postmenopausal breast and colon cancer and diets high in saturated fats. Lowering fat (down to 20 percent of the diet) corresponded to a decrease in breast cancer, but that observation has yet to be confirmed. Although it may be ideal, rigidly sticking to a 20 percent fat diet can be tough. Another approach is to focus on drastically reducing your intake of *saturated* fat. (See pages 34–40.)

Iron. After menopause, your need for iron lessens if you are no longer menstruating. If, however, you are on hormones that cycle and induce monthly bleeding, the iron loss persists.

ELDERLY WOMEN

As we age, our body functions change, and so do our nutritional needs. Although one-fifth of our population is expected to be over sixty-five by the year 2030, we have no current nutrition policy designed specifically to meet the needs of America's eldest. And many of the health problems of age relate directly to diet.

Over our adult years, our fat-to-muscle ratio increasingly favors fat; we tend to slow down physically, our metabolism slows in response, and we need fewer calories for sustenance. Tiny women may need as few as 1,000 calories a day, and fitting adequate amounts of protein, vitamins, minerals, and fiber into such a meager diet can be difficult. Some elderly also have problems with absorption of the nutrients they ingest. Because of vision and hearing losses, arthritis, and other disabling conditions, the elderly often have trouble shopping and cooking. Consequently, some elderly actually suffer from nutritional deficiencies, a problem we thought did not exist anymore. Conversely, levels of vitamin A (not beta-carotene) that are safe in younger adults may be toxic in older people because the liver loses its capacity to clear the vitamin from the body.

If you are elderly or are caring for an elderly woman, make sure to consult a doctor about a multivitamin, and ask if the diet in question is sufficient. Think young about your diet; you need the same basic elements we discuss throughout this chapter—perhaps in smaller quantities, but in balance. A gentle exercise program is also a good idea.

WHEN YOU ARE ILL

Just as we tailor our diet for prevention of disease when we are healthy, the diet has to be modified, often radically, when we are ill. If you have heart disease, you will be very concerned about your fat intake; your nutritional concerns will be quite different if you have renal disease (when too much protein is dangerous), hypertension (salt may or may not be a concern), or diabetes (you must constantly regulate sugar). If you have an illness, whether it be short-term or chronic, you must ask your doctor whether or not your eating habits should change in response to that illness and how permanent the change should be. If your doctor doesn't know or doesn't speak with the authority that gives you confidence, ask another.

WOMEN AND FOOD: SOCIETAL, EMOTIONAL, AND SPIRITUAL ISSUES

It's a simple act and a very short trip to load up a fork and traverse the distance to the mouth. Yet this act encompasses the cultural, biological, psychological, emotional, and habitual—as well as physiological—ramifications of exactly what is on that fork. Women are historically the food gatherers, the nurturers, the givers of nourishment, the food preparers, so food holds for us a special significance.

From the beginning of time, food has been a cause for celebration—an organizing concept around which relationships were sealed, disputes ended, and the soul and spirit ritually celebrated. Food is very much symbolic of the culture, cohesiveness, and spirit of the family or community, whether it be Thanksgiving, a seder feast at Passover, a Sunday dinner, or a wedding banquet. Only recently has food become the enemy or something to be grabbed on the run or zapped in the microwave—something, for many women, to be conquered, not savored.

American society has created a generation of women who can no longer enjoy the historical and spiritual connection with food as a life force. Young girls fight food—half of all high school girls are currently "on a diet" when most don't need to lose a pound. Media images everywhere promote impossible feminine bodies; even with the media's recent shift to emphasize muscular—not skinny—bodies, a woman's natural, widely variable shape has yet to be celebrated. There can be no one ideal model for all women's bodies, and the notion that there is can be downright dangerous.

EATING DISORDERS

Eating disorders have existed for hundreds of years but have become widely recognized only recently. Perhaps in another time, a deeply disturbed young woman would have exhibited different symptoms; in today's society, with such a huge focus on food and weight, she exploits this obvious means of making an obsessive and, for her, destructive statement.

Anorexia and bulimia are serious mental illnesses, to be distinguished from a young girl's culturally inspired fixation on weight. A young anorectic girl literally starves herself, sometimes to death, out of an obsessive fear of getting fat. A young bulimic woman's obsession with eating, body image, and weight becomes evident in bizarre eating patterns, gorging and then purging by either vomiting or using laxatives; with bulimia her body weight is usually normal.

An estimated five million people, 95 percent of them young women, suffer from anorexia nervosa or bulimia or both. As many as one in five college coeds, most of them white, bright, upper-middle-class achievers, starve themselves, induce vomiting, or take laxatives in an attempt to lose weight. Victims view all their personal worth in terms of how heavy or how thin they are, yet they never see themselves as thin enough. They are obsessed with food and with their power to turn away from it.

Both anorexia and bulimia begin with a modest attempt to lose a few pounds, but then something goes awry. Afflicted young women see a distorted view of themselves in the mirror, and their obsession becomes an addiction requiring professional treatment. Unless treated, eating disorders can decimate the body. Victims stop menstruating and, in a state of estrogen deficiency, can lose substantial bone mass. They can also erode their teeth, rupture the esophagus, cause irreversible damage to vital organs, and suffer from major depression. Unchecked, eating disorders cause severe malnutrition, weakness, and the inability to think clearly and make rational decisions. Some of those with severe disease may actually die of their affliction, usually from suicide or cardiac complications.

Most girls with eating disorders grew up in troubled families and have deep psychological wounds to heal. (Certain characteristics of families of youngsters with eating disorders reappear frequently: they are strict, filled with conflict, very protective but not empathetic, and driven to achievement.) Treatment requires nutritional counseling, medical supervision, and psychiatric care. For the most severely afflicted, in-hospital treatment where the psychiatric care combines behavior modification, family therapy, and peer support offers the best hope. Although victims can be threatened by relapses throughout their lives, good care holds the promise of recovery for almost all.

In this chapter on nutrition, I cannot stress strongly enough that any psychological treatment program for eating disorders must be accompanied by nutritional counseling. If you or your daughter or friend suffer from this complex and compulsive disease, don't leave the nutritionist out, for the short or long term. It can be a matter of life and death.

THE STATE OF NUTRITIONAL KNOWLEDGE TODAY

As mentioned early in this chapter, 75 percent of our medical schools offer no course in basic nutrition. Despite exciting developments in research on molecular biology, human genetics, and biochemistry (all with clear nutritional implications), between 1988 and 1994 the NIH devoted less than 4 percent of its budget to nutrition. During that time also, when overall budgets increased, the percentage of nutrition-related grant requests receiving funding actually dropped from previous years. With little physician training and even less government-supported research, how are tomorrow's physicians going to learn to respect and advocate the importance of nutrition? And how can disease prevention through nutrition gain the national focus it needs?

The principles that drive our current federal nutrition policy are inadequate, poorly coordinated, and weakly grounded in science. We cannot now defend with hard science some of our most basic nutritional practices, like feeding vitamins to our kids or giving them—and ourselves, for that matter—low-fat milk. Committees and task forces have been created to study nutrition as it affects specific diseases such as diabetes, heart disease, hypertension, cancer, and obesity. But most of these studies only pull together existing, often inconclusive studies and fail to call for the fully coordinated clinical and basic research effort directed at nutrition and health that is urgently needed.

WHERE WE HAVE TO GO

We simply must learn more about nutrition and women. We must shift our national focus from avoiding nutritional deficiencies to understanding the preventive miracles proper nutrition offers. We must commit to doing dietary studies even though they are difficult to conduct and easy to criticize. The validity of nutrition as a legitimate scientific discipline can no longer be questioned. Here are just a few of the questions we must answer:

• What is the complete relationship between nutrition and hormonal status at different stages of a woman's life? How, for example, do oral contraceptives or hormone replacement therapy affect dietary needs?

• We need major clinical trials to further explore how nutrients protect against disease. For example, we now know that broccoli does prevent cancer—it contains the chemical *sulforophane,* which causes the liver to produce an enzyme that appears to block carcinogenic activity. Sulforophane, also present in cabbage and brussels sprouts, stimulates the immune defense system. How else might nutrition improve our ability to combat cancer? To resist infection? To fight off diseases like AIDS?

• What other naturally occurring remedies can we find in food? A preliminary 1993 study suggests that collagen found in the breastbones of chickens can suppress the swelling and crippling pain of rheumatoid arthritis. Other studies have touted the healing properties of shark cartilage for cancers. These are just two examples; when herbs, extracts from animals and plants, and other food substances are considered, the potential is vast.

• What damage, though, can "natural" remedies do? Some herbal remedies, now so prevalent, may be useless or even harmful. We must learn which have real benefit, and precisely for whom and for what.

• What is the clear relationship between brain function and food? We know amino acids can influence sleep, arousal, muscle performance, anxiety, and more. Tryptophan (found in milk and turkey) induces sleep; tyrosine (in cheese and wine) may relieve stress. The military is considering adding such nutrients to food rations and snack bars. Where can all this go? Will designer food be the wave of the future for us all?

• How should we regulate fad diets, or should we? First, can they do real damage? Do we have the means of assessing the damage?

• How does the body utilize nutrients? Are there simple methods—like drinking orange juice with our calcium supplements—through which we can improve the amount of a nutrient that our body can actually absorb? We know a little, but far from enough.

• What is the relationship between diet and breast cancer? The Women's Health Initiative should answer that directly.

• What impact does one nutrient have on another? We suspect, for example, that too much zinc combined with too little copper may contribute to heart disease.

• What is the relationship between heredity and nutrition? Are we prewired genetically to draw special benefits or incur special risks from certain foods?

QUESTIONS FOR YOUR DOCTOR

When it comes to nutrition, I can assure you that your physician needs your help. Most of us had virtually no nutritional training in those seemingly endless series of classes and lectures during medical school and residency. As specialists we learn about nutrition within a narrow band of the illnesses we treat. Cardiologists can tell you plenty about fat and cholesterol, and rheumatologists are great on calcium and vitamin D. The cancer specialists keep up with the latest on fiber and fat. And obstetricians and gynecologists can tell you about folic acid. They are all confused about vitamins. How often does your doctor ask you about what you eat, even in passing, let alone in detail?

Doctors need your help to sensitize them to the importance of providing you the latest in nutritional information and doing so in the context of your total health, not just as it relates to a notable disease. Staying on top of the latest nutritional headlines—however confusing or conflicting—and bringing them to your doctor's attention are sure ways to get the message across.

Ask your doctor questions about nutrition; embarrassed by any lack of knowledge, he or she will learn more about the subject in no time, I can assure you!

- What is your doctor's diet, and is she changing what she eats in response to the latest information on vitamin E or broccoli?
- What about calcium? Do you need supplements? What chemical form seems best?
- Should you be taking vitamin supplements? If so, which ones?
- Are there any problems with your diet? (Review it together.)
- How should your diet change if you have a chronic illness?
- What should you do before embarking on a weight reduction diet?
- Based on your blood chemistry test results, do you need to modify your cholesterol intake further?
- Does your doctor have a list of registered dietitians you can consult with directly if you are (or someone in your family is) facing any kind of illness (or if you just want routine advice)?

WHAT WOMEN CAN DO PERSONALLY AND POLITICALLY

Women play a special role in our fight against disease, since we are highly represented in the fields that primarily influence lifestyles—ranging from pediatricians, nurses, and nutritionists to kindergarten teachers, and moms. I challenge you to recognize yourselves as the true leaders in this regard, working through the school boards and the corporate boards; in the garden clubs and in the downtown business clubs; in the local community action committees and by bringing pressure on the congressional appropriations committees.

One thing the recent debate on health care reform has shown us is that individuals and the organizations they work through can have a big impact on America's agenda. You can exert pressure on your elected representatives through phone calls, faxes, computer networks, and so forth. And don't forget the White House, which oversees all those federal agencies like the NIH, the Centers for Disease Control and Prevention, the FDA, and the entire Public Health Service, including the Office of the Surgeon General. If more of your like-minded friends make their opinion known, your message will have a greater impact. One thing all politicians do well is count! Don't overlook the power of local and national nonprofit organizations such as the American Heart Association, the American Red Cross, the American Cancer Society, the American Dietetic Association, the Juvenile Diabetes Foundation, and the American Diabetes Association to have a major effect on local and national policy as well as on public education.

During my years as director of the NIH, I had many formal and informal discussions about the field of nutrition with my friend and colleague Dr. Darla Danford, who was the director of nutrition in the Office of Disease Prevention at the NIH. She told me that her office was on the verge of being abolished on more than one occasion and that the battle to make nutrition a scientific and health priority was wearing her down (since she and I both left NIH, her office was, sadly, demoted). We worked to make nutrition a high priority in the 1993 NIH Strategic Plan and coined the term "bionutrition" to attract more interest and dollars to a cooperative research effort incorporating molecular biology and human genetics into the field of nutritional sciences. These NIH efforts show just how difficult the task can be. The medical community, the food industry, public health agencies, and the public at large must see the American diet as a matter relating to both quality and quantity of life. To achieve this vision, we need to do some public consciousness-raising as well as demand more solid nutritional information, tailored to the needs of the individual.

I hope you will recognize throughout your life that women are uniquely susceptible to chronic diseases and that at least half of these diseases can be mitigated by what you eat. Eat less fat and more complex carbohydrates, more plant protein and less animal protein; aspire to the simpler diet of our ancestors. But your individual healthy diet is only a part of your mandate: because scientists have neglected the study of nutrition and because the consequences are being felt disproportionately by women, we must insist on more medical research and greater awareness of the subject in the medical community. The world should have done better by our mothers; now we can and must do better for our daughters.

THREE

REPRODUCTIVE LIFE
Power and Vulnerability

No woman can call herself free
who does not own and control her body.

—M A R G A R E T   S A N G E R ,
W O M A N   A N D   T H E   N E W   R A C E ,   *1 9 2 0*

The disease that is love brings into conflict
our conscious intelligence and our basic will.

—A N D R É   M A U R O I S ,
S E V E N   F A C E S   O F   L O V E ,   *1 9 9 4*

She was seventeen and she wanted to keep her baby. It was 1968. She
did not want to marry the infant's father, for, young as she was, she
knew that to pay for her one passionate mistake with an even greater
mistake, a lifetime with an uncaring man, was a penance neither she
nor her child deserved. Abortion had not been a consideration for her.
It was illegal, and the methods forced by illicit circumstances could
quite possibly have mutilated or killed her. Besides, she was a devout
Catholic and probably wouldn't have opted for it anyway. At that
place, in that time, her only alternative was to give her baby up for
adoption, but she somehow created a choice where choice did not exist. Unlike the other Crittenden girls—the "bad girls" whose families
could scrape together enough money to send them away to the Flo-
rence Crittenden Home to wait out their pregnancies, getting good
care but far from the shaming eyes of the righteous public—unlike all
those numb and frightened young women, this one was fiercely determined. Social workers, nurses, doctors all tried vigorously to convince

her to avoid scandal and shame and change her mind, before and after her son was born. They isolated her, fearful that her maternal instinct would poison the other girls' resolve.

I met Ellen on my obstetrical rotation at the Boston "Lying In" Hospital; I wasn't much older than she. I too tried to change her mind; the life she was choosing seemed so hard to me, and we all knew what was the "right thing" to do. (I certainly didn't suspect that I would, a little more than a decade later, face a similar challenge, divorced and raising my infant daughter alone!) But when I made my rounds the day after her delivery and found Ellen sitting up in the chair by her bed feeding her infant, I became silent. She told me of her plans to go back to school and to raise her son with the help of her widowed father, who ran a small grocery store in their neighborhood. This was no teenager indulging in a whim, but a woman, one of the most profoundly powerful and committed women I think I've ever seen. I recognized in that moment that what was proper for the time had little to do with what was right for this girl-woman. Her image is with me still.

In every woman's experience of her sexual and reproductive life lies the story of her constant choice making, her decision to be complacent or unaware, or to recognize, protect, and responsibly employ the immense and awesome power she carries in her body and soul. The unorthodox choice of a pregnant seventeen-year-old girl in the sixties who seemed willing to face a difficult life and social stigma to raise her child highlights a monumental saga of social and scientific change. We look at sexuality, contraception, pregnancy, and childbirth through a very different lens now. But regardless of the era, there is a timeless, unchanging dimension to the difficult decisions every woman inevitably faces, and to the unique way each woman views the private power of her sexual self and how she safeguards or subverts it. The forces now buffeting us may take more subtle forms than the outright restrictions and prejudices that backed Ellen and her peers into such hard corners, but in many ways women today are just as vulnerable as ever, even if in a different way.

POWER AND VULNERABILITY AND HEALTH

A woman's reproductive life is not just about nine months but, rather, a lifetime of love, companionship, and human relationships. It is in our attentiveness to our reproductive health and well-being throughout our lifetime that we most definitely claim our power as women. How a woman thinks about her reproductive life becomes a critically defining element of her sense of herself and her long-term happiness. Wise, self-aware decisions in love protect our spirits. Caution and precaution in our sexual choices shield us from the dangers of sexually transmitted diseases. Knowledge of our bodies and sexual needs and desires keeps us fulfilled and whole. Treating our bodies as our ultimate domain may even provide some of the incredible strength we need to leave abusive relationships. Viewing pregnancy as a health-affecting gift we give ourselves and our spouses liberates us from the feeling of being enslaved by our maternal capabilities.

The scope of a woman's reproductive life is mammoth. Accordingly, I have divided this chapter into four parts, defining the crucial stages in most women's reproductive lives: love and sexuality; contraception; conception and infertility; and pregnancy and childbirth.

LOVE AND SEXUALITY

Though we can reproduce without love, few women do so by choice. Love is a reality and a risk in our world; I would wager that love gone wrong may be among the greatest causes of women's health problems—and love gone right, one of our greatest gifts.

PSYCHOLOGY OF LOVE
AND LOVE GONE WRONG

We all, male and female, seek to bond, to link with another human being, generally with the purpose of fulfilling our biological imperative: to reproduce. I find particularly credible two related theories of how and why we carry out this quest. The first stems from evidence that despite the changed role of women and the supposedly increasing enlightenment of our culture, our evolutionarily imprinted compulsions still run strong within us. According to Dr. David Buss, a psychologist at the University of Michigan, women, whether in rich or poor countries, regardless of political system, religion, race, or educational level, place a higher value on a mate's financial well-being than do men. Women instinctively look for strong providers and protectors to feather the nest through the external foraging and competition. Once a mate is found, women focus on perpetuating and solidifying the relationship.

Men, across cultures and continents, consistently place a higher value on youth and beauty than do women, presumably as biological markers of fertility and therefore desirability (specifically, thin waists, bigger hips, good skin, full lips, lustrous hair, and bright, clear eyes). Dr. Buss did find universal qualities on which both genders placed a high priority: kindness, intelligence, love, and mutual attraction. He and other evolutionary theorists attribute these seemingly universal findings in the face of dramatic social and cultural differences to an inescapable throwback instinct to carry on the species, a behavioral pattern that is in all likelihood tied up in our genes. As Dr. Buss puts it, we all carry with us today the desires of our successful forebears.

The second theory explaining our urge to pair-bond comes from the psychologist Dr. Dorothy Tennov, in her book *Love and Limerence: The Experience of Being in Love*. She distinguishes between the two types of erotic love (erotic love being, according to psychoanalyst Erich Fromm, the "craving" for one particular person, apart from other forms of love, such as motherly love or spiritual love). Dr. Tennov believes love begins as "limerence," a word she coins to describe the head-over-heels feeling of being "in love," with a fever or compulsion that can consume us even independently of our wills; an emotional drive distinct from sex, liking, or affection. Some individuals are more susceptible to Cupid's arrow than others, and, as most know, these feelings can be felt whether or not they are reciprocated. The intense emotional charge of limerence typically lasts between six months and three years; it then either decays or blossoms into the second stage of love, what Tennov calls "affectional bonding." This love forms the foundation of lasting relationships, different and deeper than, but not as intense as limerence, based firmly on what Fromm would call "acts of will," involving reason, faith, courage, and discipline.

I do not in any way find Dr. Buss's findings of the two genders' preferences disheartening or sexist; they provide an explanation of the emotional patterns defined in Dr. Tennov's work. The limerent state is likely a gift from our ancestors too. We are all composed of biological and evolutionary impulses that make sense for the species. Perhaps thrusting us into the passion of limerence encourages us to pair off with a mate; but we each have within us the reason and wherewithal to filter those impulses through our self-conscious minds, and seek affectional bonding in our permanent mates.

Limerence is not without its dark or pathological side, the obsessions that can rob a woman of her power and identity, driving her to unhealthy extremes. When it is combined with poor self-esteem, a woman can succumb to an irrational limerence that enables her to tolerate pathological bonding, as for example seen with spousal abuse. This horrifying type of attachment is poorly understood, often secret, and highly destructive. Somewhere between two and four million women a year in this country allegedly are battered by spouses or lovers; conservative estimates suggest that 25 percent of women will have experienced abuse by a significant other in their lifetimes.

Although as a society we bemoan the high divorce rate, separation and divorce are almost always the only option for an abused woman and her children. Children raised in abusive homes are at high risk of becoming abusive adults. We must warn our daughters about the dangers of abusive "love" relationships, and we should all be alert to signs of a possible abuser: a man who has a violent temper; who exhibits a strong, dominating, controlling personality; who cannot accept independence in his significant other; who is rigid in his world view with little tolerance for disagreement by his partner; who is abusive to those who are weak or dependent (even to animals), and shows contempt or low regard for women in general. Erratic verbal abuse alternating with remorse should be seen as a red alert; the man who threatens, screams, and rails for little reason is a possible batterer. Battering men are often charming and manipulative early on in relationships—don't cling to that memory as a rationalization for tolerating aberrant behavior. The psychological as well as social and economic forces can be incredibly strong to keep women locked into abusive relationships.

Falling madly in love is a treasure, but an even greater treasure is a woman's ability to evaluate the object of her passionate affection through her conscious mind. Accept limerence for the fleeting pleasure it is, but place a higher value on the universal and conscious qualities that bond us to our mates, and which require self-awareness rather than an absence of will.

SOCIOLOGY OF LOVE AND SEX

It is in the physical manifestation of love and bonding that we have seen the line between power and vulnerability in women become most blurred and confused. Throughout much of Western history, without education and economic or political clout, women had few means beyond allure to take charge of their lives. Lack of birth control made sexual experimentation a risk not worth taking for many women; most

STUDIES WE NEED: ON LOVE AND LIMERENCE

Emotions—such a vital part of our lives—have received very little attention in scientific studies of the brain or clinical studies of behavior. One reason is that the major agencies that would fund this kind of research (both the NIH and the NSF) often take a dim view of the "softer" social sciences as compared to the "harder" sciences of chemistry, molecular biology, and physics. We may be seeing some turnaround as we learn more about the biochemical basis of mood in general, but recently expressed concerns of organizations like the American Psychological Association that their field is given too low a priority in the context of its importance to the nation's health are, to my mind, quite legitimate. Love gone wrong is a major contributor to many women's health problems, short- or long-term, such as those involved in unwanted pregnancies, abortion, sexually transmitted disease, spousal abuse, child abuse, and some aspects of depression.

Understanding the psychology of human relationships is a health issue. The human yearning to form bonds and the form that desire takes are a reflection of the character of a community—of the times as well as the individual. The psychology of love may seem unimportant when a society functions smoothly. But in a society where one in two marriages ends in divorce, where there is an overwhelming illegitimacy rate, where alcoholism and drug abuse are increasing, and violence and depression and social isolation are on the rise, we do need to think about "love" as a human emotion that is in trouble. It is especially important when this state of "love" becomes intrusive, eclipses rational thinking, affects good judgment, and poses a risk for bad health or criminal actions.

others were taught that sex had no place outside of marriage. And marriage itself was an economic necessity, not a choice of the heart.

All this changed staggeringly in our own recent past. What is considered appropriate sexual behavior for both single and married women has been shifting dramatically. First the Pill allowed women to be active sexually without the fear of an unwanted pregnancy; then the early woman's movement suggested that a woman who wanted to succeed outside the home had to be just like a man—on the job but also in bed, meaning she had to want the kind of unattached, brief sexual flings that have had such extensive if superficial appeal for men. Popular lore had stigmatized young women for being "experienced" in the 1950s and early 1960s, but almost ridiculed them for their virginity in the 1970s and 1980s. In the 1950s, married women gave sex as a duty; in the 1980s, the popular lore was that a good wife must lust nonstop and engage in goofy Saran Wrap and whipped cream antics. Shere Hite's infamous 1976 *Hite Report* suggested that women had greater numbers of sexual partners than their older sisters and more casual sex, were more open about their sexual behavior, had more frequent sex (whether married or single), and were pleased to be free from much of the secretiveness and inhibitions that they had seen in their mothers.

But there was a dark side to the new freedom. Although most women surveyed by Hite believed that, on balance, the sexual revolution was good, many women she surveyed expressed concerns that they were being harmed, not helped; they felt on occasion powerless, not powerful, caught up in something they could not control. In this context, Hite noted, though the change was labeled sexual freedom, in fact "it has not so far allowed much real freedom for women. . . . It has merely put pressure on them to have *more* of the same kind of sex. . . . You cannot decree women to be 'sexually free' when they are not economically free; to do so is to put them into a more vulnerable position than ever, and make them into a form of easily available common property." As one of Hite's respondents said: "What revolution? There has been no real revolution. It makes women feel they *have* to have sex and can't say no." Other comments: "The sexual revolution was late sixties bullshit. It was about *male* liberation, women being shared property, instead of private property." Much of the media coverage of the *Hite Report* focused on more risqué revelations, while this undertow of women's discontent stemming from a whole new set of social pressures in the tumultuous sixties and seventies was largely ignored.

Now, in the middle part of the last decade of this topsy-turvy century for women, things seem to be changing yet again. Some women are recognizing that, though the outgrowth of our revolution must be viewed as positive overall, socially accepted sexual freedom without a clear sense of inner guidelines and entrenched moral values means unhealthy choices, leading to lowered self-esteem and a vast increase in both sexually transmitted diseases and unwanted children.

But the messages are more mixed than ever. Women are told through every form of media to exploit their own sexuality and desirability in the most primitive and male-pandering ways. The one consistent theme we get from the popular culture is that women are not only sexual objects, but willing and thoughtless sexual objects.

Nor do we have to go back into history to find socially sanctioned brutality against women based on a woman's role as wife, mother, and reproductive vessel. Just turn on CNN. Reports of bride burning, female genocide, wife beating, and polygamy are accepted and unpunished social behaviors in many parts of our world today. In the guise of marital stability and of purity, young girls in many cultures are subjected to genital mutilation—either *clitoridectomy,* whereby a girl's clitoris and labia minora are partly or completely cut out, or *infundibulation,* whereby after her clitoris and labia minora are removed, her labia majora are sewn together, leaving only a tiny opening for urine and menstrual flow—often under painful, unsterile, and inhumane conditions. Genital mutilation is intended to control a woman's sexual pleasure, control her reproduction, and surgically brand her as acceptable goods. The stamp placed while she is still a helpless child of nine or ten is an almost inhumanly brutal abuse marking her as chattel.

Please be aware that this is not a rare event. Although it has been outlawed in many countries, there are easily some hundred million or more women worldwide who have undergone clitoridectomies. The only way to deal with these severe social assaults on women is to change what is socially acceptable, through publicity and calculated outrage expressed in the media and public world forums like the United Nations and the World Health Organization, as well as within individual countries.

In America it seems that, no matter whether the mood of the nation be conservative or liberal, we are conflicted, if not schizophrenic, about sex. Graphic public displays of sexual behavior are rampant in entertainment, whereas serious studies of sex that could educate and provide important health information have been labeled perverse and squelched. While I was at NIH, both the Democrat-controlled Congress and the Republican White House banned the organization from funding the National Health and Social Life Survey (discussed on page 81) and a survey looking at teenage social behavior, including sex. The opposition to the study was based on the intimate and sometimes "dirty" words used in the questionnaires—never mind that the interviews were to be done by medical professionals, in a medical context, for medical purposes, and with informed consent, including that of the parent if the person to be questioned was a teen. Private money came to the rescue. Ironically, the work has told us so far that America in private is more sexually restrained and conservative than imagined from public displays.

The 1994 National Health and Social Life Survey, conducted by Drs. Edward Laumann, John Gagnon, Robert Michael, and others, found a general movement toward more fidelity, more monogamy, fewer sexual encounters, and a differentiation of male and female sexual behavior. Women have fewer partners than men do, become sexually active later, and exhibit less homosexuality, though they still show a pattern of adventurous sexual behavior in marriage that was not found in years gone by. Perhaps the conservative shift was prompted by fear of AIDS—or perhaps women have finally just had enough.

I see only one path for any woman today to take amidst all of this conflict: use your own heart, mind, and common sense to make decisions that are right for your peace of mind, physical health, and carefully thought-out moral or ethical values. The answers are not going to come from society or Congress. Neither a man's desire for a virgin bride nor the false freedom of liberation without self-control should dictate your actions; your own personal values and choices, tempered by your knowledge of your own health requirements, must be your rule.

Remember how far we have come these past hundred years. Suffrage is about being able to say "no," not just "yes."

THE PHYSIOLOGY OF SEX:
WHAT LITTLE WE KNOW

A woman's power in her sexuality is derived from two sources: her strength in making hard choices based upon her self-awareness, personal values, and commitment to protecting her health and reproductive capability, and a knowledge of her own body and how it derives sexual pleasure. Unfortunately, this latter understanding is not easy to gain. Yes, experience can be an adequate teacher, but objective scientific studies of feminine sexuality, potentially an equally powerful source, have generally been avoided by researchers like the plague.

We know that the emotion of sexual love is quite different from most other moods and emotions, in that it is tightly linked to a particular physiological response: sexual behavior. Most of what else we know about the female sexual response we owe to researchers Masters and Johnson, who in the 1960s took to the clinical laboratory to study directly the sexual function of thousands of paid human volunteers and came up with answers—some predictable and self-evident, some questionable (since their subjects, almost by definition, were not your average Janes), and some critical in debunking existing dogma.

In their sex laboratories, Masters and Johnson used video cameras, probes, and their own observations to monitor heart rate, blood pressure, muscle contraction, tone, skin color, secretions, and other physiological variables before, during, and after sexual intercourse, foreplay, and masturbation. Based largely on their work and that of the few other sturdy souls who followed, we have learned that there are several discrete physiological phases of a sexual encounter, each powerfully tied to an emotional response. These phases include desire, arousal, orgasm, and resolution. Before I detail them, let me remind you that they should not be taken out of the context of emotional bonding and a trusting relationship. The morning after is either hideous or glorious, depending on the emotional and human relationship, not on the success of the physiological performance.

SEXUAL DESIRE (LIBIDO)

Libido is one of the many primitive drives that are crucial for survival, such as appetite for food or the desire to sleep, which originates in the hypothalamus, within a section of the brain called the *limbic system*. (You will read more about this part of the brain in chapter 7, since it is also critical to mood.) A combination of higher cortical function (which restrains or encourages) and the lower limbic drive or instinct produces feelings of desire, particularly when attention is captured by an external love object. Testosterone is the hormone that plays a major role in sexual drive for women as well as men. (Endocrinologists have shown that levels of testosterone in the blood actually correlate with a woman's interest in sex, her responsiveness and satisfaction.) The amount of testosterone circulating in the bloodstream of a woman is about 8 to 10 percent that of men, suggesting that not much testosterone is needed for libido. Since the hormone is produced by the ovaries and the adrenal glands of women, the adrenal glands continue to produce it even after a woman's ovaries are removed or stop functioning at menopause. Testosterone and other sex hormones (LH, FSH; see below) surge at mid-cycle, before ovulation, presumably to stimulate the libido just at the fertile period. But there is considerable variability in sex drive from woman to woman, surely based on a complex mix of genetically set brain and hormone function, modified heavily by early conditioning, external situations, and emotional relationships.

AROUSAL

Arousal, or sexual excitement, describes a specific physical and emotional response to a sexually stimulating event; this may be a movie or a photograph or music as well as a person or a sensation; it does not necessarily imply a sexual encounter with another. Although the brain controls sex drive and the decision to turn excitement into an overt sexual act, many of the physiological manifestations of arousal are primitive genital reflexes stemming from the lower spinal cord. The higher brain can override the physiologic response by consciously turning away from the stimulating circumstance and substituting some other mental or physical activity—exercise, food, work, or whatever. If the setting is deemed socially appropriate, however, arousal proceeds unchecked and prepares the body for a sexual encounter. Thus, a person's psychological and intellectual response to arousal determines the final outcome; this stage is the critical moment of saying "yes" or saying "no."

When a woman becomes aroused, the first physiological change she experiences is a sweatlike secretion from the lining cells of the vagina, which acts as a lubricant for sexual intercourse. Her vagina then dilates, and her uterus, labia, and clitoris become engorged. As arousal continues, her uterus moves up and back in the pelvis, and the muscles at the opening of the vagina tighten. Her breast nipples may become erect, and the blood vessels in her breast tissue dilate, causing breast swelling and flushing of the skin on her arms and chest. Her heart rate increases to over 100, and her blood pressure rises as much as 20 to 30 percent. The arousal stage generally lasts around ten to twenty minutes for a woman (whereas a man can move from arousal to orgasm more quickly, generally taking two to five minutes).

ORGASM AND RESOLUTION

If the sexual excitement phase is allowed to proceed unfettered, the next stage is orgasm, a climax of emotional and physical excitement. This area of human physiology has had limited study, and for a time was yet another arena in which women were made to feel inadequate. The truth is, women experience orgasms in very individual ways; some achieve them with every sexual encounter, others rarely do, and many women fall somewhere in the middle. Women are likely to describe a sexual experience as satisfying with or without an orgasm, whereas men seem to require an orgasm to be sexually satisfied. Women take a longer time to achieve orgasm than men. On the other hand, women are capable of multiple orgasms within the same sexual encounter, and men usually are not.

Masters and Johnson were able to debunk a myth about female sexuality that pervaded much of this century: the Freudian notion of two types of female orgasms, clitoral and vaginal. Freud held that women often experienced orgasms only through the clitoris—and that these orgasms were infantile, lesser versions of the male, penile orgasm. A true womanly orgasm, he said, was vaginal and rare. The truth is, an orgasm is an orgasm, for a woman or for a man. No matter where a woman's orgasm originates, it always involves all the genital parts in an integrated whole. The intensity may vary from encounter to encounter, depending on the surrounding circumstances, her partner, her own psychological readiness—but penis envy has nothing to do with it. Physiologically, when a woman has an orgasm, it is accompanied by a feeling of intense emotional release along with reflexive and rhythmic contraction of muscles within the vagina, and sometimes the uterus. Skin flushing reaches its peak, and many muscles of the body momentarily contract. The orgasm lasts a matter of seconds, after which comes a period of resolution, in which the congestion or swelling of the tissues in the pelvic region decreases rapidly. Complete resolution of the physical changes takes fifteen to thirty minutes, during which a feeling of calm and relaxation ensues and often sleep takes over.

SEXUAL DYSFUNCTION IN WOMEN

Because true scientific studies of both sexual function and dysfunction are sorely lacking, I'm afraid I cannot say definitively how many women are truly "dysfunctional" sexually, or even provide a good definition of sexual dysfunction. Though there are certainly women whose bodies do not respond physiologically in the ways described above, I suspect that most suffer less from dysfunctioning bodies than from psychological blocks arising out of a society that tells a woman to be both virgin and whore; from relationships that demoralize her rather than support her individuality or value her as a person; and from a simple lack of sexual education. Different women also have different drives for sex, as do men—and a woman's level of desire will vary throughout her lifetime.

CAUSES

Whether it is due to "dysfunction" or, more likely, stymied function, the most frequently reported sexual problems of women are the failure to have an orgasm and "frigidity," or a lack of desire for or strong dislike of sex. Both complaints generally are thought to involve one of the following factors:

Interpersonal Problems

Most disorders of sexual function are believed to stem from problems in the relationship with the partner—lack of communication or information, emotional distance, distraction, unmatched needs, or lack of love or bonding. Serious discord in an intimate relationship is going to be reflected sooner or later in sexual dissatisfaction. Trust, security, and shared values are key elements in making an intimate physical relationship satisfying over the long term.

Psychological Problems

Sexual dysfunction may stem from deep within a woman's psyche. Some women, despite great love or affection for their mate, are not interested in sex, find it an ordeal, do not enjoy it, or are generally inhibited about intimate behavior. This may be due to early upbringing during which girls were taught that sexual satisfaction was not theirs to have. Sometimes a woman has been traumatized by a frightening sexual encounter, sexual abuse, or rape, leaving her with negative feelings about sex in general.

Biological Bases

There is a curious but largely silent gender gap in research into the physiological causes of sexual dysfunction. Whatever the reason, suffice it to say that, since "impotence" is seen largely as a man's affliction, we know much about the biological causes of impotence in men and how to treat it—yet we know almost nothing about the biological causes of sexual dysfunction in women.

We've found that during pregnancy and menopause a woman's level of desire can shift drastically (see pages 82 and 183), but the research books are blank when it comes to a solid assessment of possible biological bases for abnormally low sex drives not related to hormones, or for clearly unresponsive bodies. We also know very little about the effect of medications on women's sexual behavior. For example, drugs like beta-blockers, certain antidepressants, antihypertensive agents, and cholesterol-lowering drugs are known to decrease libido and potency in some men, but, though I suspect we would find similar side effects in women, the questions don't seem to surface. We do know that testosterone and other androgenic hormones given to women before menopause (sometimes to treat such problems as endometriosis) and after (sometimes prescribed for decreased libido) are reported to increase sex drive.

TREATMENT

It's pretty difficult to claim your sexual power as a woman when you face sexual difficulties and no one really has any answers. Nonetheless, you must try. If you are unhappy with your sexual functioning, first assess your relationship, ideally with the help of a qualified psychotherapist. I suggest you first talk with your gynecologist, who might suggest a Ph.D. psychologist trained in treating such problems, rather than rushing to consult a marriage counselor or sex therapist. (See page 309 on picking a therapist.) Sexual problems can have so many origins; your first job will be to determine whether you simply need education and advice, couples counseling, or more in-depth help. If this turns out to be the approach you need, a sex therapist can be very helpful in educating you and your partner, explaining to you both what to expect, how to enhance sexual pleasure, and how to reduce anxiety and inhibitions through relaxation techniques and other exercises.

Your primary care physician or gynecologist will help you sort out whether you may be experiencing a biological problem and review any medicines you are taking that may be contributing factors. For sexual issues that arise during pregnancy and menopause, your physician will most likely be both your first and last stop in getting help, by providing clear advice and reassurance during pregnancy, and lubricants and hormonal therapy during menopause.

CONTRACEPTION

No advance in the history of modern times has given more power to individual women than readily available and legal contraception. A woman who can decide when she wishes to become pregnant can control her own destiny. We should not forget the intense battles that were waged so that women could win access to birth control.

Nor must we forget how recently the tide has turned. Although contraceptive devices, potions, and techniques have been around throughout history, they have for the most part been folk secrets passed among women, largely outside the realm of traditional society. As recently as the early part of this century, it was illegal virtually all over the world to provide, print, or distribute information about birth control.

We can so easily obtain birth control today largely thanks to the efforts of one woman, Margaret Sanger, an obstetrical nurse who faced the horrors of botched illegal abortions, an epidemic of infant and maternal mortality, and the horrible secrets of syphilis and gonorrhea. Sanger initiated her birth control crusade in the early 1900s. For regularly defying the laws against disseminating information, she was arrested several times, subjected to criminal indictment, and on at least one occasion sentenced to a workhouse for thirty days. She and her colleagues persisted, however, debating the issue as a matter of medicine and science that would save maternal and infant lives.

By the mid-1930s, court rulings finally prohibited the government from seizing contraceptives in interstate commerce, and gradually public opinion shifted to the view that married couples should be able to decide about contraception for themselves. But it wasn't until 1965, a mere thirty years ago, that the Supreme Court declared as unconstitutional a Connecticut law that made contraception illegal, thus rendering it legal throughout the United States. In the landmark case *Griswold* v. *Connecticut*, the court spoke of a "zone of privacy" protected from government intrusion. "We deal in a right of privacy older than the Bill of Rights," the court asserted. That privacy right has been the basis of most reproductive freedoms afforded women since.

A little more than a year after the Griswold decision, Margaret Sanger died of a heart attack at age eighty-eight, her job done.

CONTRACEPTION TODAY

We may not have the perfect contraceptive, but many choices are available to women today, and there is almost no reason for an unintended pregnancy to occur. About 90 percent of all women who do not wish to become pregnant do in fact use some form of birth control, and the vast majority of the unintended pregnancies that occur each year develop in the 10 percent of sexually active women who do not practice contraception.

Contraceptives can be divided into three general approaches: hormones that interrupt ovulation; mechanical approaches that chronically block fertilization or implantation; and acute barrier techniques that keep semen from moving into a woman's reproductive tract. *Note that only barrier techniques protect against sexually transmitted diseases.*

HORMONES

ORAL CONTRACEPTIVES

Today, oral contraceptives ("the Pill") are the most popular reversible contraceptive in the United States, used by almost 30 percent of all women. The Pill was discovered in 1956 and introduced for general use in 1959; within five years it became the most commonly used contraceptive in America.

The Pill contains the female hormones estrogen and progestin, or progestin alone, hormones that normally escalate when a woman becomes pregnant. Very small doses trick a woman's body into believing it is already pregnant, and thereby stop the ovaries from producing and releasing eggs, just as they would cease their production during pregnancy.

Long-term health consequences have been a concern since the Pill was introduced, but time has proven the Pill to be remarkably safe (although, very rarely, the Pill has been linked to hypertension and embolic stroke in smokers, blood clots in the leg veins, and, most equivocally and controversially, breast cancer). It also brings secondary and unanticipated health benefits, such as protection against ovarian and endometrial cancer and a decrease in pelvic inflammatory disease. The major exception: the Pill is dangerous for smokers, contributing to their significantly higher death rate at middle age and beyond and greater incidence of stroke and heart attack. Accordingly, the only "absolute" contraindications to the use of the Pill pertain to smokers over the age of thirty-five, and women with a history of a stroke or heart attack, severe hypertension, or active liver disease. Contrary to decades of standard practice, most gynecologists now believe that a woman who is not a smoker and is without heart disease can take oral contraceptives beyond the age of thirty-five through her fertile years. It is generally recommended that a woman stop taking the Pill at least three months before she becomes pregnant.

The failure rate of the Pill ranges from 1 to 6 percent, but failure results mostly from not taking the Pill regularly or as prescribed. Side effects include occasional nausea and breast tenderness during the first month or so of use, irregular bleeding, weight gain, occasional increase in migraine headaches, and premenstrual symptoms of bloating or irritability. Most of the side effects are due to the estrogen component of the Pill, most often ethinyl estradiol. In earlier formulations, this synthetic estrogen was given in doses of 50 to 100 micrograms; now the dose is lower, in the range of 30 to 35 micrograms.

DEPO-PROVERA

In use worldwide for more than thirty years, depo-provera was only approved in the U.S. market in 1992. This delay tells the story of government regulations gone overboard. A few studies had shown a relationship to cancer in animals, but the ten million women using the drug had no such problem—and actually showed a decrease in endometrial cancer as a result of using it.

This progestin, medroxyprogesterone acetate in its long-acting, slow-release form, suppresses ovulation for three months after it is injected, and is associated with irregular menses or no menses in many women. It is extremely effective, with a failure rate of .04 to .05 percent, and carries few side effects, although a small number of women report increased nervousness, decreased libido, and weight gain, and for some, irregular bleeding may become troublesome.

NORPLANT

The Norplant implant, introduced in the United States in 1990, is both the most effective and the least used hormonal contraceptive now available. Consisting of six flexible capsules filled with a progestin, each about the size of a matchstick, the implant can last five years. The capsules are usually implanted in the inner arm below the armpit; their failure rate is as low as depo-provera's, and after removal up to 86 percent of women are able to conceive within a year. So why is it so unpopular?

Perhaps because it was introduced to a market saturated with established contraceptives. It is also "visible" and palpable under the skin, and is initially expensive, ranging up to seven hundred dollars (although five years' worth of the Pill, condoms, or spermicide could easily add up to that amount). The implant can at first disrupt menstrual cycles. Up to 7 percent of women discontinue use because of persistent bleeding problems and have the capsules removed before five years are up. Some have complained that removal is difficult, giving Norplant recent negative publicity.

MORNING-AFTER PILLS

The morning-after birth control pill is one of the better-kept secrets of medicine. Some view the approach as, in effect, an abortion pill, which makes many drug companies leery about promoting it or getting FDA approval for it as such. Its mechanism of action, however, is to make the womb unreceptive to implantation by an egg that might be fertilized, and is therefore similar to the intrauterine device (see page 91). In the United States, it is usually reserved as an emergency measure after rape or incest.

The actual content of the pills is in fact easy for any woman to duplicate using already approved and readily available contraceptive hormones, and many gynecologists privately provide these to patients on request. (However, any user must be warned by her doctor that they are not approved in the United States and have not undergone the kind of rigorous long-term testing that would be expected for any newly introduced medicine.) As they are used abroad, the approach usually involves two Ovral pills (an oral contraceptive containing 1 mg of synthetic progestin, norgestrel, and 50 to 100 micrograms of ethinyl estradiol) taken at twelve-hour intervals for twenty-four hours within seventy-two hours of unprotected sexual intercourse—that is, a total of four contraceptive pills taken in the course of half a day. This hormonal treatment will prevent an embryo from attaching to the uterus about 95 to 99 percent of the time. Alternative approaches use high-dose estrogen (such as 5 mg of ethinyl estradiol per day or 20 to 30 mg of conjugated equine estrogen—i.e., Premarin) taken for five days after unprotected intercourse or three oral contraceptive tablets of 35 micrograms of ethinyl estradiol taken at twelve-hour intervals, again within seventy-two hours of the sexual exposure. The main side effects of these approaches are nausea and vomiting in about half of users.

Different formulations of these hormones are marketed in Europe and other countries as "emergency contraceptives." Also available in Europe is mifepristone (RU486), the latest emergency contraceptive, which is reported to have fewer side effects than estrogen and progesterone and virtually universal effectiveness. RU486 is at present not available in the United States for other than research use.

No morning-after pill or combination of pills should be used as a routine method of birth control, since studies of the long-term dangers of their repetitive use have yet to be done and answers are likely a long way off.

LONG-TERM MECHANICAL INTERRUPTION

INTRAUTERINE DEVICES

There are two IUDs on the market today. One, made of copper, can be used up to eight years. The other, which releases progesterone, can be used for up to one year. Once a popular method of birth control, the IUD is now quite limited in use. This T-shaped device inserted into the uterus can be very effective when it stays in place. IUDs are thought to work by interfering with implantation of a fertilized egg: in essence, a morning-after device.

IUDs present several problems, however. The device may not stay in place. As a foreign body in the uterus, it creates irritation and inflammation, and is associated with a higher incidence of pelvic inflammatory disease and subsequent infertility, although not nearly as much with current devices as with the earlier IUDs like the Dalkon Shield. IUDs are now used predominantly in older women in a monogamous relationship who are at low risk for sexually transmitted disease. They are not prescribed for women who wish to have more children. (On a recent trip to mainland China, I was informed that, six months after the birth of a first child, it is mandatory for a woman to have an IUD implanted, regardless of her age or her personal wishes.)

TUBAL LIGATION

Tubal ligation in women and vasectomy in men are forms of sterilization that have become the most common approaches to irreversible contraception among married couples who have no desire for future children. Close to 40 percent of all contraceptive activity in the United States involves one of these two surgical procedures. About twice as many women have tubal ligations as men have vasectomies. Interpret this as you will, but the numbers suggest a certain chauvinism, particularly since the expense, risks, and complexity of tubal ligation is greater for women than is vasectomy for men. About 0.1 to 0.2 percent of vasectomies fail, as do 0.2 to 0.5 percent of tubal ligations.

There are several different ways to perform tubal ligations, and *all* should be seen as permanent actions. Nonetheless, for women under thirty, a spring clip placed on the tubes creating a mechanical obstruction is usually advised, since these offer the best chance of reversal if a woman changes her mind. Other approaches involve destruction of the tubes at several points along their course, using an electric cauterizing knife or the placing of Silastic bands around the tubes. Many women undergo tubal ligation as a routine elective outpatient procedure, or at the time of a cesarean section or delivery.

BARRIER METHODS

DIAPHRAGMS, CERVICAL CAPS, AND SPONGES

Diaphragms and *cervical caps* are round, concave discs that are inserted into the vagina and placed over the cervix before intercourse. The diaphragm, which is larger, *must* be removed eight to ten hours after intercourse, whereas the smaller cervical cap, which fits snugly over the cervix, is designed to stay in place for as long as forty-eight hours. Both devices should be filled with spermicides (foams or jellies that contain chemicals, such as nonoxynol-9, that destroy both sperm and bacteria) before they are inserted. These barriers, in conjunction with the spermicides, appear to offer some protection against sexually transmitted diseases. The incidence of urinary tract infections is higher among diaphragm users, probably because mechanical pressure from a diaphragm's rim can irritate the urethra.

Both the diaphragm and the cervical cap can be obtained through your physician, who will fit you to determine the right size. Be sure to get your diaphragm refitted if you gain or lose more than ten pounds, and to replace your diaphragm or cervical cap every few years. Overall failure rates range from as low as 5 percent to as high as 20 percent, but are far lower if the devices are correctly measured, properly and faithfully used—and always used with spermicide.

Sponges, an over-the-counter barrier method, are not as reliable as the cap or diaphragm. These polyurethane discs, about two inches in diameter, expand when inserted into the vagina to cover the cervix and the upper part of the vagina. They are soaked in spermicide with a high concentration of nonoxynol-9. Sponges must be left in place for at least six hours but for no longer than twenty-four hours. Some women have difficulty placing or removing the sponges, and as many as 1 or 2 percent develop allergies to them. Note that they may disappear from the drugstore shelves: the FDA is concerned about the production standards of the principal manufacturer.

CONDOMS

Condoms for men provide substantial, but not complete, protection against pregnancy and a number of STDs, most notably AIDS. Though they have a failure rate ranging from 2 to 16 percent, most of the failure stems from inexperience and inappropriate use: condoms, which must be applied in the passion of the moment, can be mishandled, torn, or poorly placed. Studies show that experienced users have a failure rate of 1 percent or less.

In 1994 the FDA approved a female condom, called Reality, for general use and over-the-counter purchase. This fairly bulky device consists of a polyurethane liner or pouch attached to a ring, inserted into the vagina much like a diaphragm, except that the liner drapes outside of the vagina to cover entirely the lower vaginal walls and the external genitalia, where it is held in place by a second ring. Its major advantage is that, used properly, it protects against not only pregnancy but also STDs, including HIV infection. However, it is awkward and noisy during intercourse, and expensive. Used as intended, it can be highly effective, but the failure rate has been reported to be as high as 25 percent in a year of use. Several other female condoms are likely to follow Reality, including the Bikini condom and Woman's Choice, which use latex and different modes of insertion.

Although they may not yet be perfected, the principle of a female condom is sound, in that it gives women potentially more power and protection against STDs. However, their use may convey the destructive message that men don't have to be responsible sexually or that the risks are not equally shared.

NATURAL METHODS OF CONTRACEPTION

Only about 4 percent of couples now rely on rhythm or coitus interruptus as their regular method of birth control—quite a change from most

STUDIES TO WATCH FOR: CONTRACEPTIVE VACCINES

A contraceptive vaccine is now in clinical trials in many parts of the world, and others are on the horizon. In one approach being tested at India's National Institute of Immunology in New Delhi, Dr. G. P. Talwar and colleagues are using antibodies to human chorionic gonadotropin, the hormone that sustains the embryo from the time of implantation (see pages 102–103). The vaccine stimulates the antibodies for a limited period of time (generally several months), and while the antibodies are present they neutralize the needed hormone and prevent implantation of a fertilized egg. Over time, the antibody levels fall and fertility returns. Methods in development in Europe and the United States include reversible vaccines targeted against other hormones, such as gonadotropin-releasing hormone or FSH, both critical to ovulation (see page 101), and vaccines against certain proteins on the surface of sperm or on the zona pellucida, the membrane that surrounds the egg.

Still in their early development, vaccines represent an entirely new approach to contraception that may turn out to be safe and highly effective for individual use and general population control, and without the use of implants or continuous hormones. The biggest theoretical problem with the vaccine is that, once administered, it has a defined period of effect that cannot be shortened if a woman changes her mind about becoming pregnant earlier. However, for now the research challenge is to extend the effectiveness of these vaccines beyond a few months, rather than abbreviate their effect.

of our history. In the rhythm method, couples try to figure out when the woman is ovulating (see pages 101 and 108), and simply avoid having intercourse at that time. This can be very tough if the woman's periods are irregular, but all things considered, the failure rate of the rhythm method is relatively low, in the range of 10 to 15 percent. Withdrawal or coitus interruptus just before ejaculation is another natural approach, but one that has a far higher failure rate. Even if the man manages to withdraw before orgasm, minute amounts of semen will often leak from his penis and into the vagina during intercourse anyway.

ABORTION

As I emphasize so often in this chapter, a woman's fate as a powerful or vulnerable sexual being rests on her individual choice to protect her own health. The core question in the debate on first trimester abortion, in my opinion, is whether the decision to have one should lie with a woman, her doctor, and her God, or with the state, and be legally outlawed under most circumstances. To me there is only one answer to this question that respects the privacy, conscience, and health consequences that no one but a pregnant woman can assess for herself. The matter must be in her hands, not in the hands of some congressman or government official, her next-door neighbor, or the national pollsters.

I revere human life and well-being. For whatever reason an abortion is performed, it remains a tragic event for any woman to face. I respect and understand the diversity and deeply held views about abortion, even of those who aggressively (but legally) protest against my views. Neither I nor most women who are called "pro-choice" celebrate abortion—any more than being against prohibition is the same as celebrating alcoholism. Abortion raises deep moral concern for me and for many people—but that is not the same as saying that the procedure should be criminalized and women deprived of a profoundly personal choice. I've seen too many of the health consequences of illegal abortions to feel that the state should control how a woman uses her body.

Let us never forget what went on in America before 1970.

ABORTION YESTERDAY

I have seen the consequences of botched illegal abortions. My first unforgettable experience occurred when I was a third-year medical student on a surgery rotation. I was called to meet my new admission in the emergency room: a screaming, terrified young woman thrashing about in pain and soaked in blood. I had never seen such uncontrolled hemorrhage, so much blood gushing out of a wound, obscuring everything, making it difficult to begin to assess the damage done to her.

She was a college student who had found herself pregnant. She panicked. A friend referred her to an abortionist, who did not use coat hangers or dirty instruments but, working out of her own house, dispensed "magic" tablets: potassium permanganate, a kind of lye, which when inserted into the vagina would, she claimed, induce an abortion, and leave a woman pain-free after two days of bleeding. But it didn't work that way for this young woman, whose life was saved only by numerous blood transfusions and extensive surgical repair of the burns that had eroded parts of her vagina, cervix, and rectum.

Her boyfriend brought her in and then did his best to disappear. She refused to tell us her parents' names, dreading their anger and disappointment. There was a subtle sense among some of those treating her that she somehow deserved what had happened to her.

This was the reality of women's health before *Roe* v. *Wade* (the Supreme Court decision made in 1973 that struck down antiabortion laws and stated that it was a woman's personal and private right to chose an abortion early in pregnancy). Not all the victims of illegal abortions were as "lucky" as this young woman, doomed only to a lifetime of difficulties in reproductive and sexual function but alive. It is unimaginable to me that we could ever consider going back.

ABORTION TODAY

Abortion is not a form of birth control, and most women do not view it that way. Although far too many (more than 1.5 million) abortions are performed among U.S. women of all ages each year, more than two-thirds of the women who have an abortion do not have another. About 90 percent of abortions are performed during the first trimester. Many studies show that first-trimester abortion has no appreciable effect on subsequent fertility, ectopic pregnancy, premature birth, or low–birth weight children. Dilatation and evacuation, the procedure used to end a pregnancy beyond the first trimester, slightly increases the overall risk of premature delivery and low birth weight when subsequent pregnancies are carried to term. Very recent studies have suggested an unexpected risk of abortion in any trimester: breast cancer (see page 237).

The psychological consequences of abortion on a woman have

been debated back and forth but invariably, I suspect, they are highly individual based on a woman's personal values and religious beliefs. And whatever a person's views on the legality of abortion in the United States, under most circumstances abortion carries a stigma.

This is not the case in many other countries. In Russia, for example, abortion is an accepted routine: two out of three pregnancies end in abortion, and it is common for women to have seven to eight abortions in their lifetimes, since contraception is not readily available. The adverse health consequences (such as infection and infertility) of this unfortunate neglect of women's health are now just coming to light.

METHODS OF ABORTION

Surgical Approaches

Most abortions are performed during the first thirteen weeks of pregnancy, using suction evacuation of the uterus. Only very rarely are there any major complications, such as heavy bleeding or perforation of the uterus, and these occur primarily in later abortion (affecting fewer than 1 percent of all abortion patients).

Further along in pregnancy, dilation of the cervical canal is needed, along with more extensive suctioning of the uterine lining. Sometimes a physician may administer hormones (prostaglandin or oxytocin) to induce uterine contraction, or directly inject into the uterus a combination of saline and prostaglandin. These methods often need to be followed by a suctioning of retained tissue. For all abortions, antibiotics are routinely administered to cut down the rate of infection.

Medical Approaches

Mifepristone (RU486), an orally administered drug, induces abortion by acting as a blocker of the hormone progesterone, which is needed to sustain early pregnancy. (See page 91 about the use of RU486 as a "morning-after pill.") RU486 is available in Europe, where it has been shown, in a substantial number of studies, to be both safe and effective, although no more so than currently available abortion procedures. If it is approved in the United States, its primary impact will be to change the nature of the procedure from one that requires a variety of special instruments and a sterile environment to one that requires no more than a quiet doctor's office, thereby enabling complete privacy.

RU486 is not a simple pill, however. Its use involves a multistep procedure over several days, has a failure rate of 5 percent or more, can only be used in early pregnancies (no more than nine weeks since the last period), and entails complications. Three days after it is administered, a small amount of prostaglandin is given in the form of a vaginal suppository or via injection. In a matter of hours, the prostaglandin induces the expulsion of the embryo, which is already considerably weakened by the RU486. If RU486 is used alone, abortion occurs in 70 to 80 percent of instances; with the addition of prostaglandin, about 96 percent of the women undergoing the procedure have a successful abortion. RU486 is not a home abortion kit. The procedure must be conducted in a doctor's office or clinic, and it does carry risks. The drug's side effects include minor pain, cramps, and nausea. About one in a thousand women experiences bleeding sufficient enough to require transfusion, and RU486 is dangerous for smokers.

The Population Council of New York is attempting to shepherd RU486 through the U.S. approval procedure. It is helping to support a study jointly with Roussel-Uclaf, the French manufacturer, and sponsored clinical trials are being conducted at sites throughout the country.

Some of the sites are doing the research anonymously. Abortion has been an incredibly public issue, and even a dangerous one, ever since it became legal. It is not clear to me how we will find our way out of this contentious debate that all too often pits good people against each other, or becomes the sole litmus test of political and social acceptability.

Maybe the wisdom of the great first-century Talmudic scholar Hillel, slightly paraphrased, might be a worthy place to start: "Do not judge your fellow woman until you have stood in her place."

CONCEPTION AND INFERTILITY

Simone de Beauvoir's classic treatise on women, *The Second Sex*, was *the* book most avidly consumed by young women in my college days, back in the 1960s. De Beauvoir hit a deep chord in that preemergent phase of the woman's movement, diagnosing the "basic problem" of woman as the long-standing difficulty of reconciling her reproductive role and her role in the workplace. "The fundamental fact is that from

THE MOTHERLESS CHILD

Thanks to modern technology, many women who would have been unable to bear children even twenty years ago can and do today. But the same technology may abuse the great gift it provides. As I write this chapter, the NIH is embroiled in the debate over whether or not to fund the conception and growth of human embryos in a laboratory petri dish, solely for the purpose of scientific experimentation. Two scientific panels have supported this action; President Clinton has just stepped in and vetoed any specific funding for developing new embryos for experimentation, but has left the door open to projects experimenting on embryos "left over" from in-vitro fertilizations. Where will the line be drawn? Now the panels propose that all new fetuses will be destroyed after two weeks of use for research—but only maybe and for the time being. If we experiment on a two-week-old embryo and we find science compelling us to go further, how soon will it be before we allow a fetus to grow four weeks, or six, or eight, or to cross into the territory where it could have survived on its own?

Yes, these concerns may seem alarmist to some, and to others maybe even "antiscience." But I believe the time to express the contrarian view is now, before the work goes too far. To me, growing human embryos in the laboratory as some kind of subhuman research-slaves is morally repugnant, and such actions could ultimately corrupt the goodwill that exists between the public and the medical science community. I support wholeheartedly the research using donated postmortem tissue from aborted (nonliving) fetuses, which would otherwise be discarded, provided the research never influenced the decision either to conceive or to abort; I believe just as wholeheartedly that living human embryos should be neither conceived nor nurtured solely for the purpose of science and experimentation.

the beginning of history what doomed woman to domestic work and prevented her taking part in the shaping of the world was her enslavement to the generative function."

No longer "slaves" of our own ability to bear children, we can determine when, how, and if we wish to take advantage of this miracle only a woman's body can carry and nourish. We no longer have to acquiesce to a societal view denying any route to acceptance and achievement other than becoming a wife and mother. Now we can participate in all the choices of childbirth, from the moment we attempt to conceive to the selection of anesthesia in the birthing room. (But there are new issues on the horizon that threaten to divorce women from the birth process entirely; see page 99.)

We must strive to appreciate the wondrous power we have to give birth, and teach society to treasure it as well; but they and we must see it also as a part of the whole woman, whose choices—consciously made—to mother full-time, never to bear a child, to work full-time, to shoulder both work and child raising, can never diminish her value to society.

CONCEPTION

THE BIOLOGY OF THE REPRODUCTIVE CYCLE

A woman's ability to bear a child is not a function assigned to a single organ, such as the ovaries or her womb; it involves the totality of all she is, mind and body together. It is a ballet of cycles within cycles, involving her brain, her glands, her hormones, her tissues, and her organs. Although the biological terms may seem dry and a tad technical, to understand what goes right or wrong in a woman's reproductive cycle and, more important, to be able to discuss and question any possible treatments your doctor may propose, you need at least a passing notion of what this complex ballet is about.

The Hypothalamus

The hypothalamus—the part of our brain that functions as a central processor, which controls mood (including elation and depression), appetite, sleep, thirst, body temperature, and blood pressure, as well as libido—is the conductor in the complicated reproductive dance. Every month it releases pulses of gonadotropin-releasing hormone (GnRH), thereby signaling the pituitary gland to release at the appropriate time several gonadotropins, critical among them FSH and LH, which in turn stimulate the ovaries to function in their reproductive capacities.

This loop—between the hypothalamus in the brain, and our reproductive organs—can explain to some degree how the reproductive cycle can affect or be affected by emotional states. Gonadotropin release is affected by other brain chemicals, such as norepinephrine (which stimulate it), and serotonin and dopamine and the brain opiods (which inhibit it). When these brain chemicals shift, so can your cycle.

The Pituitary Gland

The pituitary gland manufactures several gonadotropins, including two key ovarian-stimulating hormones, *follicle-stimulating hormone (FSH)* and *luteinizing hormone (LH)*. First FSH stimulates the fluid-filled sacs on the surface of the ovary, called the follicles, to develop around the immature egg, and the cells of the follicles to produce *estrogen,* which bathes the egg and prompts it to mature. LH surges mid-cycle, stimulating ovulation, or the release of the egg from the follicle. After ovulation, LH takes on a new role, stimulating the follicle to produce *progesterone* as well as estrogen, which prepares the lining of the uterus for the egg in the event of fertilization. In its new role as progesterone producer, the LH-affected follicle is called the *corpus luteum,* which is why the last two weeks of the menstrual cycle are often called the *luteal phase.* If the released egg is not fertilized, the message gets back to the hypothalamus, which signals the pituitary to drop the LH levels; the corpus luteum disintegrates, progesterone and estrogen levels fall, and, without their stimulation, the lining of the womb breaks down and is sloughed off (menstruation).

The pituitary also produces *prolactin,* which stimulates the breast to make milk, and stores the hormone *oxytocin,* which spurs uterine contractions during delivery and facilitates the flow of milk as the infant sucks.

The Ovaries

Approximately two million immature eggs are present in the ovaries of newborn girls. They stay there quietly until the time of menarche, when the menstrual cycle starts. Then, triggered by the gonadotropins discussed above, hundreds of ovarian follicles containing eggs start to mature each month, but usually only one follicle completes full development, leaving the others by the wayside to disintegrate. The fully matured egg in the follicle breaks loose, is taken up by the hydralike opening of the fallopian tubes, and makes its way down the tubes toward the uterus in search of sperm. Why one follicle makes it and several hundred others disintegrate is still something of a mystery (which can't be mimicked by fertility drugs that stimulate the ovary; that's why fertility drugs often result in multiple pregnancies).

The Uterus

The uterus is always in some stage of preparing for the fertilized egg (or *embryo*), and it is the embryo, or the lack thereof, that signals back to the whole line—the hypothalamus, the pituitary, the ovarian follicle, and the uterus—that pregnancy has or has not started.

During the first half of the cycle, when the follicle is just developing, the growing levels of estrogen cause the lining of the uterus to thicken. After ovulation, under the influence of increasing progesterone, the uterine lining matures and becomes ready for the implantation of the few-days-old embryo. (As we've seen, without fertilization the progesterone levels drop, the lining is sloughed off, and the entire exquisitely timed cycle begins again.)

The Embryo

Once the egg breaks out of the ovarian follicle and starts its journey down the fallopian tube, it has about a day to be found and penetrated by a sperm before it starts to disintegrate. Meanwhile, only a small fraction of the millions of sperm that are deposited in the vagina during sexual intercourse manage to swim upstream through the cervix and the uterus and into the fallopian tubes. Once a sperm has penetrated the egg, the fertilized egg seals up and will accept no other; it immediately begins to grow and continues to move down the fallopian tube into the uterus; by about six days after fertilization, the embryo has implanted itself into the endometrium of the uterus.

The implanted embryo forms an attachment plate, or *chorion*, which becomes the placenta. Thus, the embryo forms its own home: a sac that is filled with amniotic fluid. This entire process, or "full implantation" of the embryo in the endometrium, is completed in around two weeks.

With incredible speed, the embryo, through its placenta, takes over as command central to sustain its own existence. The placenta first starts to produce *human chorionic gonadotropin (HCG)*, which prevents the corpus luteum of the ovary from disintegrating and stimulates it to keep producing the progesterone and estrogen vital to early pregnancy. After a while, the placenta makes its own progesterone, estrogen, and many other hormones that affect the mother and the developing fetus. It also becomes the interface between the mother and the growing embryo, extracting any and all nutrients needed by the fetus from the mother's bloodstream.

DIAGNOSING PREGNANCY

Gone are the days of waiting for the rabbit to die. HCG, a clear marker of pregnancy, can now easily and inexpensively be detected in the urine, sometimes as early as a week after a missed period, and definitely within a week of full implantation of the embryo. The marker HCG is what shows up in those drugstore kits. Of course, no test is perfect. If the test is positive, it virtually always means pregnancy; if it is negative, it may be wrong—either defective or too early.

INFERTILITY AND FECUNDITY

In popular language, fecundity means fruitfulness and productive power, including intellectual creativity and inventiveness. At its origin is a feminine phrase that speaks to the power of women to procreate— the "power of producing offspring" (a word that comes from the Latin *fecundus*). In medical jargon, "fecundity rate" means the chance of becoming pregnant after a designated period of attempting to become pregnant. The fecundity rate among American couples overall is in the range of 85 to 90 percent after twelve months. For individual couples, though, as many as 30 percent or more will experience at least one twelve-month period in which attempts at achieving pregnancy fail.

When fecundity is impaired for a period of twelve months, a couple may be deemed "infertile," which does not necessarily mean they cannot conceive, only that conception has not occurred and there may be a problem. It is a bit ironic that infertility has afflicted some five million women in America and is growing; at a time when we are taking more control over when we have children, some of us find that, for a variety of reasons, we cannot.

Although the numbers are fraught with imprecision, it is likely that the growing rate of infertility is due both to baby boom women's choosing to delay pregnancy until later in life, when fecundity drops naturally and fertility problems tend to arise (see below), and to the sexually transmitted diseases that have become epidemic for women during the past twenty years. (See chapter 4.)

CAUSES OF INFERTILITY IN WOMEN

When a couple has trouble conceiving a child, about a third of the time the problem can be traced to the man, two-thirds to the woman. Although a discussion of male infertility falls beyond the scope of this book, keep in mind that such problems as endocrine abnormalities, inadequate sperm numbers or function, or anatomic or physiologic problems of the male genitalia must be evaluated as a possible cause when you are exploring the reasons you are not conceiving. Female fertility problems fall into classifications similar to a man's: endocrine disorders, primary problems with egg production, and anatomic or physiologic disorders of the reproductive system.

Endocrine Disorders

The endocrine system refers to the complex interplay discussed above between the hypothalamus, the pituitary gland, and the intricate cycle of rising and falling hormone levels. Obviously, a system this complex can and does malfunction. The problems outlined below together contribute to half of all cases of female infertility.

POLYCYSTIC OVARY SYNDROME (POS)

Sometimes the pituitary hormones become imbalanced—typically, too much LH and not enough FSH is produced—and the ovaries function improperly. With polycystic ovary syndrome the ovaries produce uninterrupted estrogen and increased amounts of androgenic hormones including testosterone. A range of disorders may ensue, including the suspension of ovulation, amenorrhea (absence of periods), irregular menstruation, dysfunctional uterine bleeding, and infertility. Women who have this syndrome may also have excess body hair and a male pattern of body fat distribution (a shape more like an apple than a pear). Polycystic ovary syndrome is not uncommon; some estimate that as many as 5 to 6 percent of women of reproductive age may have it in some form, and others suggest the numbers may range as high as 20 percent.

HYPOTHALAMIC DYSFUNCTION

Dysfunction of the hypothalamus is, aside from pregnancy, the most common cause of interruption in the normal menstrual cycle. As I mentioned above (see page 101), brain chemistry can have a strong impact on fertility. The release of gonadotropin-releasing hormone by the hypothalamus can be thrown off track by stress, anorexia nervosa, or other causes of a sudden drop in body weight, excessive exercise, or tranquilizers and antidepressant drugs affecting brain neurotransmitters, particularly serotonin (see page 286).

Other hormonal problems may also interfere with this system. For example, thyroid hormone is known to influence the function of the ovaries: too much thyroid hormone or too little can impair normal ovulation. In some women with infertility who are found to have low thyroid function, treatment with thyroid hormone corrects the problem.

Problems with the Reproductive Organs

An infertile woman's reproductive organs may themselves be scarred or otherwise damaged, but the impact of such injury on fertility varies considerably.

ENDOMETRIOSIS

Occasionally cells from the lining of the uterus can migrate to areas outside the uterus, including the immediate pelvic region (fallopian tubes, uterine surface, ovaries) or even places outside the pelvic cavity. One theory suggests that endometrial cells are shed into the fallopian tubes at the time of menstruation and passed along out into the pelvic cavity, a kind of "retrograde menstruation." Wherever it has taken residence, this transported endometrial tissue continues to be stimulated to grow and slough off under the influence of estrogen and progesterone, which can lead to scarring of surrounding tissues. Some women's own immune system may react more vigorously than others against the abnormally placed endometrial cells, increasing the localized inflammatory reaction and the associated problems. Genetics may have a hand in the development of endometriosis: the condition tends to run in families.

Endometriosis is a problem of women of childbearing age, and its prevalence increases with age. An NIH study estimated that up to 25 percent of women in their thirties and forties may have endometriosis. A third of all women with endometriosis may have some difficulty conceiving a child. In fact, close to a third of all infertile women show some evidence of the disease. In other words, having endometriosis does not mean you won't be able to conceive, but if you can't conceive, there is a one-in-three chance you have endometriosis.

Since endometriosis is less often seen in women under the age of twenty-five or thirty, and is more common in women who have not had children or who have delayed their childbearing, it used to be known as the "career woman's disease." Not so very long ago, some gynecologists preached that endometriosis was natural evidence that women were meant to start having children early in life and to do otherwise was either selfish or unhealthy or both. This argument seemed to assume, however, that a woman's greatest concerns about having a child were the biological factors below her neck. Education, waiting for the right spouse, being emotionally ready and even economically able to care for a child—these counterarguments were left out of the next breath. What is the commonsense answer? Fear of endometriosis should not push a woman into motherhood before she is ready, but as a woman moves into her thirties, she obviously has to factor her age and age-related decreases in fertility, of which endometriosis is only one, into her decision about when to have a child.

FIBROIDS AND OTHER UTERINE FACTORS

The uterus itself can be scarred by a number of factors, but many gynecologists believe that such damage has little impact on fertility. Nonetheless, you should be aware that such problems exist.

Up to 40 percent of all women have benign fibromuscular tumors called *fibroids* in their uteruses. Fibroids, more common in black women than in white women, can be painful and can instigate uterine bleeding. Sometimes too, scarring within the endometrial cavity from previous surgical currettings of the lining (as might be done for heavy bleeding, after a spontaneous abortion, or for an abortion) may impair implantation of the embryo, but only if the damage is extensive. Congenital abnormalities of the uterus, such as are seen in some offspring of women who took diethylstilbestrol (DES) for threatened abortion prior to 1970 (see page 259), may also impair fertility.

DAMAGE FROM SEXUALLY TRANSMITTED DISEASES

This epidemic can clearly take its toll on fertility, in several ways. STDs can scar and close the fallopian tubes, or scar the ovaries themselves, and thereby prevent the egg from moving down the tube after ovulation. They can also damage the cervix, through infections and sometimes through cancer, impairing a woman's ability to conceive or, if she conceives, to carry a baby to term. (See pages 142 and 166.)

PREMATURE OVARIAN FAILURE

The ovaries lose their ability to produce eggs at menopause, which generally occurs around age fifty. Sometimes menopause comes very early; if it hits a woman before she turns thirty-five, it is termed "premature" and has consequences beyond infertility (see page 176). We don't know what causes this spontaneous premature ovarian failure, though it is speculated that some women may carry a genetic tendency for it, or for some kind of autoimmune disorder in which the body's immune system attacks the ovaries.

Smoking is known to bring menopause on a few years early; it is possible that other external factors may also lead to premature ovarian failure. The most definite causes we can point to are those rare instances of premature ovarian failure in women who have had anticancer treatments, including radiotherapy and chemotherapy.

IMMUNOLOGIC PROBLEMS

Although we do not know why, both men and women can develop antibodies to sperm, and in some cases these appear to cause infertility. Certain kinds of antisperm antibodies (ASAs) coat the surface of the sperm and interfere with its ability to swim. Normal sperm can be immobilized or damaged by antibodies to either the sperm body or its tail. Such antibodies may form in cervical mucus, thereby creating a barrier for sperm entry into the reproductive tract.

DIAGNOSING INFERTILITY

Since we do have a good idea of the many possible causes of infertility, determining your specific problem may be time-consuming but at least not mysterious. Your doctor will systematically consider all possibilities, first taking a detailed history and doing a complete physical examination to determine into which of the above general categories your problem probably fits.

One of the first steps in any infertility study is to document and assess whether you are ovulating and your pattern of ovulation, and determine if the corpus luteum is doing its job. You'll be asked to keep track of your daily body temperature on awakening, looking for the one-degree increase in temperature that occurs at the time of ovulation and remains until the corpus luteum disintegrates some two weeks later. You may also be asked to pick up at the drugstore a simple kit that can predict your ovulation with great certainty and precision. Such kits detect the surge of LH coming from the pituitary gland that occurs just twelve to twenty-four hours before ovulation.

Transvaginal ultrasound of the ovary can also detect follicle rupture at mid-cycle and pinpoint the exact time of ovulation. Progesterone levels document that ovulation has occurred and how long it continues to support the endometrium. Progesterone-effect may also be determined from biopsies of the endometrial lining of the uterus. Analysis of the cells in the biopsy can precisely define the stage of the reproductive cycle and whether the endometrium is appropriately responding in the luteal phase, in which implantation occurs.

If your doctor suspects hormonal abnormalities, a battery of blood tests to evaluate hormonal function, including levels of FSH, LH, and thyroid hormone, is in order. If you are clearly not ovulating, your doctor will perform specific antibody screens or look for other autoimmune problems that might explain early ovarian failure.

If your physician believes your problem is anatomically based, the diagnostic test she recommends will vary with the specifics of the problem. Tubal obstruction and dysfunction are evaluated by a special radiological examination called *hysterosalpingography*. A catheter is inserted through the cervix, and dye is introduced into the uterus and tubes while X rays are taken. The X rays precisely define abnormalities in the structure of the uterus or the tubes, and will show sites of narrowing or obstruction. (Both radiation exposure and dye are damaging to a developing embryo, and absence of early pregnancy must be assured before the test is performed.)

To detect ovarian cysts, scars around the tubes, or abnormalities in the opening of the tubes, or endometriosis, your physician will use a technique called *laparoscopy*. Under local anesthesia, a fiberoptic viewing tube is inserted into the abdomen, through which your doctor can directly and clearly examine and diagnose your ovaries and fallopian tubes, and, when appropriate, can perform minor surgery through the laparoscope.

TREATMENT OF INFERTILITY

The decision to embark on infertility treatment, and just how far to walk along that road, is not simple. For example, some drug treatment may prove to be risky, and assisted pregnancies (such as in-vitro fertilization) can be very expensive, uncomfortable, psychologically draining, and ultimately ineffective. Determining whether or not to stop trying can drag on and on, and lead to depression. Some women will not be able to bear children even after a clear diagnosis of the cause of infertility, and after many attempts at treatment. This inability represents a real and very painful loss, one that must be recognized, respected, and appropriately mourned (see page 290).

All that said, the fact is we do have more choice in combating infertility than ever; you don't have to accept infertility as a permanent diagnosis until you have exhausted a number of treatment options— options that would have been considered miracles merely a decade or so ago.

Hormone Treatments

A wide range of hormonal therapies is now available to women who are infertile for reasons of hormonal problems, or problems in the endocrine system (see page 104).

CLOMIPHENE

If you are ovulating unpredictably or not at all, the odds are your doctor will prescribe *clomiphene citrate* to stimulate ovulation. Clomiphene is an antiestrogen agent that binds to estrogen receptors and tricks the hypothalamus into pouring out higher pulses of GnRH, which, as we've seen, prompts the pituitary to release more FSH and LH. In almost all instances of hormonal dysfunction, ovulation can be induced with clomiphene, but the actual pregnancy rate is closer to 40 percent. This suggests that in some cases the clomiphene may negatively affect other key players in conception; for example, it may interfere with the functioning of cervical mucus or endometrial lining cells.

Clomiphene is prescribed with increasing frequency—sometimes, I believe, with too much haste, before a true fertility problem is diagnosed. A powerful drug, it has in some recent studies been associated with a slightly increased risk of ovarian cancer. This association is not firmly proven at this time, but this may be due in part to the relatively short time the drug has been in use, and the long period between the introduction of a cancer-triggering element and the actual development of the cancer. Clomiphene can be a miraculous answer to a devastating problem, and I urge you only to discuss it carefully with your doctor before embarking on a program, and then to use it in moderation for limited periods of time. (See pages 253 and 258.) The drug's immediate side effects, though minimal, may include enlargement of the ovaries and, in as many as 10 to 12 percent of pregnancies, multiple births.

GONADOTROPINS

Gonadotropins, human chorionic gonadotropin (HCG), or human menopausal gonadotropin (Pergonal) may be used by women for whom clomiphene has been unsuccessful, or who have infertility of unknown cause, and as part of assisted pregnancy techniques (see below). Pergonal is a powerful hormone that maximally stimulates the ovaries, leading to marked ovarian enlargement, and requires close monitoring, often including frequent transvaginal ultrasound and repeated blood samples to measure hormone levels. Another regimen involves clomiphene administration until the physician determines that ovulation is ready to occur, at which time HCG is given to mimic the mid-cycle LH surge. When these drugs are used, ovulation occurs about 90 percent of the time. The spontaneous abortion rate is also high, however, as is the chance of multiple births. Whether the use of these particular ovary-stimulating hormones increases risk for ovarian cancer, and, if so, whether the effect can be countered by subsequent use of birth control pills (see page 258) need answers.

Surgery

When your fecundity is hampered by anatomical disorders, surgery may be an effective option. Previous sterilization with tubal ligation can sometimes be successfully reversed using microsurgical techniques, and laparoscopic surgery can remove ectopic endometrial tissue, dissolve scars and adhesions, and repair obstructions in the tubes. When endometriosis is being treated, surgical therapy to remove the abnormally seeded tissue may be combined with a subsequent period of hormonal suppression of ovulation, using oral contraceptives or other agents, with the hope of decreasing further endometrial cell seeding after the operation.

Assisted Pregnancies

It was not very long ago at all, well within all of our memories, that the scary and impersonal futuristic term "test tube baby" was used colloquially to describe what has now come to be a group of common and accepted treatments for infertility. This family of techniques, through which ova (not yet fertilized eggs), sperm, or fertilized eggs are extracted and prepared outside the body before being reintroduced to achieve pregnancy, are now called "assisted pregnancies." Advances are constantly being made in this field—some exciting, some disturbing (see page 99).

In any case, most assisted pregnancies are conducted at clinics whose physicians specialize in this area only. Study carefully before selecting one. Clinics use differing statistics to suggest "success" rates. Enlist the aid of one or two gynecologists you respect as you research both the clinic and the fertility specialist.

ARTIFICIAL INSEMINATION OF SPERM

Artificial insemination is the oldest of assisted reproductive technologies, first performed in the United States back in 1866. This relatively inexpensive method is used in a variety of circumstances—as, for example, when the father has a low sperm count (and the sperm can be concentrated in a test tube outside the body and then inseminated) or has preserved sperm before chemotherapy or radiation treatment for cancer has rendered him infertile; when a doctor suspects the ejaculate is not reaching the uterus and tubes because of a problem with cervical mucus; or when anonymous sperm donations are used for pregnancy. It is most often done through intrauterine insemination, in which sperm is placed directly into the uterus with a catheter during a woman's fertile period. This allows the sperm to bypass infections and antibodies in the vagina or cervix that might otherwise destroy it. (Sometimes follicles are stimulated with drugs to assure ovulation at the time of insemination; or sperm is "washed" if an antibody problem is suspected, to eliminate any antibodies in the fluid of the semen.)

IN-VITRO FERTILIZATION WITH EMBRYO TRANSFER

In-vitro fertilization (IVF) is a long and expensive process with a relatively low success rate. But when it works, a miracle seems to happen. It is used when women have severe tubal disease or blockage, or sometimes when artificial insemination has failed. IVF involves four steps. First, hormones are used to stimulate follicle development, and multiple eggs are recovered, using one of two methods: either a laparoscope (for viewing) and a catheter are inserted through the abdomen and the eggs are removed through the catheter, or the catheter is inserted through the vagina and the eggs are removed while an ultrasound is used for viewing. Next, the recovered eggs are placed in a culture and fertilized with sperm. Third, embryos that result are incubated for up to seventy-two hours. Finally, one or more embryos (it is assumed that only one or two will take) are implanted in the uterus with a small catheter, and the pregnancy is supported by the administration of progesterone or HCG for about two weeks. Since multiple eggs are usually retrieved, healthy fertilized eggs that are not implanted are frozen and stored for future use—by the parents, or for donation for use by other infertile couples. (The consequences of freezing and thawing human embryos on long-term development are not known, nor will they be for a long time. There are some animal studies that have at least raised some concerns. It should also be pointed out that many states in the United States and several countries throughout the world regulate the preservation and/or donation of human embryos as well as their use in research.)

The success rate of deliveries per retrieval of eggs still hovers around 15 percent, although some centers consistently claim results of 20 percent or more. Women who are over forty have lower success rates, generally under 10 percent.

GAMETE INTRAFALLOPIAN TRANSFER

A variation of IVF called *gamete intrafallopian transfer (GIFT)* is a simpler procedure. The eggs are removed from the ovaries, as in IVF, and mature eggs are selected and placed, along with sperm, into the fallopian tubes with a catheter. Fertilization takes place within the fallopian tubes, not in test tubes. GIFT has a pregnancy rate of close to 30 percent, but it can only be used by women with healthy fallopian tubes.

EGG DONORS

When, for one reason or another, a woman is unable to produce eggs, they can be obtained from another woman, and the IVF or GIFT technique chosen would be the same as if the eggs came from the woman hoping to conceive. However, some experts believe that there may be an additional complication to this procedure—tissue rejection. The immune system of the woman receiving the egg may mount an attack on what it perceives as foreign tissue. Donor matching and tissue typing can minimize this possibility.

I would add a strong caveat here: egg donors must understand fully the potential risks to their own fertility and possibly of ovarian cancer that they face without any biological benefit. Egg donations also raise some thorny ethical issues. One that troubles me is the solicitation of egg donors through college newspaper in-search-of columns, using monetary lures that may overshadow a financially strapped student's sense of immediate or long-term risk.

ASSISTED CONCEPTION BEYOND MIDLIFE

With the advent of IVF, the biological clock may not be ticking so loudly for many women. When a 1990 issue of the *New England Journal of Medicine* reported successful assisted pregnancies in four postmenopausal women, its editor, Dr. Marcia Angell, commented, "The limits on childbearing years are now anyone's guess; perhaps they will have more to do with stamina required for labor and 2 A.M. feedings than with reproductive function." For those who delay childbearing to the point of ovarian failure, IVF may seem a blessing. Needless to say, though, the long-term health consequences for egg donor and recipient are as yet unknown.

PREGNANCY AND CHILDBIRTH

However conception is achieved—accidentally, planned and naturally, or helped along through modern technology—once the healthy fetus starts to grow, it will develop in the same way. A baby is a baby, thank goodness.

Normal pregnancy lasts about thirty-eight weeks, or forty weeks from the first day of your last missed period—although a birth date of anywhere from thirty-eight to forty-two weeks from your missed period is well within the range of normal, and few babies pop out exactly on schedule. The forty weeks of pregnancy are generally viewed as three approximately three-month-long trimesters. Most of the action in terms of development occurs within the first trimester, by the end of which the embryo (now called a *fetus* and in fairly well-defined human form), though only about one ounce in weight and a few inches long, contains functioning versions of virtually all the organ systems of the body.

During the second trimester, the organ systems develop almost fully and the fetus grows to about one and a half pounds and eight or so inches. Except for still immature lung development and very little body fat, fetuses by the end of the second trimester are close to being able to sustain independent life.

In the last trimester, the fetus mainly grows in weight and puts on fat. From thirty-four weeks on, the baby is pretty much able to survive separate from and fully independent of its mother.

PROBLEMS IN PREGNANCY

Most pregnancies result in healthy, happy bouncing babies with exhausted and exhilarated moms. Occasionally, there are problems; unfortunately, the space I must devote to each can overwhelm the reality—namely, that the vast majority of births are straightforward. My main reason for discussing problems is to inform and alert women to what they can do to minimize these difficulties if they should happen. (We'll discuss risk factors for these problems later in the chapter.)

PROBLEMS IN INHERITED CHROMOSOMES

Some 2 to 3 percent of infants are born with a congenital malformation of some kind, about a quarter of which are caused by defects in chromosomes. Egg cells and sperm cells (called *germ cells*) each have twenty-three chromosomes, whereas all other cells in our bodies each have forty-six. When the egg is fertilized by the sperm, each of the twenty-three pairs up with its matching chromosome. Occasionally in the process of cell division leading to egg or sperm formation, errors occur involving increases or decreases in the total number of chromosomes. Sometimes the chromosomes themselves become abnormal because of deletions or breakages, or because of translocations, whereby part of one chromosome splits away and hooks on to another, producing a hybrid. Since these chromosomal abnormalities occur in the germ cell line even before fertilization, every cell in the developing infant's body will contain the same errors.

Chromosomal defects are often associated with mental retardation, distinctive physical abnormalities, and malformations of internal organs. One of the most common chromosomal problems is trisomy 21 (and, less frequently, trisomy 18 and 13), also known as Down's syndrome. "Trisomy" means that when the egg or the sperm was originally formed, two copies (rather than one) of the chromosomes were incorporated into the cell. If the egg carries the extra chromosome of DNA, three copies of the chromosome result when it fuses with the sperm—not two, as is normal. Children with Down's syndrome have characteristic physical features, generally mild but varying degrees of mental retardation, a high incidence of malformations of the heart and intestinal tract, and frequent ear problems, and are susceptible to early-onset Alzheimer's disease.

DEVELOPMENTAL ABNORMALITIES AND TERATOGENS

Even if the chromosomes passed on to the fetus from the mother and father are normal, in the process of developing into a complex human the one-celled fertilized egg goes through billions of cell divisions as it moves from embryo to fully formed fetus, and errors may occur. The fetus is at greatest risk for such errors during the first trimester, when most cell division is occurring. These defects may occur spontaneously, because of internal exposures to infections such as a virus like rubella (German measles), or to external toxins called *teratogens,* such as radiation, that alter the normal course of development (see "Hazardous Exposures," page 121). The vast majority of developmental abnormalities, however, cannot be related to specific maternal exposures but seem to occur sporadically and without identifiable reason.

ECTOPIC PREGNANCY

In about 2 percent of all pregnancies, a fertilized egg can implant itself outside the uterus. Most of the time, this *ectopic* pregnancy occurs in a fallopian tube (ectopic pregnancies are often called "tubal pregnancies"), but in 5 percent of ectopic pregnancies the fertilized egg manages to implant itself elsewhere—in the abdominal or pelvic cavity, or in the cervical canal.

The number of ectopic pregnancies in America has skyrocketed over the past twenty or so years—about sixfold, according to a 1995 report from the Centers for Disease Control and Prevention (CDC). They estimate that more than 100,000 women a year face an ectopic pregnancy. Many factors have contributed to this surge, particularly the explosion in sexually transmitted diseases, such as chlamydia (see page 151), which damage the tubes. Also contributing may be the growth of infertility therapies, both hormonal and surgical, which alter the normal timing of reproductive events.

Suspicion of an ectopic pregnancy comes when there are symptoms of early pregnancy (nausea, fatigue, breast enlargement, missed or delayed period) and then the development of lower-abdominal pain that is stabbing or cramping, becoming progressively more severe. Shoulder pain can result from leakage of blood into the abdominal cavity. Vaginal bleeding usually occurs.

Ectopic pregnancies are a threat to the life of the mother, but, given the earlier means of detecting pregnancies now available, we can usually detect and treat ectopic pregnancies early enough to stem severe damage. Blood levels of human chorionic gonadotropin produced by the developing placenta are quantified, and when the level fails to rise as it should (double within 48 hours) it signals problems with implantation or survival of the embryo; rising levels may be abnormal in both ectopic pregnancies and early miscarriages. An ultrasound at this stage is able to define precisely the location of the embryo, including its dangerous presence within a fallopian tube, which will lead to destruction and rupture of the tube.

Although treatment usually requires an operation to remove the fetal material (which is invariably disintegrating by the time of diagnosis) and sometimes the tube, there is now growing interest in the use of certain chemicals to end the ectopic pregnancy, such as the anticancer drug *methotrexate,* administered either through a laparoscope or by intravenous or oral therapy over a one- to four-day time period.

EARLY MISCARRIAGE

Miscarriages (also called spontaneous abortions) are both distressing and quite common, almost always occurring in the first trimester of pregnancy. Somewhere between 20 and 40 percent of all women will experience a miscarriage, although often the problem occurs before she even knows she is pregnant. Many people believe miscarriage is nature's way of ending an unhealthy pregnancy; I find there is much truth in this, for 50 to 70 percent of miscarried fetuses carry chromosomal defects.

Signs of an impending miscarriage include bleeding and sometimes cramping pain; if the cervix dilates, miscarriage is inevitable. Bleeding alone doesn't always lead to miscarriage, however; if the cervix doesn't dilate and the bleeding stops, the pregnancy may well go to term, and the bleeding episode is not associated with a greater chance of congenital abnormality. There is no treatment for first-trimester threatened miscarriage except watchful waiting. If the miscarriage occurs, typically it does so over about a three-day period. Although it has been almost routine to perform a dilatation and curettage (D&C) once it is clear that a miscarriage is occurring to accelerate the process and/or remove any retained tissue from the uterine lining, this procedure is now being questioned. D&Cs have complications, including damage to the cervical canal and infection. In a recent study from Sweden published in the *Lancet*, Drs. Sven Nielsen and Mats Hahlin showed that in about 80 percent of their patients the miscarriage completed itself naturally without a D&C. Watchful waiting led to no increase in symptoms or complications and only a one-day increase in days of bleeding, which overall was about a week.

Having one miscarriage does not place a woman at any greater risk of having another. After three, however, she falls into the category of being at risk of habitual fetal loss, and she should undertake further tests, including genetic studies of herself and her husband, and evaluation of her genital tract, endocrine system, and ovarian function, including the corpus luteal phase (last two weeks) of the menstrual cycle, which is important to the sustenance of early pregnancy (page 102).

MIDTERM MISCARRIAGE

Once a pregnancy has advanced into the second trimester, spontaneous loss is rare. When miscarriages do occur, the problem is usually maternal rather than fetal, and due to *cervical incompetence*, whereby without warning, the cervix dilates, the membranes surrounding the fetus rupture, and the fetus is lost. Signs are bleeding or cramping, which a pregnant woman must always bring to her doctor's attention immediately. Women who have had damage to the cervix at the time of a previous D&C, or surgical excision of part of the opening of the cervix (conization) for carcinoma in situ (see page 248), are at greater risk for this problem.

It is almost impossible to anticipate cervical incompetence that provokes a second-trimester abortion, but if the problem is detected early, three-quarters of threatened midterm miscarriages can be saved. Treatment involves suturing the cervix and placing the mother on bed rest for the duration of her pregnancy.

INFECTIONS

Throughout your pregnancy, your obstetrician will keep a careful watch for certain infections which can prove particularly dangerous to you or your baby. Virtually all infections of pregnancy can either be prevented or treated.

It is not uncommon for *streptococcus group B* bacteria to be found in the vagina at various times throughout pregnancy, but this is dangerous only during delivery, when the newborn can contract the infection and develop a serious pneumonia. Many obstetricians screen for the infection just before delivery and if it is present treat it during delivery.

Rubella is a well-known virus that causes measles, a onetime infection that leaves you with lifetime protection against a second attack. Rubella during pregnancy causes major congenital defects, including deafness, mental retardation, heart defects, pneumonia, and blood abnormalities. Before 1969, when a vaccine was developed, many women who developed rubella early in pregnancy opted to have abortions, and many who planned to get pregnant purposefully exposed themselves to rubella to put that risk behind them and develop immunity. All this disappeared when the vaccine arrived, and since that time the incidence of congenital defects from this infection has fallen by 95 percent.

Toxoplasma gondii is a parasite that is contracted by eating raw meat or from having contact with infected cats. (The parasite resides in the intestine of about 1 percent of cats, and its eggs are excreted in their feces, contaminating their litter boxes. Usually it is seen in outdoor cats.) If a woman gets an acute infection during pregnancy, she faces a high chance of transmitting it to her developing infant, with devastating results. The diagnosis is made by a blood test for antibodies to the parasite, or by culturing amniotic fluid. If acute infection with toxoplasmosis is detected in the developing fetus, many doctors recommend pregnancy termination, for the damage can include central nervous system defects, eye infections, hearing deficits, and mental retardation. Treatment with antibiotics can help. The best advice is for pregnant women to avoid cats and their litter boxes during pregnancy, not eat raw or poorly cooked meat, and wash their hands thoroughly after contact with either.

Most of the *sexually transmitted diseases* are transmissible to the fetus and lead to major and often long-term illness in the infant. These are discussed in detail in chapter 4.

PREECLAMPSIA, OR PREGNANCY-INDUCED HYPERTENSION

There is a reason why, as we'll see below, routine prenatal exams rigorously track weight gain, blood pressure, and urine protein. These three measures monitor the development of preeclampsia (once called toxemia, now called pregnancy-induced hypertension), a serious complication of pregnancy. About half the time, this condition develops in the last trimester of pregnancy, but it can also develop at the time of or right after delivery. It is believed to result from spasm of the maternal and fetal blood vessels related to increased sensitivity to the powerful blood pressure hormone, angiotensin, discussed in chapter 9. (Normally, pregnant women become *less* sensitive to this hormone.)

With preeclampsia, high blood pressure develops, fluid is retained so the mother visibly swells in the hands, feet, and sometimes the face, and she leaks protein into her urine. She may also have blurred vision or headache, nausea, and vomiting. Unchecked, preeclampsia can lead to extremely high blood pressure, mental confusion, seizures, and coma (known as eclampsia); both mother and infant are in mortal danger, and their only hope is delivery. Even then about half of the babies die, and though delivery usually leads to a complete resolution of the problem, as many as 10 percent of the mothers experiencing eclampsia develop serious lingering complications, including cerebral hemorrhage, heart or kidney failure, and even death. Women are most at risk for this complication during their first pregnancy.

PLACENTA PREVIA AND ABRUPTIO PLACENTAE

Sometimes the placenta lies across the opening of the cervix, blocking the baby's path down the birth canal. When the cervix starts to dilate

late in pregnancy, the placenta can be damaged, placing the fetus at risk of losing its blood and nutrient supply. Even if the placenta is not damaged, its inconvenient location will necessitate a cesarean section. This condition is called *placenta previa*. Occasionally even a placenta implanted well within the body of the uterus may prematurely separate from the uterine wall; this is called *abruptio placentae*.

A clear warning sign of any damage to the placenta is vaginal bleeding, which is usually painless. Although you may experience a small amount of bleeding late in your pregnancy for several harmless reasons, including the loss of your mucus plug or simple stretching of the cervix, it should *always* prompt an immediate call to your obstetrician. These placental problems pose a serious risk to mother and child. An ultrasound can quickly determine the diagnosis and an emergency cesarean is usually warranted.

PREMATURE RUPTURE OF MEMBRANES

Sometimes the membranes that surround the fetus rupture before the onset of labor and the amniotic fluid leaks out—your water breaks. (This may be a big gush or a small amount that can be missed or mistaken as urine.) If rupture occurs before your thirty-sixth week, it is a high-risk situation requiring hospitalization, for there is the threat of premature delivery and also of infection of the amniotic fluid. If your pregnancy is thirty-six or more weeks along, most obstetricians will induce delivery if it does not occur spontaneously, out of concern about infection.

POST-TERM PREGNANCY

When normal gestation exceeds forty-two weeks from the last menstrual period, it poses danger to the well-being of the fetus; the placenta starts to fail, and the amniotic fluid is not properly regulated and is often inadequate in volume. Treatment is straightforward: induce delivery; sometimes this means cesarean section.

RISK FACTORS FOR MOTHER AND BABY

A healthy pregnancy means a healthy and attentive expectant mother, but a problem pregnancy does not mean the mother has been careless. There are risks we cannot control, and those we can. A woman's power lies in taking command and avoiding risks—and in not blaming herself when an unavoidable risk results in a tragedy.

HAZARDOUS EXPOSURES

Hazards to the fetus include environmental exposures that might alter the normal course of a baby's development. *Smoking* is one of the most common hazards to a developing fetus, associated with low-birth-weight infants and an increase in miscarriages. The major risk seems to be to the blood supply to the placenta, rather than a direct toxic effect on the baby. This is in contrast to the tragedies of *illicit drug use:* we have learned, for example, about the direct fetal toxicity experienced by the crack babies filling our hospitals. Fetuses exposed to cocaine and other illegal brain toxins by drug-addicted mothers develop long-term neurological damage. *Alcohol* is another fetal toxin that has been shown to cause neurologic problems in infants exposed in utero. (see page 63.) In addition to these obvious abuses, a pregnant woman must beware of more subtle teratogenic risks under her direct control.

Although most medicines pose no known risk, any woman contemplating pregnancy should be sure to discuss her *prescribed medicines* with her doctor. There are a few in particular that your doctor may wish to stop or change, including the anticoagulant *Coumadin;* antiseizure medicines such as *dilantin;* some medicines for mood disorders, including *lithium* and the *tricyclic antidepressants;* some antibiotics; the antiacne medication *isotretinoin (Accutane);* and certain androgenic hormones, such as *danazol.* After intensive studies and more than thirty years of use, there is no evidence that oral contraceptive hormones are tied to congenital birth defects. It is generally recommended, however, that a woman be off contraceptives as well as most other medicines for three months before conceiving a child.

Most over-the-counter medicines, such as aspirin and other pain relievers, cold tablets, decongestants, antihistamines, cough suppressants, and vitamins, are not associated with birth defects, but I would still talk with your physician before taking any of them. One special case should be noted: very high daily doses of vitamin A—in the range of 25,000 IU to 40,000 IU—increase the risk of congenital birth defects.

X rays are well-known environmental risk factors; don't get any (even simple dental X rays) while you're pregnant without consulting your physician. Ionizing radiation, the kind that comes with diagnostic X-ray studies, induces abnormalities in the developing embryo by damaging the DNA of dividing cells.

This form of radiation is to be distinguished from the nonionizing radiation emitted by everyday technology such as microwaves, televisions, and computers (radio frequency electromagnetic radiation); we know very little about this, but it is nonpenetrating and, in any event, unable to reach the fetus. Although we've all heard about the dangers of electromagnetic radiation that comes from high-power lines, nothing has been proven beyond anecdotal evidence, and I'm quite skeptical. (See page 221.)

MATERNAL AGE

Women who have babies at either end of their reproductive lifespan face higher levels of many types of risks during their pregnancies.

Teen Pregnancy

Some 7 percent of teens age fifteen to seventeen become pregnant, and 15 percent by age eighteen or nineteen. It is estimated that more than a quarter of all first babies in our country are born to single teens, and the future doesn't hold much promise of change. The major societal and personal problems faced by these youngsters (who so often are doomed thereafter to lives of limited opportunity, if not poverty) also present health problems for both mother and child: fetal mortality, premature delivery, poor prenatal nutrition, and lack of prenatal health care are all higher among mothers under seventeen.

Midlife Pregnancy

Advanced maternal age has long been associated with a higher rate of miscarriages, preterm births, late-term placental problems, and children with chromosomal abnormalities, and with more complications from other illnesses, such as hypertension and diabetes. But what is "advanced maternal age"? Thirty-five used to be the cutoff, but a healthy thirty-five-year-old woman stands a greater chance of an uneventful pregnancy than does an unhealthy twenty-four-year-old. Chromosomal abnormalities are tied to the age of the mother: one out of fourteen hundred births from women in their twenties has the chromosomal abnormality of trisomy 21, or Down's syndrome; among women age forty, the number rises rather dramatically to one in a hundred; and among women age fifty, to one in sixteen. (Paternal age may also be a risk factor for chromosomal abnormalities, but this has not been well studied.) Aside from this problem, however, today women well into their late forties are having babies safely. Most doctors no longer even call having a first baby after age thirty-five an inherently high-risk pregnancy or use that rather unappealing but formerly common descriptor, "elderly primip," to describe these mothers.

COEXISTING MATERNAL HEALTH PROBLEMS

Regardless of a woman's age, if she has coexisting health problems she will face a higher-risk pregnancy. Women who have *diabetes* face a higher risk of sudden intrauterine death of the fetus in the third trimester, and require careful fetal monitoring and sometimes induced delivery at thirty-eight weeks. Preexisting *hypertension* puts a woman at greater risk for preeclampsia, and *sexually transmitted diseases* increase the risk of infection to the fetus. Other coexisting major illnesses, such as *heart disease, kidney disease,* or diseases of the *autoimmune system,* also place you at a higher risk, and your doctor will carefully monitor your pregnancy if you suffer from any of them.

PREGNANCY CARE

Although volumes have been written about how best to take care of yourself and your developing baby, for the most part it boils down to common sense and good communication with your doctor. Of course, what is "common sense" now wasn't so for our mother's generation; our mothers weren't browbeaten about the dangers of smoking, drinking, and medications, as we are. Nor were doctors as sensitive back then to the risks of X-ray exposure used in diagnostic studies.

Nutrition, we've learned, is paramount (see page 62). This means adequate calcium intake; ample protein (usually not a problem unless you are a strict vegetarian); iron-rich foods, preferably from fruits and vegetables (spinach, prunes, dried beans and peas); and the B vitamin, folic acid, important in cell division (orange juice and oranges, broccoli, asparagus, legumes). (Folic acid supplements are also important before pregnancy to decrease the risk of neural tube defects such as spina bifida.) Most doctors recommend prenatal multivitamin supplements, and sometimes additional supplements of iron and calcium. A good well-balanced prepregnancy diet will serve you just as well during pregnancy—as you get hungrier during pregnancy, eat more of the good foods you normally do, and you and your baby will be fine.

Adequate exercise is important, although it should be sensible, reviewed with your obstetrician, and, in whatever form, never to the point of exhaustion. Maintenance of prepregnancy exercise during pregnancy is generally acceptable if it is not too strenuous. Beyond this, the regularly scheduled visits you make to your doctor will include clear and sufficient tests to keep you and your baby worry-free.

During these visits your blood pressure, urine, and weight will be checked, along with your emotional well-being and your baby's heartbeat and growth. Early on, you will be screened for blood type incompatibility with the developing baby (which may prompt special attention at delivery), and for any infections that increase fetal risk.

These regular visits can be among the happiest visits a woman will ever have to her doctor, as she feels the baby grow, smiles at its heartbeat, and plans for what's ahead.

ULTRASOUND

Should any problems arise, or should you be classified high-risk for any of the reasons above, your obstetrician has a host of sophisticated means available to track and evaluate the developing baby. One device used in almost every test is a machine with which you're most likely already familiar, the *ultrasound*. Ultrasound (see page 224), which uses sound waves to transmit an image of the fetus onto a nearby video screen, may be used throughout the pregnancy to examine the fetus, if a suspicion of a problem arises. Painless and noninvasive, ultrasound enables parents and physicians to see the developing fetus with a clarity that can provoke wonder and laughter. (It should be pointed out that many obstetricians use ultrasound routinely during early pregnancy to assess the development of the fetus and confirm gestational age; in this setting its use does not imply a suspected problem.)

PRENATAL TESTING

Although tests are most frequently used by mothers over the age of thirty-five, many pregnant women are now choosing to take advantage of one of the main tests available to determine whether the fetus carries chromosomal abnormalities or certain other malformations of the nervous system. Maternal serum can be used to screen for spina bifida, a malformation of the spinal cord. Only a few fetal cells are needed to perform screens for serious health conditions present in the fetus, such as Down's syndrome. Chromosomal analysis also tells the sex of the fetus. The two primary methods used to obtain samples for these genetic screens are amniocentesis and chorionic villus sampling.

Amniocentesis, the most common, is performed after the sixteenth week of pregnancy. (In some circumstances it is possible to perform this procedure as early as thirteen weeks, but some believe with greater risk.) A needle is inserted through the abdominal wall into the uterus, usually while an ultrasound image guides the way, and a small amount of the amniotic fluid is withdrawn. This fluid contains both biochemicals and cells shed by the developing fetus. Since these cells contain the same chromosomes as the fetus, they can be screened for abnormalities. Amniocentesis is a safe and relatively painless procedure, although some momentary discomfort may occur. The risk of miscarriage or early rupture of membranes is less than 0.5 percent.

Chorionic villus sampling is performed in the first trimester, at about the tenth week. It is a more risky test, however, with a 1 percent chance of causing spontaneous abortion and reported to be linked, rarely, to fetal injury, including malformation of the jaw and limbs. (Because of such risks, some obstetricians are abandoning this approach. In any event, make sure the doctor who is going to do the test is experienced: it takes more skill than amniocentesis.) The chorion, a membrane covering the outer embryo, projects minuscule branches of tissue and vessels into the placenta. Using ultrasound to see inside the womb, the clinician takes samples of these "villi" (which are generally the same tissue as the fetus) by inserting a thin suction tube through the abdomen and into the space between the uterine wall and the chorion. The cells of the villi are cultured and studied for abnormalities.

Another approach is employed in the setting of *in-vitro fertilization.* Special methods have been developed to remove one cell from an eight-cell preimplantation embryo for chromosomal testing. If it is normal, the embryo can be implanted in the uterus.

Methods of *maternal blood testing,* obtaining minute amounts of fetal protein and fetal cells from the mother's blood for the same kinds of genetic and other analyses that are performed on amniotic fluid or chorionic villus samples, are also on the horizon. Such tests, using a special laboratory amplification technology called PCR, will probably eliminate the need to invade the uterus with a needle, will be virtually risk-free, and should be substantially less expensive.

Though some of these procedures have become commonplace in the practice of obstetrics, they also, quietly but surely, raise some fairly powerful ethical questions. In the future, we may well be able to test easily for a wider range of potential health problems, such as genes for breast cancer, Alzheimer's disease, manic-depressive illness, alcoholism, or heart disease, or maybe even human traits such as short stature, obesity, or even IQ or personality. Will some couples use this information to try to produce the "perfect" child, casting off all others? How many healthy children might be lost in an attempt to weed out some theoretical long-term risk or "undesirable" human trait? As a society, we soundly reject the notion of eugenics, but what about individual couples trying to "design" their own offspring? These ethical, social, and personal dilemmas will surely confront us and our children as we unlock the secrets of the human genome.

TESTING LATE IN PREGNANCY

If you have a history of stillbirths, or health problems that may compromise the fetus (heart disease, preeclampsia), or you are two weeks beyond your due date, or some other concerns arise about the fetus, your doctor may conduct special tests to assess fetal health late in your pregnancy. The commonly used tests assess the growth and nourishment of the fully formed fetus and the health of the placenta, with ultrasound (and sometimes echo Doppler, a special form of ultrasound that is able to measure blood flow). In the *nonstress test,* the mother signals whenever she feels fetal movement, and the baby's heart rate is monitored to see if it speeds up as a result. The ultrasound also reveals other physical profile measures including fetal movement, such as breathing, fetal tone, and gross body movements, and enables your physician to assess the volume of amniotic fluid. Abnormalities on the nonstress test prompt other studies to define fetal distress more precisely. In the *contraction stress test,* for instance, fetal heart rate and sometimes placental blood flow in the fetal umbilical artery are monitored during uterine contractions (occurring normally during late pregnancy or induced by Pitocin) to see if the placenta is starting to fail. In the event of fetal stress, the obstetrician may decide to induce labor or, if need be, perform a cesarean delivery.

CHILDBIRTH

Despite the dramatic high-tech transformations in reproductive medicine, labor and delivery have become more "high touch." Unlike a generation ago, when fathers were excluded from what was seen as a medical event for the mother, fathers, if they choose, now have the option to help their wives prepare physically and psychologically for birth and be with them throughout delivery. Women are awake during delivery—even, most of the time, during cesarean sections. My husband—who had three grown children under the old system—told me in a reverent whisper that seeing our Marie born was the most moving experience of his life.

Modern obstetrics lets the mother, with the counsel of her doctors, make most of the decisions about the kind of delivery she wants—natural childbirth, or childbirth with anesthesia, and if so which kind; birthing room (which looks like a bedroom) or delivery room; delivery in hospital or at home; midwife or obstetrician; whether or not to include other family and friends in the delivery. At the same time, modern obstetrics has more powerful means to assure early detection of fetal distress and close monitoring of the mother's progress. The following sections touch on some of the major medical interventions used today. Since obstetrics is still mostly mother's work, the mother should learn as much as she can about her delivery before it happens, and be sure to discuss her views and feelings clearly with her doctor and others who will be helping her deliver.

FETAL MONITORING

In low-risk pregnancies, having a nurse regularly listen to fetal heart rate is customary. In higher-risk situations, continuous monitoring is available. Electronic monitoring of the baby's heart rate throughout labor is done by external monitors placed on the abdomen or, more reliably, by placing small internal probes onto the baby's scalp after the membranes of the amniotic sac have broken. Monitoring capabilities are especially important in long labors and high-risk pregnancies, such as in women who have heart disease, diabetes, or preeclampsia. I suggest you find out about the capabilities of the facilities available to you and choose a hospital that is well equipped.

OXYTOCIN STIMULATION OF CONTRACTIONS

If labor is difficult or prolonged or uterine contractions seem weak, a drug called oxytocin (Pitocin), a pituitary hormone which has been used in deliveries for decades, can be given intravenously to stimulate contractions and move labor along. The "pit-drip," as it is often called, is also used for *inducing* a delivery before natural labor sets in. Oxytocin-induced contractions may be stronger and therefore more painful, and increase the need for pain relief as well as monitoring.

EPISIOTOMIES

An *episiotomy* is an incision made at the last moment in the outer back wall of the vagina (into the perineal tissues between the vagina and anus) as the baby's head starts pushing out, to control tissue tearing and speed delivery by making a wider opening for the emerging baby's head. Though they were once performed routinely, most obstetricians now decide during delivery on a case-by-case basis. There are clear circumstances where an episiotomy becomes necessary, such as when the baby's head is having difficulty pressing through the vaginal opening, or when forceps have to be used. Episiotomies generally heal up within a matter of weeks, but sometimes pain or discomfort can linger for as long as three months and cause temporary difficulties with sexual intercourse.

FORCEPS AND VACUUM EXTRACTION

The metal instruments placed around the head of the infant to help rotate and guide the fetus through the lowest part of the birth canal are called *forceps*. Forceps deliveries got a very bad name for a time, because they were used either unnecessarily or incorrectly—for instance, when the baby was still too high in the vaginal canal. Now, however, with proper use, they are a helpful and sometimes necessary tool to accelerate the final push of the baby at delivery, particularly when the mother is exhausted or unable to push adequately. Forceps can make a vaginal delivery safer for a baby, protecting the fetal head from prolonged pressure against the lower vagina and its surrounding tissue.

A more recent variation on forceps that accomplishes the same goal is the *vacuum extractor,* whereby a suction cup is placed on the baby's head and suction is supplied by a vacuum pump. Though this approach is less traumatic to the mother's tissues, some obstetricians believe it may be less effective than forceps in protecting the baby's head in the last stage of delivery. In skilled hands the two approaches are probably equivalent. As in any kind of medical intervention, what you want most of all is an experienced operator with superb judgment.

ANESTHESIA AND ANALGESIA

We need look no further than the types of anesthetics used in childbirth over the last thirty years for a clear and pointed metaphorical picture of the pendulum swings in women's reproductive health: drastic shifts in physicians' and mothers' attitudes impossible to implement without equally significant medical and scientific advances.

We've moved from a time when children entered the world from mothers heavily dosed all too often with scopolamine, a drug that doesn't reduce pain but simply causes amnesia (and restlessness, and sometimes hallucinations), through the era of natural childbirth, in which women pressured to make a political statement, and feeling guilty about doing otherwise, subjected themselves to sometimes unendurable pain, to the wise and respectful perspective we have achieved today.

Central to modern obstetrics is pain control that is safe for both mother and infant—and at the discretion of each woman to take or not to take. Use of narcotics and tranquilizers is restricted, because of the effect on the baby, but some of these agents can be given in low doses in a carefully monitored setting. For example, the perineal area may be numbed before an episiotomy by the local injection of drugs such as lidocaine while the woman remains fully conscious.

For controlling the pain of labor and delivery, many women today choose to use *epidural analgesia*. When contractions become unbearable, the anesthetist will, on the woman's request, insert a small catheter in the outer, epidural space surrounding her spinal cord (not directly into the spinal canal). With the catheter in place, low doses of anesthetic agents such as lidocaine or pain-relieving opioids like Demerol can be given to the mother as needed. An epidural allows her to be awake and alert but somewhat numbed; she can move her legs and help push the baby out, but not to the degree she could without anesthetic. Though many women find the epidural to be a godsend, it is not without risks. Epidural analgesia can slow down contractions and can sometimes cause temporary drops in blood pressure; it thus requires close supervision and, most often, continuous electronic monitoring of fetal heart rate. Also, the obstetrician will often have to use forceps or a vacuum pump to assist women whose ability to push has been decreased by an epidural, and will sometimes, if rarely, resort to a cesarean section. (Some obstetricians think widespread use of epidural analgesia is responsible for part of the increased C-section rate.)

Cesarean Delivery

Cesarean section, an operation that removes the baby from the uterus through an abdominal incision rather than through the vagina, is used in almost one in four deliveries in the United States. More than a third of these operations are being done because the mother has had a previous cesarean section, which traditionally ruled out subsequent vaginal deliveries; others because of acute fetal distress, failure to deliver after a prolonged and difficult labor, and a breech birth (where the baby is positioned to come out rump first, rather than head first).

Cesarean deliveries are generally safe for both mother and child. The overall U.S. rate of C-sections is high compared with that of other countries, and variable from hospital to hospital, which may imply that at least some of these procedures are unnecessary. The surgery can create a medical problem for the mother, whose recovery will be longer and more painful, and who is denied the experience of normal childbirth. Cesareans also drive up overall medical costs. Many C-section opponents have claimed that fear of malpractice suits subtly influences some doctors to choose a C-section, because far more doctors have been sued for not resorting to a C-section when delivery becomes problematic than for performing unnecessary C-sections.

In any case, the rate of cesareans is currently on the way down, and doctors no longer insist that a woman who has had a C-section have all subsequent babies the same way. Most studies show no greater risk with a vaginal delivery after a C-section than a normal vaginal delivery—but in a carefully selected group of women. For example, the kind of incision used on the uterus in the prior C-section can make the difference: a vertical incision, which cuts across more muscle bundles, is problematic for a subsequent vaginal delivery, and some obstetricians do not allow such women to labor. One that is low and transverse, in contrast, a low risk of labor problems.

The major difficulty with prior C-sections is that scar tissue may make contractions ineffective, prolonging labor. Another complication, infrequent but an increased risk among women who have had more than one C-section already, is uterine rupture at the site of the cesarean scar. In this catastrophic event, the infant protrudes out of the tear, disrupting the placenta and fetal blood supply, and is deprived of oxygen; the mother hemorrhages internally, sometimes massively. To save the life of both, an emergency cesarean must be performed, and, depending on the damage to the uterus, sometimes a hysterectomy as well. My view is that, if you have had more than one cesarean section in the past, opt for another. If you've had just one, discuss the situation fully with your doctor and make up your own mind after hearing all the risks—and don't be pressured.

One final note on cesareans. I agree that the overuse of C-sections, where that is the case, needs to be corrected; no operation should be performed unless it is necessary. But let me be the contrarian to the current views. Cesareans are health- and life-saving; there is no doubt. And when one is needed, this is not a sign of failure—of either the mother or the obstetrician. Many otherwise healthy babies would not make it without C-sections, nor would many mothers. I hope that women and their doctors are not made fearful of resorting to this potentially health-saving procedure. You should discuss both risks and benefits with your obstetrician in advance of your delivery date, and learn his or her attitude and individual rate of performing C-sections. You want an obstetrician who is neither unduly trigger-happy about cesareans, nor so driven by the political agenda to bring down numbers that your doctor puts you at any unnecessary risk by withholding a C-section that is appropriate.

POSTNATAL AND NEONATAL CARE

A healthy delivery does not end in the delivery room. The postpartum period—or *puerperium,* as it is called—extends from the moment of birth to about six weeks thereafter, until the uterus has returned to the normal size, and is a time of special consideration for both mother and infant.

With regard to the infant, there are some issues that a mother faces immediately. The first is in the delivery room: "Is my baby all right?" The second follows right after: "Do I really want to breast-feed?" Obviously, both questions need to have been well thought out beforehand.

NEONATAL CARE

An experienced pediatrician must be standing by in the delivery room to assess the health of your infant immediately. Your obstetrician usually arranges for this, but I suggest that you ask about it and even meet the pediatrician ahead of time. Find out if the hospital has a neonatal intensive care unit in case a problem develops, or what nearby unit is available. Any health problems suspected in your newborn need thorough evaluation. Discuss findings fully with your doctor, so that you understand any problems and know what to expect. As I've said throughout this book, never hesitate to get another opinion if you are not sure.

BREAST-FEEDING

Sometime before delivery, every mother must decide whether she intends to breast-feed. She is going to hear a range of opinions from family and friends, and may feel conflicted, if not pressured, about doing one thing or the other. My advice is to do what makes sense for mother and baby. Often, however, a mother cannot really decide until she tries, at least for a while. And trying it does not mean she is committed for any set period of time. If she is not sure, she can see how it goes, and then decide.

Breast-feeding offers many pluses. Mother's milk contains antibodies that enhance a baby's immune system; this benefit comes after only a few weeks of breast-feeding, since the protective immune factors are most concentrated in the earliest milk. Babies are unlikely to be allergic to their mothers' milk, and if breast-fed generally have fewer digestion difficulties. For the mother, the hormones that bring in milk also cause the uterus to contract back to its normal size and tone sooner than otherwise. Women who breast-feed have been shown to run a slightly lower risk of breast cancer. And, of course, the experience can be emotionally satisfying to both mother and baby. It's also inexpensive, it's convenient, and it's warm and cozy. But it's not for every woman.

Some mothers enjoy breast-feeding; others find it stressful. Some do so easily; some simply don't produce adequate milk. Some babies seem to need more nourishment than the mother can provide in order to thrive. When babies are born prematurely or have other health difficulties, breast-feeding may be impossible. It can also become difficult if a mother works or has major demands from other children.

Practically speaking, there is no one perfect answer, and the future of your child is not dependent on what you decide. So do what seems and feels right to you. You can be a good mother whichever you do.

PHYSICAL RECOVERY

Over the six-week postpartum period, the uterus gradually returns to normal; between seven and twelve weeks, ovulation and menstrual periods return. Mothers who continue to breast-feed take longer to resume menstruation, but this is variable. (Breast-feeding is not a form of contraception since you cannot be sure when ovulation returns.) Over this time, most women gradually lose weight and return to close to their prepregnancy size, even without any kind of dieting. A gradual resumption of a routine exercise program—with the advice of your doctor—will speed the transformation along. As for resuming most other activities, including sexual intercourse, listen to your body. Although six weeks is often the defining time period for recovery from childbirth, this is not a magical milestone; some women find themselves entirely back to normal weeks earlier, or the process may take longer.

THE POSTPARTUM BLUES

Most women feel a bit blue after delivery. This may be an old wives' tale; but there are good reasons for it. The new mother is exhausted; her bottom hurts; she may have temporary difficulty with urination or hemorrhoids; her newborn gives her no sleep and has now become the real center of attention; and of course her hormones have been on a roller-coaster ride. My advice is to expect it and pamper yourself as much as possible. An understanding husband, family members, or close friends can provide needed adult communication and support. A new mother must also find some measure of quiet time each day, to read or go out or focus on something of special interest to herself. In rare instances, a degree of postpartum depression may set in that requires professional attention. This is discussed in detail in chapter 7.

Throughout the postpartum period, a woman must remember she is not medically alone with regard to her physical and mental well-being. She should not hesitate to call her obstetrician for advice or counsel, even before the usual postpartum visit of four to six weeks.

THE POSTPARTUM BRIGHTS

Babies are magnificent little creatures, and they bring a joy like no other. Regardless of what you may or may not do in your life, don't forget: this could be your finest accomplishment, a miracle, a gift to the world and to future generations. Whatever the demands on your life, whatever your other responsibilities, whatever your personal circumstances, keep in mind that you have just done something truly wonderful!

QUESTIONS FOR YOUR DOCTOR

Your reproductive life spans a long time. Find a gynecologist that you are comfortable with and stick with her or him. A good gynecologist often serves as a primary care doctor for many women, picking up on a wide range of mental and physical problems early, and providing advice and referral. Make sure you are comfortable with your physician, and do not hesitate to ask any of the following questions.

- Discuss with your doctor any concerns you have with your love or sexual relationships that are presenting mental or physical health problems for you. If you detect changes in your libido, discuss it with your doctor. Are you taking any medications that may be causing a problem? Even if your doctor cannot deal with your concerns herself, she will give you advice on a next step.
- Your doctor should know about any pathological relationships, including physical abuse. Breaking the silence is often the first step toward curing the problem.
- Contraceptives are changing and, often, so is your need for them. Ask your doctor what contraceptives are now available that are most suitable for you, given your sexual activity. What is their long-term impact on any future decisions about pregnancies?
- What are your doctor's views about abortion? Do those views influence her practice, and if so, how? If, after much conscious consideration of alternatives and their long-term implications to you personally, you have decided to have an abortion, ask about what is the best method, and what effect it might have on future pregnancies, and your overall health.
- What about endometriosis? Do you have it? Are there ways to prevent it? Is it a concern for future pregnancies?
- If you are facing infertility, what steps does your doctor recommend for evaluation and treatment of possible infertility of both you and your spouse? How experienced is your doctor in handling infertility? Understand precisely what your doctor believes the problem to be before embarking on any treatments.

- If you are being treated for infertility, what are the risks and uncertainties involved? What are the side effects of any medication you are taking? Set a timetable for yourself, with your doctor, for how long to "try."

- If you are advised to embark on in-vitro fertilization, you need to do your homework carefully. A second opinion is a good idea. Find out your doctor's success rates for assisted technologies for your particular problem. What are the costs going to be? What happens to the spare embryos? How does in-vitro fertilization compare with GIFT? What is the chance of multiple pregnancies resulting from IVF or GIFT?

- If you are pregnant, find out what the views of your doctor are about delivery, fetal monitoring, anesthesia, episiotomies, and forceps. What are the indications for cesarean section? How many does your doctor (and the group that she is part of) perform? Ask these questions early in your pregnancy.

- Who is on call to back up your doctor if she is unavailable? You should meet with any other member of the group who might be caring for you at delivery. A hospital tour is also a good idea.

- Does the hospital your doctor uses have a neonatal intensive care unit? Or is such a unit available nearby? Will there be a pediatrician in the delivery room? Who?

- If you are thinking about a home delivery, learn and carefully weigh all the risks. How do you obtain emergency care? Who is on standby for the baby?

WHAT WOMEN CAN DO PERSONALLY AND POLITICALLY

I have placed the subject of this chapter within the broader context of power and vulnerability; ironically, women are now both as powerful and as vulnerable sexually as they have ever been. We have birth control, sexual freedom, and safe childbirth—and we have conflicting forces ready to influence or override an individual woman's personal autonomy about what is right for her and her own health. We have terrorists threatening and even murdering innocent people at Planned Parenthood clinics across the country, manipulating fear to deprive women of a protected right granted to them under the law. We see abusers somehow feeling freer and freer to express their anger in violence against women. There is much to be done.

- Each woman must assess for herself her feelings about whether or not she and her daughters should be able to make decisions about their reproductive life free from government intrusion, and make her voice heard, however she feels. Your voice needs to be heard at the local, state, and federal levels, whether through letters to congressmen, opinions expressed in local newspapers and radio, or support of groups that adequately represent your views.

- There has been considerable neglect of contraceptive research over the years, as well as delays in the introduction of contraceptive medicines and devices into the U.S. market. Women must be informed of the current and emerging contraceptive options; we must place pressure on elected officials and federal agencies that oversee these activities, at both the research and regulatory levels, to assure that the work continues. It is difficult to comprehend why the staunchest opponents of abortion don't take up the cause of better and improved contraception.

- Domestic violence and spousal abuse have not been taken seriously by many law enforcement authorities. Women themselves need to acknowledge these often secret problems, and support efforts within their communities to address them. We must give support and attention to local shelters or counseling services for battered women. And we must teach our sons and daughters about these risks, and where to turn if these problems develop.

- We can also encourage our health professionals to play a more assertive role, to become forthright about directly asking a woman with obvious trauma—depression or anxiety, suicide attempts, unexplained head or neck injuries—whether she has been abused.

- Parents should take an active interest in what is being taught their children in sex education classes in school, and be frank and supportive in helping them at home as they embark on early boy-girl relationships. Consider strong encouragement of abstinence for health reasons at the least, teaching the dangers of teenage sex with as much concern as the dangers of smoking or illicit drugs are taught.

- Research and development work being done on human embryos and other approaches for assisted pregnancies are posing new medical dilemmas for ourselves and our daughters. Ask yourself, for example, where we should draw the line on growing embryos in federally supported laboratories for research or other purposes. Should we be questioning the solicitation and use of college students as hired egg donors? Such issues will only loom larger in the years ahead and need full airing.

- Think about the psychology of human relationships as a health matter that reflects the character of our communities, our times, and each of us individually. Gaps in our knowledge of human bonding, and unwillingness to support certain kinds of research either because it is "soft," unworthy science or because it delves into delicate areas of human behavior, should be reconsidered. We have a lot to learn and much to support.

- In this particular area of women's health as in no other, we need openness to one another's views and personal choices. This includes reproductive choices and sexual preferences, the choice to stay home and raise a family full-time, to be a full-time careerist, or to struggle (however imperfectly) with both. Throughout the ages, intolerance toward those who are "different from us" has ultimately brutalized women more than anything else. All women have a personal and political stake in fighting the disease of intolerance.

Ellen Chesler, in her 1993 biography of Margaret Sanger, recounts the toast given to Mrs. Sanger by the writer H. G. Wells: "Alexander the Great changed a few boundaries and killed a certain number of men but he made no lasting change in civilization. Both he and Napoleon were forced into fame by circumstances outside themselves and by currents of the time, but Margaret Sanger made currents and circumstances. When the history of our civilization is written, it will be a biological history, and Margaret Sanger will be its heroine." What Wells knew and we must remember is that Sanger's kind of heroism not only made life bearable for millions of women, but affirmed the right of women everywhere and for all time to determine our reproductive health and happiness. This is now our power, and our sacred responsibility.

FOUR

SEXUALLY TRANSMITTED DISEASES
The Silent Plague

In the supreme moments of danger, alone woman must ever meet the horrors of the situation. . . . The talk of sheltering woman from the fierce storms of life is the sheerest mockery, for they beat on her from every point of the compass, just as they do on man, and with more fatal results, for he has been trained to protect himself, to resist and to conquer.

— ELIZABETH CADY STANTON,
  THE SOLITUDE OF SELF, *1892*

In this chapter you may be overwhelmed by statistics, medical lingo, and graphic language. But what is really overwhelming is the gravity of the problem, faced by all women. Sometimes the figures don't mean much until you encounter the human tragedy linked to the medicalese—in this case the plight of a young woman who suffered from one of the largely unknown sexually transmitted diseases (STDs) afflicting women. Let me tell you about Jenny. Though she is gone, she has many sisters still out there.

Jenny, a beautiful brunette from the Midwest who looked like a young Jane Seymour, lived with her boyfriend after college. He had been her only "real" boyfriend, but they were not yet ready to get married. She was from a deeply religious family, and the living arrangement led to a pretty big strain with her parents. A diligent young woman, Jenny was trying to move along in the tough world of a major Chicago architectural firm. She worked hard through school and as a young associate, and neglected her annual visits to her gynecologist. When she finally went for a checkup, cancer cells were present on the Pap smear. The cells indicated that she had a dangerous strain of a sexually transmitted infection, HPV, the human papilloma virus, as well as extensive invasive cervical cancer. She endured major surgery; the loss of her reproductive organs; radiation therapy. But the cancer spread to involve her bladder and intestines, and she was faced with more chemotherapy, intractable pain, and progressive debilitating weakness. The architectural firm kept her on, even after she started missing more and more work, until she couldn't leave her small apartment. Along the way, her boyfriend left her, unable to stand living with this dying young woman. Though he was undoubtedly the one who had given her HPV, that was now her problem, not his: he was not at risk for cancer. Her girl friends rallied to help; her parents kept a vigil at their dying daughter's bed. Her firm helped as long as they could. A promising architect, a lovely young woman, she died before her thirtieth birthday.

She never married, never had a child; her parents lost their child, her friends their friend. Such a silent, tragic, brutal loss may be obscured in the statistics. But, unlike most illnesses, this one did not have to happen. If she had only known that her relationship with this young man was lethal, she could have protected herself.

Even as I write this, tears are in my eyes—of frustration, of sadness, for her and for those we do not know. We rally to the tragedies of violence on the street, brutality in Bosnia, famine in Mogadishu. What will it take to rally to educate our daughters and our sons about this stealthy violence lurking in the shadows of growing up, before it is too late? Why have we failed to get the message out to the more than six million young women a year who contract these diseases?

Women today can be deeply grateful for the opportunities that the women's movement brought us, but they should not be blind to the dangerous situations their freedom sometimes places them in. Quite apart from gender equality in education and in the workplace is the medical reality that, when it comes to sex, women are not just like men and can never equal men in their so-called sexual freedoms. When it comes to sex, women are much more vulnerable than they, or their partners, like to hear.

STDs: FROM MEDICAL SECRETS TO SILENT PLAGUES

In 1913, the U.S. Postal Service refused to deliver the issue of the *New York Call* that wrote about a "medical secret," telling women, in strong and vivid words, to protect themselves and their children from the ravages of venereal diseases. The article cautioned women against ignorance of this life-threatening problem, and decried the double standard of sexual behavior which allowed men to be sexually promiscuous while keeping women in the dark about their own health risks.

And a double standard it was. The government, even as it stifled this message to women, was festooning the bars and barracks of the United States and Europe with posters warning soldiers of the dangers of venereal disease—posters that invariably bore a representation of an attractive but obviously "loose" woman. The message was implicit: women give men venereal disease. There were no posters implying that the reverse might also be true. Variations on such posters reappeared during World War II, with the same message: women transmit disease.

But we have known all along that the reverse is true as well. In fact, recent epidemiological studies have shown the reverse to be more true than we would like. Women appear to be nearly twice as susceptible to STDs as men. Only with the arrival of AIDS did educational efforts such as posters, radio, and television public service announcements begin to address both sexes. However, AIDS has appropriated virtually all the publicity, and, I might add, much of the funding, for study and prevention. Little or no public education effort is being directed against the many other devastating and all too silent sexually transmitted diseases that, as you will see, are disproportionately hazardous to women. What was called a "medical secret" at the opening of this century has become a silent plague at the century's close.

WHAT ARE STDs?

What used to be called venereal diseases are now known as *sexually transmitted diseases,* an umbrella term for a group of diseases of different cause and severity which are transmitted sexually. These diseases include gonorrhea, syphilis, chlamydia, herpes simplex, hepatitis B, HPV, AIDS, and perhaps forty more diseases that are passed from one person to another through sexual intercourse or other intimate human-to-human exchanges, such as sharing dirty needles as part of the ritual of drug abuse.

For the most part, intimate means intimate—not kissing or using the same toilet seat. Sexual transmission of viruses or bacteria usually comes through exchange of fluids, including blood, vaginal secretions, and semen through vaginal or anal intercourse. Some viruses appear in saliva, and infection can occur through oral sex. Broken or inflamed skin or erosions in the genital tract facilitate transmission of the infecting organism.

STDs have been at epidemic proportions in our nation for almost a decade or longer, and yet few outside the medical community seem to know or acknowledge this, perhaps because their attention has been consumed by AIDS. Most Americans are startled when they find out how common these diseases have become. This year the nation will suffer an estimated 3 to 5 million cases of chlamydia; more than 1 million new cases of gonorrhea; 500,000 new cases of herpes simplex; 500,000 to 1 million new cases of HPV infection; 200,000 to 300,000 cases of hepatitis B; about 100,000 new cases of AIDS and about the same for syphilis. The picture for women is gruesome: 6 million cases of STDs, and half of those women are teenagers.

The figures, taken from public health reports, represent only a fraction of the true incidence of STDs infecting this nation's women. Physicians are not always conscientious about reporting cases of the diseases, perhaps thinking that it may reflect on their practice or patients, or perhaps because reporting them only adds to the paperwork that is threatening to engulf their practices. Some physicians are concerned about the privacy of their patients, which is never really assured when information gets into the hands of a government agency.

An even more worrisome reason for the underestimation of the figures is that STDs all too often go undetected, especially in women. These diseases are often "clinically silent," which means that the women do not yet have symptoms. When minor symptoms arise, STDs are the last thing that occurs to most women. In a society that openly discusses and depicts sex to the point of obsession, sexually transmitted diseases, aside from AIDS, are seldom mentioned, as either threat or reality.

THE ANATOMY OF A WOMAN'S SPECIAL PROBLEM

BIOLOGICAL VULNERABILITY

STDs are distinctive as women's diseases, and women face unique susceptibility in transmission. Women are infected far more readily than men. Men are exposed to the organisms that cause the disease, but women are injected with them. In addition, whereas men's genitalia are exposed to the elements—such as cold temperatures and soap and water—creating an unwelcome environment for bacteria and viruses to take hold, the vagina provides a warm and protected environment that allows them to grow and flourish. The vagina also provides an inlet to the pelvic cavity; such an inlet does not exist for a man. Perhaps because the infection is internal, the early symptoms in a woman are often less severe or apparent than they are in men. Because many women are asymptomatic, they are less likely to seek early diagnosis and treatment.

HEALTH CONSEQUENCES

There may be no better example of gender bias in the annals of medicine than the neglect of STDs in women and the ignorance surrounding the consequences of STDs to their health. For most of this century, venereal disease clinics were for men only and VDs were the diseases loose women gave to men. STDs in men had fairly minimal long-term consequences if treated, and could be quietly and definitively handled as a medical secret.

Nothing could be further from the truth when it comes to women, who face far more severe consequences for virtually every form of infection. As discussed in greater detail below, these may include infertility, ectopic pregnancy, spontaneous abortion, destruction of parts of the reproductive organs, genital cancer, and death. The child of a mother with an STD can face developmental deficits (particularly of the nervous system), blindness, or laryngeal warts, and may die. The burden such diseases place on a woman is made heavier when she realizes that only she can transmit an STD to her newborn children.

SOCIAL CHANGE

Today's epidemic of STDs has roots in the 1960s, the decade in which postwar baby boomers came of age and then passed on their newfound freedoms to their children. A group known for their turmoil within and without, they were a generation of revolution. As with all revolutions, no one anticipated its coming, and no one could foresee its consequences.

Coincidentally, birth control pills came into widespread use and with them the abandonment of condoms, diaphragms, and other barrier contraceptives, which offered a degree of protection against disease. The Pill and, a few years later, greater access to abortion facilitated the sexual revolution. Women became just as "free" as men. Free to ex-plore and experiment, many did both with a passion, as if trying to cast away centuries of repression within a decade; indeed, for some, sexual liberation became the symbol of women's liberation. These so-cial changes may have seemed to transcend health, but they became a major determinant of women's health. (Ironically, despite seeming sexual equality, a woman still faces a greater stigma when she is in-fected with an STD than a man does, often making her reluctant to ad-mit she has the disease and to seek treatment early.)

MEDICAL COMPLACENCY

As women were being lured into believing that they could be just the same as men, the medical profession of the era was being lured into complacency by its successes in repressing "venereal disease." Peni-cillin and other then new antimicrobial agents had cut rates of syphilis and gonorrhea, and the consequences of infections such as chlamydia and HPV were not yet known. No tests had been found that would de-tect them with any degree of reliability. Even in the 1980s, a medical school student was lucky to get four hours of lectures on STDs during a four-year medical education, since the STD problem was thought to be on its way to extinction. Many of us back in training in the early 1970s thought that the medical specialty called infectious diseases was also on its way to extinction.

Then, suddenly, AIDS burst onto the scene in the early 1980s. STDs were reborn in a more lethal and dramatic form, and the nation woke to the danger and threat they posed. But AIDS, with its mystery, wasting deterioration, and inevitably fatal outcome, drew most of the nation's attention to itself, leaving other sexually transmitted diseases to con-tinue to spread in silent obscurity. Nonetheless, all STDs are part and parcel of the same kind of devastating disease, carrying similar patterns of risk and spread. Before delving into the specific forms of infection, I will discuss the risk factors that apply generally, to all of them.

RISK FACTORS FOR STDs

When epidemiologists label age, economic status, drug use, race, and sexual activity as risk factors for STDs, they are speaking about the opportunity for infection, not susceptibility. They are saying that women with certain characteristics are more likely to be exposed to disease, not that they are more vulnerable. Any woman involved in a sexual relationship with a nonreliable partner is at risk.

PATTERNS OF SEXUAL BEHAVIOR

Many of the new sexual standards created during the 1960s remain, and may have become permanent aspects of our culture. A woman need not be promiscuous by today's standards to acquire a disease that could destroy her life. A woman alone does not control her risk or even know her risk, which lies within the life and body of her sexual partner. In a momentary encounter, she and her future baby, if she should get pregnant, are being threatened by all the serious and possibly lethal diseases that her sexual partner has been acquiring for years.

The risk to a woman who has sex with a man infected with one or more STDs depends on the specific organisms he carries (some, as we will see later, are more infectious than others) and on her frequency of unprotected sexual intercourse with him. A pretty good estimate is that a woman faces at least a one-in-three chance of getting an STD from an infected partner with each sexual encounter. Obviously, the risk of transmission is increased as the number of different partners increases.

A current psychosocial phenomenon that lulls many women and especially young girls into believing they are safe from disease is *serial monogamy*. Sometimes women think of themselves not as having multiple sex partners but, rather, as sleeping with only one man or boy, who will be with them forever. Two months later, they are sleeping with another man or boy, who will also be with them forever. All too often what remains forever is a disease.

Patterns of sexual behavior are complex, sometimes unpredictable, and very much a matter of culture, family views, religion, and peer pressure. Sexual behavior is driven by a healthy compulsion of the species to continue, and satisfies deep personal needs for intimacy, companionship, and pleasure. My concern, however, is that women may be uniquely vulnerable by virtue of their sexual behavior without knowing how or why. As a physician and a professional, I am not being judgmental, but trying to offer sane advice where ignorance frequently cancels out competing pressures to say "No" or "Let's wait" or "What are my risks?" Although I am respectful of differences surrounding sexual behavior, there are no differences among women when it comes to their health and their vulnerability to the ravages of STDs. As I often say, we are all the same in a hospital gown. Ultimately each woman will decide for herself about her own pattern of sexual behavior, but such a decision should be well informed and must factor in her own self-esteem, her deeply held values, and her hopes and dreams for a future healthy life.

YOUTH

When epidemiologists cite age as a risk factor for STDs, they really mean that youth is the risk. Being young in America very often connotes sexual activity, a lack of sophistication, and a lack of maturity, all of which predispose individuals to contracting STDs. They infect those who have multiple sex partners; those whose naïveté, ignorance, and lack of judgment preclude the recognition of risks or efforts to avoid them; those who think they are immortal.

Adolescent girls face a particular biological risk as well. During the early stages of puberty, the inner-surface lining of the uterus—called the *columnar epithelium*—extends into the vagina and lacks the protective coat of mucus the canal will acquire when the epithelium retracts into the uterus as the girl matures. The columnar epithelium is particularly susceptible to infection by gonorrhea and chlamydia. One of the most insidious aspects of these infections is that in their early stage they remain internal—and therefore invisible—infections that quietly fester. This assures the silent spread in the next sexual encounter.

ENVIRONMENT

Although the prevalence of sexually transmitted diseases in women cuts across all groups, and bacteria and viruses recognize no class distinctions, entrenched poverty contributes to the spread of diseases that are deeply rooted in many poor inner-city populations. Most human diseases pursue ignorance, poverty, and squalor wherever they can find them. When a social environment does not value human life, does not promote personal responsibility, self-esteem, discipline, human dignity, and decent education, and offers a limited sense of opportunity or hope for the future, then we see the breakdown of the family, a high illegitimate birthrate, sexual promiscuity, and rampant sexually transmitted diseases. Promoting a healthy environment requires more than medicine; it means promoting a healthy society.

DRUGS

Drugs (including alcohol) and sexual disease are eternal companions and have been since the dawn of civilization. Bacchus is never depicted drinking wine and reading a book. The epidemic of illicit drug use and the epidemic of STDs have expanded together. Drugs impair judgment and amplify sexual desire; the use of them is sometime a collective indulgence that draws participating individuals together in a shared experience. The combination of all these factors virtually assures sexual relationships and the transmission of disease.

The use of crack cocaine has added a new facet to the STD epidemic. Sex and crack cocaine are practically synonymous in many communities. The drug is extremely addictive, and provides a more short-lived high than other drugs. Addicts never get enough, and never have enough money to get the drugs they desire. Crack's highly addictive nature practically demands that users exchange sex for drugs when they lack the funds to buy them, and it also appears to enhance sex drive. The combination is deadly. In young crack-using women, the rate of gonorrhea is thought to be twenty-five to fifty times that of their non-crack-using peers.

Blood-borne diseases such as AIDS and hepatitis are also transmitted when needles are shared. Heroin addiction, AIDS, and hepatitis coexist just as crack and gonorrhea do. This nation will probably never rid itself of sexually transmitted disease if it does not also rid itself of the drug epidemic.

COEXISTING SEXUALLY TRANSMITTED DISEASE

STDs travel together. It is common for multiple sexually transmitted diseases to be found in the same individual. The presence of one—gonorrhea, for example—raises the suspicion of the presence of chlamydia, herpes, HPV, and other even more obscure organisms. In up to 50 percent of cases, the tests for concomitant diseases will be positive. Many STDs create open sores on the external genitalia and within the vaginal tract, which are open doors for other infections, including the AIDS virus.

IGNORANCE AND SENSE OF NOT-ME

Cultural biases serve to spread the disease. Heterosexuals think only homosexuals suffer the consequences of STDs. The clean and sober think only drug users suffer STDs. The wealthy feel that such disease is a problem concentrated among the poor. Many in the majority think it is a problem that afflicts minorities. The educated feel that these diseases strike only the uneducated. People who live in towns think the epidemic is concentrated in the city. Those in rural communities think it lies within towns. It is always someone else's town, someone else's school, someone else's daughter, someone else. "It won't happen to me" may be the five most dangerous words a woman can utter.

UNDERSTANDING THE DIFFERENT STDs

Although in many instances the symptoms of STDs are subtle, it is important that women be alert and prepared to recognize their appearance. *The only way to confirm an STD is to visit a physician or clinic and be tested for the specific infection.* Self-diagnosis and self-treatment invariably fail and frequently carry more serious consequences. The initial symptoms of many STDS are all too often transient; in their natural course the symptoms come and go. A woman may be deluded into thinking the disease has been cleared up when it is actually progressing. This delays diagnosis, delays treatment, spreads the disease, and enhances the severity of the disease once it reappears full-blown. Also, reappearance of the disease is assured if the infected partner goes undetected. If a woman is infected, her sexual partners should be treated as well.

GONORRHEA

Gonorrhea has been around for thousands of years. Dr. Rudolph Kampmeier, a specialist in infectious diseases, noted that among the ancient Greeks gonorrhea was seen as the "woman's disease" that led to "running of the penis." Throughout history, gonorrhea became the marker for STDs, including syphilis, because of its visible effect on the male urethra, causing a continuous discharge or leakage. Although the bacterial nature of the infection was not known until this century, the disease early on was associated with brothels and whores, not considered a problem for "nice" women.

Similarly, changes in the incidence of gonorrhea (now known to be an infection caused by the bacterium *Neisseria gonorrhoeae*) reflect the rise and fall of other STDs in America as well. Its incidence rose about 13 percent a year through the mid-1970s (thought to be partly due to soldiers' bringing it home from Vietnam), when between 900,000 and 1 million cases were being reported annually. The number of cases stabilized during the 1980s, showed a 22 percent drop between 1986 and 1989, and is now again on the rise. Just as a portion of the drop may be attributed to safe sex practices adopted because of the fear of AIDS, perhaps a portion of the subsequent increase can be attributed to complacency about AIDS, which has led to an abandonment of safe sex practices. Public health officials surmise that in 1995 an estimated 1 million or more Americans will contract gonorrhea.

SIGNS AND SYMPTOMS

Only about half of the women with this infection have any initial symptoms of infection. When these do occur, they include heavy vaginal discharge, abnormal vaginal bleeding between periods or excessively heavy menstrual flow, and slightly painful and frequent urination. In up to one-half of women with genital infection, the anorectal area becomes involved from local contamination (even in the absence of anal intercourse), causing rectal discomfort, itching, a yellow or slightly bloody rectal discharge, and in severe cases sharp and throbbing rectal pain. (By contrast, anorectal infection in a man almost always means he has acquired his infection by anal intercourse with an infected partner.) In some women, the disease may produce a skin rash and fleeting stabs of arthritis-like pain in the joints of the arms and knees. Many of the symptoms of gonorrhea can also be produced by chlamydia, which coexists with gonorrhea in up to half the cases seen today.

CONSEQUENCES

The bacteria grow in the cervix, urethra, anal canal, and pharynx. If undetected, the infection can spread from the cervix to the lining of the uterus and into the fallopian tubes. Here it causes acute endometritis (infection of the lining of the uterus) and salpingitis (inflammation of the fallopian tubes), the latter of which can cause abscess formation and in the long term damage the tubes irreparably. Acute tubal infection brings abdominal pain and abnormal menstrual bleeding. If the infection progresses unchecked, it spreads into the pelvic cavity, where it leads to a severe generalized illness called *pelvic inflammatory disease* or *PID* (see page 164).

Sometimes gonococcal infection can disseminate into the bloodstream and lead to such dire consequences as infection of the lining of the brain, meningitis, or of a heart valve, endocarditis. Gonococcal infection in a pregnancy is dangerous to both mother and child and is associated with retarded growth of the fetus, premature rupture of the membranes (i.e., her "water" breaks early), and premature birth. When gonorrhea is transmitted to a newborn, it can cause a type of conjunctivitis that may lead to blindness. (Administering silver nitrate drops, topical antibiotics, or other antibacterial agents to the eyes of newborns prevents this infection and is a legal requirement in the United States and many other countries.)

DIAGNOSIS AND TREATMENT

The bacteria are cultured directly from the cervix or another visibly infected site, such as the urethra or the rectum. A swab is taken of the discharge from the infected area, and the material is placed in special culture medium to grow, a process that takes more than a day. At the same time, the discharge can be examined under the microscope with special stains, and the bacteria, with their characteristic shape and staining properties, may be spotted, enabling immediate treatment. Growing the organism in a culture helps the physician identify which antibiotics are most effective in curing the infection. Some organisms become resistant to many antibiotics; the number of drug-resistant cases of gonorrhea rose from fewer than ten thousand a year in 1985 to nearly sixty thousand a year in 1990. (Drug resistance means newer and more powerful antibiotics must be used to cure the infection, not that it is incurable.)

Gonorrhea can be eliminated by one or more of several antibiotics, many in the penicillin, tetracycline, or erythromycin family. One of the most common regimens that has proven effective is a combination of ceftriaxone and doxycycline. (Sexual partners need to be treated also.) If treated early, gonorrhea can be cured without any residual problems. What cannot be cured, however, is the damage and scarring that smoldering infection causes in the reproductive tract.

SYPHILIS

Once called the "great pox" or the "French disease," syphilis has been a recognized medical scourge for hundreds if not thousands of years. It was epidemic in Europe in the fifteenth century. In the spirit of always pointing to some other group, the voyages of Columbus are sometimes blamed for bringing this disease into Europe from the West Indies in the late 1400s.

Wars were often the vehicle for spreading venereal disease—in the early years because of rape and pillage, and later because of increased prostitution servicing soldiers away from home. But it was the last world war that led to its control. With the birth of penicillin during World War II, and the subsequent routine screening and treating of the adult population at the time of military recruiting, marriage, child-birth, and even hospital admission, syphilis was headed for the history books. In 1943 there were almost 600,000 cases reported; by 1953 the figure had plummeted to about 6,000 cases. But that has now changed. Syphilis has had a comeback. In this decade, so far, more than 100,000 cases of early syphilis are being reported annually, the highest since the end of World War II. The rate of infection jumped 59 percent between 1985 and 1990 alone.

The bacterium causing syphilis, *Treponema pallidum* (a corkscrew-shaped bacterium called a *spirochete*), is one of the more insidious members of the hidden army of STDs in North America. A single bacterium, a small dot under a microscope, is sufficient to cause infection in a woman, and experiments have shown that fewer than 100 bacteria—a minuscule quantity—will cause the disease in about half of those exposed.

SIGNS AND SYMPTOMS

In the early phases of syphilis, the signs of infection are rather modest and often missed. The first appearance after infection, called primary syphilis, is usually a single painless *papule* or raised area of the skin that ulcerates and forms a chancre. The papule or chancre appears at or near the site of the initial infection, usually the cervix or labia, and lasts for a few weeks. The lymph glands of the groin may become tender and swollen. Meanwhile, the bacterium is lurking and quietly spreading throughout the body; the next phase, called secondary syphilis, will occur within weeks or months.

Though secondary syphilis is more obvious, it can still be easily dismissed as some nonspecific illness. The woman may have a pale red or pink rash around the waist, chest, arms, and legs, and also on a site unusual for any rash, the palms of the hands and soles of the feet. Other symptoms appearing for the first time include fever, weight loss, fatigue, loss of appetite, headache, depression, vomiting, or constipation.

CONSEQUENCES

If the disease remains unrecognized and untreated, it goes underground, moving into a long latent period. In some patients the infection will spontaneously resolve, but in others, syphilis in its third stage will emerge ten to thirty years later, with dire consequences: central nervous system degeneration and cardiovascular disease affecting the aortic heart valve and the central artery, the aorta.

Syphilis is dangerous to pregnant women and can infect a fetus at any stage of pregnancy. Some 40 percent of infected pregnant women will lose their children—if not to a spontaneous abortion, then to a stillbirth. Other consequences include premature delivery, neonatal death, and congenital syphilis, a condition in which there are lifelong malformations of the teeth and skeleton or a brain infection that leaves the child with a seizure disorder or impaired brain development.

DIAGNOSIS AND TREATMENT

The diagnosis is made by clinical signs and a blood test for antibodies to the infecting bacterium. If the disease is in its early form, where there is a rash or a chancre sore, the spirochete can often be detected in scrapings from the involved skin sites. Once the diagnosis is made, the treatment is straightforward: antibiotics in the penicillin or tetracycline family. Early detection allows quick resolution of the first stage of the disease and the prevention of its transmission to sexual partners and unborn children. Testing all pregnant women for syphilis is part of standard prenatal care. Once the disease goes into its advanced, third stage, causing heart or brain damage, treatment of infection is minimally effective: the damage has been done.

CHLAMYDIA

Chlamydia, an unusual bacteria unable to survive on its own outside a living host cell, will affect from three to five million Americans this year. It is believed to be the most common *bacteria* being transmitted sexually in the United States today. This estimate is broad, because in many states chlamydia need not be reported to state health officials, because laboratory testing is not uniform, and because many with the infection have no symptoms of illness. The highest rates of infection are in people under the age of twenty-five. Although the disease may be concentrated in impoverished areas, studies at university clinics have found that one in ten women patients was infected with chlamydia.

SIGNS AND SYMPTOMS

The majority (75 percent or more) of women infected with the organism *Chlamydia trachomatis* will remain asymptomatic until the disease is well established. Even then symptoms may not appear, or may be so vague as to elude diagnosis. The infection begins in the cervix and, if unchecked, moves through the lining of the uterus and the fallopian tubes, and into the peritoneum, the lining of the abdomen. As it progresses, it can cause a number of problems, including cervicitis (inflammation of the cervix), endometritis, salpingitis, peritonitis (inflammation of the lining cells of the abdomen and pelvis), and urethritis (inflammation of the urethra, the outlet of the bladder.) Patients may also experience a fleeting arthritis similar to what may occur with gonorrhea.

A thick cervical discharge containing pus is evidence of cervicitis. Sometimes the infection causes abnormal cells on the Pap smear, incorrectly suggesting a precancerous change in the cervix. Urethritis is indicated by painful and frequent urination. Endometritis causes abnormal vaginal bleeding and abdominal pain; salpingitis, abdominal and pelvic pain. Nausea and vomiting, abdominal tenderness, or generalized abdominal pain may indicate either endometritis or peritonitis. Low-grade but persistent fevers may occur with any of these inflammatory conditions.

CONSEQUENCES

This insidious infection may lead to ectopic or tubal pregnancy from scarred tubes, spontaneous abortion, chronic pelvic pain, or pain on sexual intercourse. It has been estimated that chlamydia is a causative or contributing factor in as many as 75 percent of all cases of infertility caused by scarred or blocked tubes. The longer chlamydia goes undetected, the more likely that scarring and pelvic disease will occur. It can be harsh on pregnancies too, leading to stillbirths, or to pneumonia and blindness (from conjunctivitis) in a newborn.

DIAGNOSIS AND TREATMENT

Until recently, we knew very little about this disease, because we had no way to diagnose it in the laboratory. It is difficult to grow in the laboratory, since it will only survive inside cells. (Most bacteria grow as independent clusters on the surface of a culture medium.) Detecting antibodies in the blood provides limited help, in that it means an infection has occurred at some time but does not pinpoint active infection, and can yield false positive or negative results. Though we now know how to culture this organism in the laboratory, in special cell lines maintained in culture, it is expensive and takes time. A newly developed test using a direct antibody stain of secretions is rapid and reasonably sensitive. Even newer methods are in development, using the latest techniques of molecular biology including a highly powerful method called *gene amplification* (the technical term is *polymerase chain reaction*), which will make a diagnosis faster and surer.

Chlamydia is one of those diseases for which treatment is a lot easier than diagnosis. If it is found early, it can be cured with a standard antibiotic regimen of doxycycline, ofloxacin, erythromycin, sulfa, or related compounds.

HERPES SIMPLEX

Genital herpes, typified by recurrent ulcers in the genital area, will infect between 200,000 and 500,000 Americans this year. An estimated thirty million Americans carry this virus—about 10 percent of our population, and about one in every five men and women between the ages of fifteen and forty. Genital herpes simplex, usually caused by the type 2 strain of the virus, is to be distinguished from the herpes that occurs around the mouth and nose as a cold sore, usually caused by the type 1 virus. (These distinctions are not perfect: 10 percent of genital herpes is caused by type 1, and 10 percent of oral herpes is type 2.) First exposure to herpes type 1 typically comes in childhood, whereas exposure to type 2 comes later on, with sexual activity.

Genital herpes is transmitted mostly by ignorance, often ignorance that an individual is even infected. The disease is highly contagious when there are herpetic sores. Many who infect their partners have the sores but don't recognize them as herpes. Furthermore, a few days before the blisters appear the virus is present in the region and may be transmitted through contact with infected surface cells or secretions before any signs or symptoms of the disease are present. When recurrent disease brings only a few small ulcers and few if any symptoms, or if the herpes ulcers are not readily visible to the eye (as, for example, when on the cervix), disease may be transmitted unwittingly. Moreover, sexual transmission has been shown to exist even when there are no visible ulcers. Invariably, however, it takes intimate contact to contract the infection, since the virus itself is not very hardy, dying at room temperature or outside the body.

SIGNS AND SYMPTOMS

Herpes is the most common cause of genital ulcers in women. It usually shows itself within a week after the initial infection, and that first infection is the most severe and potentially dangerous. With primary herpes, painful vesicles or blisters appear that contain fluid with active virus. The blisters crust over and then become raw, round, oozing yellow craters that are very painful. These sores may involve the external vulva area, the vagina, or the cervix and are associated with discomfort and a burning sensation and irritation and swelling of the surrounding tissue. In the majority of women the first illness after infection, i.e., the primary infection, is the worst, and often leads to fever, headache, generalized weakness, intermittent sharp shooting pain or tingling sensations (neuralgias) in the genital area, and swollen lymph nodes in the groin. The entire illness lasts two to three weeks, as the sores gradually heal over.

With that first or primary episode of herpes, however, the disease is only beginning. The virus moves from the skin cells along the surrounding sensory nerves to the nerve roots coming out at the bottom of the spine (called the *sacral root ganglia*). There the herpes virus takes up permanent residence and becomes what we call a *latent* infection. In some women the symptoms may never reappear, but these are the luckier few. For 80 to 90 percent of those infected, there will be recurrence on the site of the original sores. The herpes ulcers reappear for no apparent reason, or may be initiated by fever, menstruation, or physical and emotional stress. Over time the recurrences will become less severe and less frequent in number.

CONSEQUENCES

Herpes infections have been implicated in cervical cancer. Genital herpes has also been linked to cancer of the vulva, an aggressive tumor that can be treated only with extensive and disfiguring surgery. Most often, however, herpes is a source of pain and disfigurement, and a reminder of some questionable past sexual encounters.

Herpes may be mostly an irritation and an embarrassment to adult women, but it is devastating to their newborn. From four hundred to a thousand cases of neonatal herpes simplex are reported annually. Sixty percent of these babies will die; among the survivors, roughly 90 percent are left with serious health problems, including skin and mouth ulcers, eye infections, and encephalitis (infection of the brain) and may be left with major developmental disorders.

DIAGNOSIS AND TREATMENT

The diagnosis is made mostly by the appearance of the herpes sores. Viral cultures taken from an active lesion confirm the diagnosis; microscopic examination of tissue scraped from the sore will show fairly distinctive cells. It is difficult, however, to know if someone has genital herpes when the disease is in its latent phase, with no visible sores.

The current recommended therapy for herpes is acyclovir taken three to five times a day for five days to a week, and starting as soon as the blisters seem to be erupting. Acyclovir will decrease symptoms, the period of infectivity, and the healing time by about twenty-four hours, but it will not eliminate the virus from the body. Long-term acyclovir in lower doses as a preventive measure can reduce the frequency of recurrence of herpes in those who are faced with repetitive bouts of the ulcers. As yet, there is no cure for the disease.

Pregnant women with herpes need special attention. If the disease is latent, most babies can be delivered safely. But if herpes ulcers are present in the genital region, cesarean delivery is the only way to decrease the risk of infant exposure; the baby must not pass through the birth canal if it is riddled with open sores bearing virus. A pregnant woman infected with herpes should tell her obstetrician, and together they should monitor its status very carefully. A pregnant woman never infected by this virus should avoid sexual contact with a partner who has herpes, since a primary infection near the time of delivery has the greatest chance of being transmitted to a newborn.

These precautions to protect the unborn have been publicized extensively, but somehow this neonatal disease goes on. Tragically, neonates are infected in at least one in every twenty-six thousand live births in the United States each year. Some 70 to 80 percent of these babies are born to mothers who have no memory or history of infection but have had sex partners with a history of herpes. This silent plague thus not only conspires to rob women of their health and sometimes their motherhood, but also maims or kills thousands of their babies—a disastrous price for any woman (or man) to pay for risky sexual behavior.

HUMAN PAPILLOMA VIRUS

HPV infects the DNA of the skin and lining cells (epithelium) of the external genitalia, the urethra, the perianal area, the vagina, and the cervix. Transmitted during sexual intercourse, the virus gains access through small erosions in the tissues of the lower genital tract that may occur as a result of the sexual contact. There are up to forty known strains; some cause genital warts, called *condylomata acuminata*. Some half-million new cases of genital infection caused by HPV are thought to occur annually. Furthermore, it is estimated that about twelve million people harbor this virus in the United States without even knowing it. Public health officials surmise that, with newer screening and testing technologies that are more sensitive to the presence of the virus, we will discover the number of cases to be nearer thirty million.

This disease is so widespread because it is so readily transmitted. Some experts say the risk of transmission is more than 70 percent—that is, if you have sexual intercourse with someone carrying the virus, you have a very good chance of becoming infected.

SIGNS AND SYMPTOMS

Perhaps two months after the initial infection, warts often start to appear. (The latency period, from the time of infection to the first sign of the disease, may be as long as six months, however.) The warts are usually small and occur in little clusters which can be flesh-colored, pink, or pigmented like light moles. As the warts shed their superficial layer of infected cells, they spread the virus at the same time, either to other sites within the genital area or to a partner during sexual intercourse. Warts spontaneously disappear in response to the body's immune system, but may recur later.

Not all forms of HPV infection cause warts. In fact, only about one-third of women with HPV show visible signs of warts. Nonetheless, the virus is there in the lining cells, spreading disease for a period of six to nine months, until the body's immune system suppresses it.

CONSEQUENCES

Certain strains of HPV infection cause or promote cancer. Two strains in particular (HPV16 and HPV18) and possibly a few others (HPV31, 33, and 35) have been closely linked to cervical carcinoma. HPV has also been linked to cancers of the vagina, vulva, and anus (and in men, rarely, to cancer of the penis). These HPV-related cancers are seen most often in younger people and are very aggressive. Some studies have suggested that herpes infection plus HPV increases the chance of getting a genital cancer.

As with most STDs, actively infected pregnant women can transmit the infection to their offspring. HPV can infect the respiratory system. Respiratory warts can cause breathing problems for infants as well as interfere with their vocal cord motion, and sometimes the warts must be removed surgically.

DIAGNOSIS AND TREATMENT

If warts are present, they can be removed by freezing the tissue or with mild acid treatments, but either treatment is merely cosmetic: the virus still lurks within many other cells in latent form and can come back at any time.

A diagnosis of HPV calls for close, continual monitoring and routine Pap smears to detect cancer early if it appears. There are newer tests for screening for the virus. Cells on a Pap smear can be tested by a technique called DNA hybridization which identifies viral DNA and the specific strain of HPV. Called the Virapap, this procedure is gradually moving into clinical practice, and holds the promise of being able to identify women with the more virulent and cancer-linked infections for closer monitoring. Unfortunately, as with most viral infections, there is no cure.

Doctors can control the acute flare-ups. A variety of cell-toxic agents similar to cancer-treating drugs are used locally to destroy viral warts. Podophyllin, a naturally occurring resin from a plant, is applied directly to the warts and destroys them, but can cause severe local inflammatory reactions. The anticancer agent 5-Fluorouracil, used topically in cream form, controls the warts in about 80 percent of instances. Interferons, immune system proteins that have antiviral properties (and are also used in cancer treatment), are approved for use in the therapy of advanced warts, in combination with local removal of the warts.

If a pregnant woman has active genital warts, cautery is generally recommended, since these cell-toxic agents can harm the fetus. Only if the warts are very large is cesarean section indicated.

HEPATITIS B

We used to think that the hepatitis B virus, which causes an acute liver infection (formally called *serum hepatitis*), was primarily transmitted by a contaminated blood transfusion or through needle sticks with contaminated blood. We now know better. Up to half of all new cases of hepatitis B are transmitted through sexual encounters. Hepatitis B might even be called the mystery STD, since, even though transmission through sexual intercourse has been well established, the public does not generally recognize that in many instances it is a "venereal disease."

In infected individuals the virus is present in saliva, semen, and vaginal secretions as well as blood. Hepatitis is about a hundred times more contagious than the human immunodeficiency virus (HIV), the virus that causes AIDS, and can readily be transmitted through open sores or any site of broken skin or erosions in the mucosal lining of the mouth or the genital tract. (In the hospital setting it is not uncommon for health care workers to contract hepatitis from accidental needle sticks or contact with blood or body fluids of infected patients. In contrast, HIV is very rarely contracted in this manner.)

More than one million people in the United States are infected with hepatitis B, and some 300,000 are infected annually. Many carrying the virus are unaware they have the infection and may innocently transmit it to a sexual partner. During the past ten years, the incidence of infection has increased by almost 80 percent in the highest risk group: young, sexually active heterosexual men and women. Indeed, about three-quarters of all hepatitis B occurs in people between the ages of fifteen and thirty-nine. At the same time, we have seen a decrease in transfusion-acquired transmission of the virus, since blood products are routinely screened for hepatitis by blood banks.

What distinguishes the hepatitis virus from many of the other sexually transmitted pathogens is that it is especially hardy, able to survive for several days on surfaces such as sinks and toilets. Some have suggested that the sharing of toothbrushes, razors, or other personal articles might spread the virus, but the risk from these and other objects is simply not known.

SIGNS AND SYMPTOMS

Half of those infected with this virus will be asymptomatic, that is, show no signs of illness with their acute liver infection going unnoticed, and the other half will develop symptoms within 45 to 160 days following infection. The symptoms include a mild, flulike illness, nausea, vomiting, malaise, appetite loss, abdominal pain, skin rashes, and jaundice (yellowish skin and yellowed whites of the eyes). Some 20 percent of those with symptomatic hepatitis will become very ill, with complications that require hospitalization.

CONSEQUENCES

In a small number of those infected (less than 1 percent) hepatitis B leads to its worst consequence, a fulminant hepatitis: the liver literally collapses because of the death and dissolution of masses of liver cells. With the loss of the many proteins normally manufactured by the liver, numerous processes throughout the body become deranged. For example, the blood ceases to form effective clots, causing bleeding into the skin and the gut. Brain toxicity develops, and some patients lapse into hepatic coma. Failure of the kidneys often follows, and then general cardiovascular collapse. Most people with fulminant hepatitis die; a lucky few survive to good recovery.

Some 10 percent of patients with acute hepatitis go on to develop chronic hepatitis after the acute episode resolves. Many of these chronic carriers will develop cirrhosis of the liver, and, not infrequently, liver cancer. Hepatitis kills some five thousand people every year directly, while another eight hundred die of hepatitis-associated liver cancer.

DIAGNOSIS AND TREATMENT

We now have relatively simple tests for present or past infection with the hepatitis B virus. Detecting surface molecules that characterize the virus or antibodies to the virus, these tests have made the screening of blood for use in transfusion and the testing of patients for hepatitis B a ready procedure. Such technology protects the human blood supply from a major threat, as the HIV screen keeps transfused blood from transmitting AIDS.

As with AIDS and virtually all viral illnesses, there is no treatment to rid the body of hepatitis B. Most treatments—for example, the administration of interferon—are geared toward controlling the proliferation of the virus into other cells.

The good news about this infection is that we now have a safe and reliable hepatitis B vaccine, administered in three doses over a period of six months. Medical personnel who are exposed to blood or blood products are now routinely immunized, and vaccination is advised for any individuals at risk for exposure to the virus, including drug users, household members of those who have or have had hepatitis, and individuals who have exposure to multiple sexual partners. For those with recent exposure to hepatitis B, a medicine called *hepatitis B immune globulin* (HBIG) is administered to help the body's own immune system fight off the virus and lessen the liver infection if it occurs. The immune globulin is given at birth to babies of infected mothers. Pregnant women can receive either the hepatitis B vaccine or HBIG if need be.

HUMAN IMMUNODEFICIENCY VIRUS

In 1980 no one had ever heard of acquired immunodeficiency syndrome, or AIDS. Thirteen years later, AIDS had taken the lives of millions of people worldwide. AIDS is caused by the human immunodeficiency virus 1 (HIV-1), an RNA virus. Once the RNA virus infects a cell, it uses special enzymes within the cell to fashion another molecule, which then becomes part of the cell's master control molecules, the DNA. In this manner the virus seizes control of the cell. HIV infects many cells in the human body but particularly the white blood cells circulating in the bloodstream (lymphocytes), which are critical to the immune system's ability to fight off infection. HIV also infects cells in the lining of the gut and certain cells in the brain.

AIDS has now claimed more than 200,000 lives in the United States alone, and will continue well beyond the end of the century if a cure is not found. Of the 339,250 cases of AIDS reported by the end of 1993, some 40,700 were in women. Early in the epidemic, AIDS was seen as a disease mostly of male homosexuals, but this is no longer the case. Heterosexually acquired AIDS now constitutes about 20 percent of all reported cases, and the incidence is growing.

The Centers for Disease Control and Prevention (CDC) notes that in adolescents the rate of heterosexual HIV transmission surpassed homosexual transmission in 1990. In the same year, 51 percent of all women contracting AIDS acquired the disease through heterosexual contact, usually with a man who is a drug user; and the rest were infected mostly through using dirty needles. By 1993, more than half of the heterosexually transmitted cases of AIDS were in women. (In contrast, most men still get the disease from homosexual encounters or from injecting drugs, and only 4 percent from heterosexual contact.) It is a biological fact that a woman is more apt to catch HIV from a man than is a man to get HIV from an infected woman. Furthermore, a woman is more likely to contract HIV if she has a preexisting genital infection such as herpes, whose open ulcers provide a gateway for the virus.

AIDS is still mostly a young person's disease, with two-thirds of the women infected being under thirty. Since the latency period of the disease is in the range of ten years, the majority of both young men and women with the disease must have acquired the initial infection when they were in their teens and early twenties. By now an estimated two million Americans—or one in every 125—carry the virus. Since most with the virus are young men, one can figure that at least one in every fifty young men is an HIV carrier. What this means for women is quite simple: beware.

SIGNS AND SYMPTOMS

The initial symptoms of infection by the HIV virus appear from six weeks to six months following transmission. These include a flulike illness, night sweats, fevers, and swollen lymph nodes, and are often dismissed by the infected woman as just a bad cold or something like mononucleosis. After the acute symptoms subside, the virus lies dormant within the body for years before showing symptoms again. Throughout this silent time, however, the virus can be transmitted, for it is present in blood, semen, and other body secretions.

Those carrying the virus but not yet sick with AIDS are the most dangerous, often unaware of their infection or in denial about it, and readily able to keep it a secret from others if they choose.

CONSEQUENCES

This notorious virus works indirectly. HIV destroys the immune system, leaving its victim open to a host of "opportunistic" infections that will eventually claim her life. These include fungal infections throughout the body, pneumonias, eye and brain infections, cancers (including lymphoma and cancers of the cervix), pelvic inflammatory disease, thrush (Candida fungal infection of the mouth or vagina), chronic fever, diarrhea and weight loss, and, late in the course of the disease, dementia and blindness. Because of their low resistance to other infections, AIDS victims often become incubators of diseases we once thought were well controlled, such as tuberculosis or salmonella. (As a result, TB has now made its reappearance in a more virulent form.)

HIV can be transmitted to a fetus during pregnancy or delivery, or through breast-feeding. Most cases of pediatric AIDS come from the mother.

DIAGNOSIS AND TREATMENT

AIDS is relatively easy to diagnose: the presence of an "opportunistic" infection such as a fungal infection or a rare pneumonia in a young person, signaling a deficient immune-protective system; abnormalities in the lymphocyte count (CD4 count); and a positive blood test for the presence of the HIV virus. The HIV antibody blood test can pick up the infection long before the disease starts to destroy the immune system. (Within six months of infection, 95 percent of patients will have a positive HIV blood test.)

Once it is detected, however, there is no way to rid the body of this virus, which lives within cells throughout the body, and there is no cure. Even the best therapies we have, such as AZT (zidovudine), have not been conclusively shown to extend life, but they do delay the onset of symptoms of the disease and decrease the chance of maternal–fetal transmission when administered to a pregnant HIV-infected woman. The specific infections and cancers are treated aggressively using standard therapy. Research is critical to stopping this disease, and it must move on numerous fronts: creating better antiviral drugs or drug combinations, uncovering better ways to treat the associated infections, discovering vaccines to prevent infection, and finding ways to rebuild the damaged immune system even in the presence of viral infection.

SOCIAL AND POLITICAL NOTES

One of the major consequences of HIV is that it has brought national attention to the ravages of sexually transmitted diseases. This attention did not come easily, but must be credited to the thousands of patients, family members, and friends who devote their energy and whatever resources they have to getting educational and research support for this disease. There are organizations, demonstrations, rallies, benefits, letters, relentless pressure, and the symbolic expanding AIDS quilt (with each patch representing another victim), which is laid out before the Washington Monument (and also is regularly brought to the NIH) every year to remind the public and their elected officials of the many who have died. The fact that the Congress has allocated 11 percent of the NIH budget for AIDS research and established a special mechanism to coordinate all government-supported AIDS research work is a testimony to the effectiveness of the political activism that has championed the AIDS cause.

But let me reiterate: there are women in that quilt too. The incidence of women contracting this deadly virus is on the rise. Any reader who thinks she can't get AIDS because she's heterosexual, or because

STUDIES TO WATCH FOR: WOMEN, CHILDREN, AND HIV

The National Institute of Mental Health (of the NIH) and the CDC have collaborated on studies to develop prevention messages geared specifically for young women concerning the AIDS risk. The Prevention of HIV in Women and Infants Demonstration Projects, at multiple sites throughout the country, study behavior patterns, contraceptive choices, and psychological factors affecting reproductive decisions in women at risk for HIV infection. The projects focus on the psychosocial factors that influence the epidemic of STDs in general, and are aimed at decreasing risky sexual behavior. The NIH, through its National Institute of Allergy and Infectious Diseases, has embarked on numerous studies of HIV infection in women, including pregnant women. In its national network of AIDS Clinical Trial Groups, women are being enrolled in clinical studies of drug treatment designed to fully reflect their rate of affliction and the unique character of AIDS in women. These studies will expand our knowledge about the different rate of progression of HIV in women, the unique gynecological complications, including cervical cancer, and the means of decreasing the transmission of HIV from a mother to her fetus.

she's female, must think again. I spoke on several occasions with the late Elizabeth Glaser, who got AIDS from a blood transfusion and saw her first child die and her other child live with HIV. She told me her hope was to survive long enough to be there for her younger child, but she didn't make it. I admired her activism until the very end. She and others—like the AIDS activist Mary Fisher, who contracted the disease from her husband—put a human and female face on this tragic illness.

OTHER INFECTIOUS AGENTS TRANSMITTED SEXUALLY

Many other infectious agents—bacteria, viruses, and parasites—may also be transmitted sexually, and often accompany more serious infections. These include cytomegalovirus, Epstein-Barr virus, *Trichomonas vaginalis, Giardia lamblia, Entamoeba histolytica, Cryptosporidium, Hemophilus ducreyi, Ureaplasma urealyticum, Mycoplasma hominis, Shigella, Salmonella, Campylobacter, Gardnerella vaginalis, Mobiluncus curtis,* and the parasites *Phthirus pubis,* or crab lice, and *Sarcoptes scabiei,* or scabies. (I cannot begin to cover all of them here, but I have listed in the back of the book sources where you can get more information on any of these specific illnesses.)

The names are not important. What's important is that these many different organisms are frequent fellow travelers moving along with the STD epidemic. Their presence may be a marker for a coinfection with a more serious form of STD in a given individual. For example, the parasitic infections *Giardia lamblia* and *Entamoeba histolytica,* which cause dysentery, acute infections of the rectum, and genital sores, may also accompany HIV infection. Moreover, each infection makes the next one easier to acquire, and in turn makes the spread faster.

PELVIC INFLAMMATORY DISEASE

Although I have spoken about the specific infections and how they uniquely cause disease, there is one generic illness, pelvic inflammatory disease (PID), which results from infection by one or more of these bacteria or viruses. The illness is defined more by the problems it causes than by the specific infection.

A women's internal organs lying within her pelvis are exposed to the outside world through the same path that a sperm takes as it winds its way into her body in search of an egg. That path of entry can also

be taken by certain bacteria, viruses, and other foreign agents. Gonorrhea and chlamydia are the two primary organisms that can make
their way into a woman's pelvis and set up PID, but not the sole invaders. It is thought that one or both of these organisms establish the
initial infection, which provides opportunity for subsequent bacteria
to introduce themselves and move from the cervix through the fallopian tubes and into the uterus.

PID spreads through the lining of the reproductive tract, causing
inflammation and sometimes abscess formation in the uterus, tubes,
and ovaries; inflammation of the urethra or neck of the bladder; and
infection throughout the pelvic cavity. The condition accounts for 10
percent of all hospitalizations in women between the ages of fifteen
and forty. About one million women will be seen with PID this year,
and 10 to 20 percent of them will be left infertile as a result.

Some forms of PID are not sexually transmitted, but these are usually far less virulent. Intrauterine devices have been associated with
PID, although new studies suggest that the risks they pose may not be
as high as was once thought. Other reports have implicated douching
as a strong independent risk factor for PID, possibly because it forces
infected secretions back up through the cervical canal.

SIGNS AND SYMPTOMS

Symptoms don't usually appear to signal an infection until it is well
established and considerable damage has been done. The initial symptom is most commonly pelvic pain, which may worsen during intercourse or other physical activity. Early on, the discomfort is usually
noticed during the first seven days of the menstrual cycle and then
subsides. As the infection progresses and spreads to adjacent pelvic
tissues, fever appears, and the pain becomes unrelenting and unbearable. The pus-filled abscesses of the fallopian tubes, ovaries, or both
can rupture into the pelvic cavity, leading to massive infection, shock,
and death.

Signs and symptoms reflect the progress of the disease. A thick yellow discharge means infection of the cervix. Painful and frequent urination is caused by urethritis. Proctitis, or infections in the anus and
rectum, causes constipation, rectal discharge, and bleeding. Salpingitis
causes lower-abdominal and pelvic pain. Peritonitis causes increased
abdominal tenderness, nausea, and vomiting—symptoms similar to
those of a ruptured appendix.

CONSEQUENCES

The two most common long-term consequences of PID are ectopic pregnancy and infertility, both resulting from scarring or complete obstruction of the fallopian tubes. The damage is often done and irreversible by the time the infection is recognized and treatment under way. It is estimated that as many as 75 percent of those with three or more recurrences of PID will become infertile. All too few young women think ahead about the potential tragic loss of a baby they may desperately want someday.

DIAGNOSIS AND TREATMENT

PID is diagnosed by the clinical symptoms described above, exquisite pain and sometimes a tender lump detected on pelvic examination, and microscopic examination of cervical or other genital secretions for signs of pus and bacteria.

Many women with PID require hospitalization, though some will respond to antibiotic treatment as an outpatient. Doctors routinely administer intensive broad-spectrum antibiotic therapy directed at a wide range of possible infections, such as gonorrhea, chlamydia, and other bacteria. This usually means at least two antibiotics, including one in the penicillin group. The therapy is usually successful, but at least one in five women will experience a minimum of one recurrence during her life.

PREVENTION: MOSTLY COMMON SENSE

Understanding STDs is the first step in prevention. In Margaret Sanger's era, the preservation of ignorance, especially in women, was deliberate. Sex and its attendant consequences were not only something women should not talk about, but something they should not even know about. Today, though sex talk is ubiquitous, the vast majority of women remain ignorant of just how the epidemic of STDs might affect them.

The diseases are "out there," but only somewhere else. Until women recognize that these diseases are right in their communities— among their friends and children, and in the persons they are thinking of going out to dinner with tonight—the epidemic is not going to be stopped, much less reversed.

SEXUAL BEHAVIOR

Total abstinence, of course, provides total protection. Although I believe this should be seen as a viable option for some, especially for teenagers, it is not going to appeal to sexually active adults. For them, monogamy offers almost the same degree of protection against sexually transmitted disease. When both partners in a sexual relationship are faithful to each other, they can enjoy sex as frequently as they wish without any risk at all. So the answer would seem to be something rather "old-fashioned"—namely, limited and carefully chosen sexual partners, and a goal of faithful and continuous monogamy. Besides its value to society as a whole, this practice has great health value for the individual.

I am in favor of an aggressive campaign to promote abstinence for our children. The good news, from all the latest surveys (see page 81), is that this now seems to be a feasible goal. I would remind reluctant souls who think I'm either square or dreaming that as a society we had *no* problem mounting massive campaigns to keep people from smoking, and with great effectiveness. We have marshaled social resources to transform the culture of the workplace, public spaces, airplanes, hotels, and many other gathering sites into smoke-free zones. Smoking has become socially stigmatized, and the pressures not to smoke have in turn drastically reduced smoking among most groups. Are we afraid to do the same for teenage sex? Or for promiscuous sex? Infidelity? Should we publicize the health costs to women and their children, as we have portrayed those for smoking? No one says, "Smoke only with a filter," or "Smoke less." Rather, the urgent demand is for abstinence, self-control, and discipline. Sexually transmitted diseases are at least as bad, if not worse, in their consequences.

MEDICAL HISTORY OF A SEX PARTNER

Sexual history is as important a part of a person's medical history as a history of smoking or drug use. Nor should such information be confined to doctors' files. Any woman contemplating a sexual relationship with a man should know his history, which could soon become her history. Like the physician, the woman should know about prior sexual activity, drug use, prior and current infections, and the character and integrity of the man and his friends and associates. Gathering such information is easier said than done, but not as difficult as it might seem, if a woman is prepared to take the time to do it. And it is worth her effort, for she is putting on the line her future life and well-being, emotional and physical. And the consequences may be irreversible.

This means taking time in a relationship to get to know the partner. Social attitudes have made it rather commonplace for a couple to have a sexual encounter on the first or second date—at a time when they likely would be unwilling even to share a toothbrush, much less dare to ask about a history of bisexuality, herpes, or genital warts. And how can a woman assess the honesty of her partner after only a few brief meetings? Perhaps the most important judgment a woman can make in any new relationship with a man is whether he is honest. Without that, the rest is meaningless. Studies have shown that many diseases have been transmitted, AIDS included, by partners who have deliberately lied about their health status. As I said, gathering a medical history is an acquired skill that all sexually active women must develop as almost the number one defense against sexually transmitted disease. But first a woman must think about her own medical history, her own behavior, her own sense of what she wants in a relationship with a man. She should put a high priority on her health and her body. A man who truly cares about her will do the same.

ROUTINE SCREENING AS PREVENTION

Some diseases are so prevalent—chlamydia, for example—that screening tests should routinely be provided to anyone who is young and sexually active. Given that half of the nation's youth have their first sexual experiences around the age of sixteen, screening teenagers for chlamydia can identify a significant number of asymptomatic infections early. Diagnosis leads to treatment and often cure, diminished spread, counseling, and, it is hoped, a more cautious approach to sex.

Screening tests have an added benefit that is seldom noted. A discussion of STDs leaves any young woman aware that she may be at risk. If she is sexually active, ordering a test tells her she is at risk. Waiting for the results gives her time to reflect on just when and how often she may have put herself at risk. King County in Washington State has one of the more effective chlamydia testing programs. Women are tested for the disease if they meet two of the following criteria: are younger than twenty-five; have had a new sex partner within the preceding two months; don't use barrier contraceptives; have a puslike discharge from the cervix; have cervical bleeding inducible by a gentle swab. Actually, almost any one of these criteria should be sufficient to indicate screening, depending on the concerns of the individual woman and her physician.

PARTNER NOTIFICATION

Partner notification is an old and established approach to preventing sexually transmitted diseases. Screening for STDs at the time of marriage—with disclosure to the parties—has only recently fallen out of favor. Many object to partner notification, since the diagnosis of an STD discloses secrets that they may have hoped would never be revealed. Physicians currently have an obligation to notify state health officials of certain communicable diseases (such as HIV), for the purpose of tracking epidemics that take their toll on a community. This does not always extend to infected persons' sexual partners. My own view is that we need to be more aggressive about partner notification for both men and women and resume STD screening before marriage. After all, children are at stake as well as the consenting adults.

CONTRACEPTIVES

Oral contraceptives do not prevent disease. In fact, I worry that the confidence they give a woman about pregnancy prevention may lull her into thinking that she is "protected." Barrier contraceptives, specifically condoms and diaphragms, provide a degree of protection, condoms more so than diaphragms. But beware. Just as those who oppose their use tend to exaggerate their unreliability, those who encourage their use often exaggerate their reliability. The truth lies somewhere in between. The condom failure rate is about 10 percent. That is high for a contraceptive—even higher if you are risking a disease that threatens your life or your future ability to have children. Condoms fail through improper use, leaks, or ruptures. Defective manufacture or storage accounts for less than 1 percent of failures. Latex condoms are more effective than natural skin condoms at preventing disease. The effectiveness of both condoms and diaphragms is markedly enhanced by the use of a spermicide such as nonoxynol-9, which can kill some organisms, including HIV. But failures are inevitable. Never forget that fact.

STUDIES TO WATCH FOR:
VACCINES FOR STDs

At present the only effective vaccine for an STD is that for hepatitis B, but NIH and several pharmaceutical companies are actively working on a range of vaccines for many of the others, including chlamydia, human papilloma virus, herpes, and HIV. Vaccines for HPV and for chlamydia, two of the most insidious and damaging infections for young women, are likely to be in early clinical testing by the mid-nineties. A vaccine for AIDS has been a major focus of research, as a means of preventing either primary infection or the advance of the disease once it has infected its host. Unfortunately, the many vaccines that have so far shown early promise have failed closer scrutiny. The work continues and can move very suddenly; stay tuned.

NEEDLE AND CONDOM DISTRIBUTION

Needle and condom distribution programs have gotten a lot of attention. Needle exchange programs hand out free sterile needles to drug addicts. Public health programs hand out free condoms in schools, and some school sex education programs teach how to put condoms on bananas. These programs must be seen for what they are: acts of desperation.

Please allow me to interject a point of view here that I realize many of my colleagues may not agree with. I fear that it is blatantly counterproductive to extol the virtues of abstinence while freely passing out condoms to teenagers. And kids see through hypocrisy very fast. We need to come to terms with the message we want to give our children. To me, these condom programs are much too far away from solving the problem. Condoms may—though this has not been shown—slow the spread of the disease, but they will not stop it, much less reverse it. They are not completely safe; when it is your life, your fertility, and your future on the line, partial safety is not good enough. Such programs also give tacit approval to the behavior, rather than trying to modify it drastically.

EDUCATIONAL PROGRAMS

Counseling and educational programs have varying degrees of effectiveness. When the full threat of AIDS became known, organizations within the gay community mounted massive and comprehensive programs that reached every member of the community and significantly slowed the spread of AIDS and a number of other STDs. There is some concern that those in the younger generation are becoming more complacent about the disease that has so devastated their elders. Awareness has not been extended to the broader epidemic of STDs, particularly as they affect the heterosexual population and women. No doubt knowledge can provide the best protection, but this knowledge must be about the gruesome details of this epidemic, infection by infection, rather than the attention being narrowly focused on teaching barrier prevention. More than one young woman, more than one parent, have complained to me that the broader, long-term message is just not getting out. *The story of Jenny is not woven into an AIDS quilt or printed on a poster.*

QUESTIONS FOR YOUR DOCTOR

- If you are sexually active, discuss concerns you have about any disease exposures, and bring up any signs or symptoms of possible infection.
- Tell your doctor about any suspicions you may have about your sexual partner. Always ask yourself, "Could my partner be infected? Should he (or she) be tested?"
- If you are pregnant, review the routine screening tests for sexually transmitted disease. If you have an STD and are pregnant, what precautions should be taken during pregnancy or at delivery?
- If you are sexually active and have changed partners, discuss this with your doctor. A new partner may alter the screening schedule for Pap smears, for example.
- Ask if there are any abnormalities on your Pap smear that may indicate HPV. Do you have the infection? If so, what strain of the virus? What should the follow-up be?
- If you have a teenage daughter, consider asking your doctor to talk with her about the risks of sexual activity. If your

daughter is sexually active, ask your doctor to help you counsel her on the hazards of her involvement and precautions she should take if the involvement is inevitable.

- If you have an STD and are being treated, how should you go about getting treatment for your sexual partner?

WHAT WOMEN CAN DO PERSONALLY AND POLITICALLY

The means for stopping and reversing the epidemic will not come from a test tube. Even though gonorrhea and syphilis were both stopped by antimicrobials once, they are on the rise again, and new, antibiotic-resistant strains have appeared. Dealing with the epidemic of STDs is going to require a massive effort at every level of society, from the highest offices of government to the living rooms and street corners across the country. And before such an effort can begin, we must first recognize that there is an epidemic and it is in our neighborhood.

At a personal level, we must all look to our own homes and neighborhoods, and be sure we have firmly and wisely counseled our children on these issues. Get involved in your local school, and become informed about what the teens are being taught in sex education. Speak up if you are not satisfied with what you learn. Politically, we should take a lesson from the AIDS activists, who have put HIV on the radar screen. But why has the effort not been broadened to include the many other devastating STDs that ravage women and their children? To fund the basic research we need on better screening, understanding of the spread of the organisms, treatment, and prevention, we must put political pressure on elected officials.

The spread of STDs among today's young women is occurring in daunting numbers. But, taken individually, each case involves a woman with a serious, chronic, lingering disease that all too often arrives in stealth and is kept in secret, whether she is a drug addict from the seedy side of town, a lawyer or a doctor with fancy letters after her name, or a naïve high-school girl falling to peer pressure. We must awaken to this plague. Remember, lovely young Jenny could be the daughter of any one of us.

FIVE

MENOPAUSE
The New Prime Time

Grow old along with me!
The best is yet to be,
The last of life for which the first was made.

— ROBERT BROWNING,
"RABBI BEN EZRA," 1864

My husband and I know a little country inn in California. We spent our honeymoon there; now just mentioning its name has become the code for a romantic respite. This year we were both asked to give lectures on the West Coast; we timed the lectures together so we could schedule a few extra days at "our" inn. At the time of our trip I was heavily immersed in preparing this chapter, so everywhere we went, I clutched under my arm a textbook on menopause. When we arrived at the inn, I waited in the elegant lodge while my husband checked in. Classical music filled the air, and complimentary wine awaited couples milling around arm in arm, starry-eyed. Suddenly I was overtaken with a queasy feeling as I looked down at my book on menopause. Without even thinking, I quickly covered it up with a dust jacket from another book, feeling somehow that the book—the subject—did not quite fit in.

A few hours later, ensconced in our room, I noticed my textbook tucked within another book's cover. My memory of concealing it rushed at me, and I was amused by my own actions. Nonetheless, on an intellectual level, I was also intrigued.

I recently celebrated my fiftieth birthday, and I feel as alive, vibrant, and feminine as I ever have. I adore my husband; we have the kind of relationship younger folks might think belongs only to them. I don't dwell on the fact that I am approaching menopause, except that I do wish we could have had more children. I don't fear being my age, if only for the fact that there is not a thing I can do about it, and it actually does beat being thirty (at least my thirty). As I look inside I find some solace and satisfaction at the long trek I've made over half a century, and eagerness about the distance I have yet to travel. One thing I know for sure is that what really doesn't change much over the years is who you are down deep or how you feel about yourself as a person or as a woman—even if the mirror or the photo albums say something different!

And yet I hid my book.

I was strongly, albeit temporarily, possessed (and I use that word quite intentionally) by the message American women have heard for decades: romance and middle age don't mix. Like so many women of my generation, I have been influenced by the cultural myths that obscure many truths about women's health. When it comes to menopause, we must fight against our own internalized misconceptions as vigorously as we must rail against long-standing societal prejudices.

Menopause of course symbolizes a loss: after menopause, we can no longer bear children. The depth of feeling this loss creates varies with each of our personalities and life experiences. For most women, it is a life passage that must be treated with respect and, perhaps, mourned appropriately.

However, the natural emotions a woman might face during menopause have become distorted and magnified—in the past and the present—by a very unnatural view of the process. Let's take a closer look at the origins of lingering myths.

MENOPAUSE, HISTORY, AND PERCEPTION

Throughout history, menopause has been associated with imminent death and decay, in large part because so few women lived long enough to go through menopause—and those who did were quite elderly by the standard of the times. As recently as the turn of this century a woman could expect to live approximately only fifty years, and many women died much younger, often in childbirth.

The lives of menopausal women have changed a great deal since then and are still changing. Our daughters will grow up in a world filled with vigorous, most assuredly alive and active menopausal women. About thirty-five million women living in America now have gone through or are going through menopause; 90 percent of all women alive today will live through menopause. In fact, most American women can look forward to another thirty years of life after menopause. If menopause is a problem, then every woman has a problem. Seen in this light, the absurdity of this negative attitude becomes clear. (As the generation caught between our mothers' perspectives and our daughters' reality, we may have to periodically remind ourselves of this truism.)

More problematic is the culturally ingrained, long-held view that women in menopause and past it are no longer women, that a woman who cannot procreate is sexually undesirable and is useless to society. Menopausal women were often labeled "the third sex": not man and certainly not woman. While, thankfully, the medical community no longer perpetuates this image, medical thinking was long influenced by the Victorian belief in the indisputable equation "woman = womb." As recently as 1970, the year I graduated from medical school, this viewpoint was espoused in a leading medical journal, which contended that women become depressed around the time of menopause because "at an age in life when a man is in the upswing of active social and professional growth, woman's service to the species is over. Professionals, including female experts, define the woman's role as one of mortification and uselessness."

Also appearing on the best-seller list that same year was a sex manual by the Harvard-trained psychiatrist David Reuben: *Everything You Always Wanted to Know About Sex but Were Afraid to Ask*. He devoted a lot of space to menopause, inappropriately using male imagery to describe postmenopausal women as being "castrated by Father Time ... a woman comes as close as she can to being a man. ... a tragic picture ... Not really a man, but no longer a functional woman." He went on to pronounce: "Once the ovaries stop, the very essence of being a woman stops."

Even more recently, in 1992, a TV reporter who was interviewing me for a piece on women's health told me that she had admitted on air that she herself was menopausal; from the control room had come a threatening male voice in her earpiece, "You've just ended your career!"

In addition, many people believe even now that menopause is the time that women go batty, either falling into the depths of depression or becoming consumed by irrational or unpredictable thinking. When I was growing up, such menopausal madness was often revealed in whispers: the aunt or older sister who ended up in an insane asylum; the lady who took to her bed just waiting to die—suffering silently rather than confiding her torment even to other women.

What I hope to accomplish more than anything in this chapter is to assure that you view menopause in its proper perspective. You're not going to be following your ovaries into oblivion, even if that is what many learned back in the sixties. Of course, however healthy your attitude may be, you'll still encounter many physiological changes during menopause, and you'll run headlong into confusion when you explore the world of treatments, particularly hormone replacement therapy (HRT). For many women, HRT is by far the most urgent and confusing aspect of menopause, and too often doctors aren't much help. We'll explore HRT thoroughly in this chapter; first, though, it's important to understand exactly what menopause is and how it may affect your body.

MENOPAUSE AND YOUR BODY

Hormones, chemicals that circulate in the bloodstream and influence vital functions throughout your body, are fundamental to menopause and, in fact, to all of a woman's reproductive functions. They lock onto hormone receptors on the surface of specific cells, thereby activating certain functions: for example, thyroid hormone stimulates cells to grow; insulin from the pancreas affects sugar metabolism; hormones from the pituitary gland regulate ovulation or milk production by the breasts. Endocrine glands produce and release the hormones. The pituitary gland in your brain is one such gland, as are the pancreas and thyroid; the ovaries, perhaps surprisingly, are another.

You're probably well aware that the ovaries contain thousands of follicles, which are fluid-filled cavities from which eggs develop monthly. The ovaries also produce many different hormones, taking signals from and in turn influencing certain hormones in the pituitary gland (see page 101). During your fertile years, prompted by the pituitary gland's follicle-stimulating hormones (FSH), the ovaries produce estrogen and progesterone, the hormones that rise and fall sequentially during the course of a menstrual cycle; additionally, they produce the male hormone, testosterone, and other less potent androgenic compounds. (Androgens in sufficient amounts produce masculine traits such as facial hair; the word *android*—"manlike"—comes from the same root. Another derivative word is *androcentric,* meaning "male-centered.")

During the eight to ten years preceding actual menopause (known as *perimenopause*), your ovaries increasingly work with less efficiency and actually begin to degenerate. The amount of estrogen produced by your failing ovaries declines steadily, and the follicles themselves begin both to wear out and to become more resistant to FSH. The pituitary gland attempts to compensate by pumping out more FSH, but ultimately, the FSH cannot counter the degeneration of the follicles, and the lack of follicles results in the cessation of a woman's menstrual cycle. FSH levels in the blood are a useful measurement for monitoring the transition from perimenopause to menopause. Premenopausal levels are 5 to 30 units, measured in International Units (IU) per milliliter of blood; during perimenopause, they oscillate between 20 and 50; after menopause, the levels exceed 100.

Even after the ovaries cease to be egg-producing organs, they continue to produce important hormones: estrogen, to a lower and varying degree, and testosterone. The hormone-producing ability of your ovaries is critical for obvious reproductive reasons, but it also benefits many of your body's other functions. Be very aware that you hold receptors for estrogen and other ovarian-produced hormones throughout your body. Your blood vessels, skin, bones, genitourinary tract, heart, and many parts of the brain—even those higher parts that deal with thinking and reasoning—all contain receptors for hormones. We don't yet know what these hormones do in many of these cases, but little in the human body exists without purpose. Even if we can't explain why, those receptors are nature's way of telling us that estrogen and other hormones circulating in the blood are communicating to the receptors for some presumably important yet still mysterious reason.

WHEN EXACTLY AM I IN MENOPAUSE?

Measuring menopause is one of those inexact sciences we doctors love to talk about with great, entirely unfounded precision. I mentioned perimenopause above. During the end of perimenopause, about one to two years before the actual and final cessation of your period, the decline in ovarian function speeds up, and the amount of estrogen your ovaries produce decreases drastically. It's at this inexact point that you're commonly said to be "in menopause" or "going through menopause," although technically the term *menopause* means specifically the time when the ovary has given up its last egg and can produce no more eggs, and you have no more periods. The precipitous drop in estrogen before your actual menopause has an impact on your body, creating many of the symptoms I'll discuss in the next section. These symptoms can be seen as harbingers of the menopause to come.

Menopause itself, by the way, is never diagnosed until after you've passed it. Your doctor will confirm it only after you have gone six to twelve consecutive months without a period.

CAN I CONTROL WHEN MENOPAUSE OCCURS?

The answer to this question is "Yes, to a small degree, but we just don't know enough to say exactly how." Natural menopause can occur anytime after age forty but on the average occurs around fifty (some women go through menopause earlier, but this is seen as premature ovarian failure). For the most part, the time your body will go into menopause is predetermined by your genetic makeup.

However, I say we can have some impact because studies have clearly shown that women who smoke go through menopause on the average one to two years earlier than nonsmokers. (Smokers also show other signs of accelerated aging such as premature vascular disease and an increase in skin aging as measured by facial wrinkles.) Certainly, smoking can't be the only external factor that has an impact. We know, for example, that women who haven't had children go through menopause slightly earlier than women who have borne offspring. It seems to me that any factor affecting the ovaries' production of eggs or estrogen—birth control pills, fertility drugs, pregnancy, illness—would certainly have some slight impact, but the studies have yet to be done to bear out that hypothesis.

THE SYMPTOMS OF MENOPAUSE

As we've seen, menopause doesn't happen overnight. During perimenopause, the gradual decline in ovarian function is signaled by a shortening cycle length, at first by two or three days. Then, when your estrogen levels begin to plummet, your cycles become irregular, and duration and intensity of menstrual flow begin to vary. Some cycles may produce extremely heavy bleeding, while others may be scant. These changes are likely due to a sputtering of ovarian hormone production.

EARLY SYMPTOMS

Your first hot flash is a clear signal that menopause is on its way and your estrogen levels are in an uproar. Hot flashes of varying intensity and duration, from seconds to many minutes, hit suddenly night or day—but mostly at night. You appear flushed or feel overwhelmingly hot; some women experience drenching perspiration, palpitations, and even anxiety. When hot flashes occur at night, they can interrupt sleep and cause restlessness and insomnia. Some women report having to get out of bed to change their night clothes.

Between half and three-quarters of women going through menopause have hot flashes. Without hormone supplements (see page 192), hot flashes typically come and go for about two years or more, decreasing gradually over time; for the most part they decrease rapidly once menstruation ceases.

Hot flashes can be quite disruptive, especially if you work in a predominantly male setting. One of my colleagues often experienced hot flashes, accompanied by visible, drenching perspiration, in the middle of stuffy, mostly male meetings. Although she could laugh about it, she still felt extremely self-conscious and sometimes panicky; there was no way her male colleagues could relate to such an alien experience.

FACTORS EXACERBATING HOT FLASHES

There is a rich folklore about what triggers hot flashes, with external factors such as stress, caffeine, spicy foods, and even sexual intercourse named as culprits. The truth is that most hot flashes are unpredictable. Only two factors have been definitively shown to increase the severity of hot flashes: smoking, which aggravates all early menopausal symptoms, and hysterectomy with ovary removal (see page 186).

A point of interest: many studies have shown that women in other cultures may not experience hot flashes. In some Asian societies such as Japan, there is not even a word for this symptom. A recent report showed that Mayan women who underwent menopause had the same hormonal profile of decreased estrogen and increased follicle-stimulating hormone as other women who had menopausal symptoms, but these women did not report hot flashes. Perhaps some of these cultures simply preclude women from reporting health difficulties they are indeed undergoing, but I suspect we may someday find a valuable lesson in whatever biological, cultural, or nutritional origins account for these different experiences. (Soybeans, for example, are high in plant estrogens, and are perhaps mitigating menopausal symptoms in Japanese women, who have diets rich in soy products such as tofu.)

CHANGES IN THE GENITOURINARY SYSTEM

Changes in the genitourinary system—the vagina, the urethra, and the bladder—are another often troublesome aspect of menopause that can begin toward the end of perimenopause and continue to worsen with time. Due to such so-called atrophic changes, the tissues in these parts of your body become thinner, weaker, drier, and less resilient. These are unpleasant symptoms. Vaginal dryness and shortening can lead to painful sexual intercourse, and urination may become difficult, uncomfortable, or more frequent, particularly at night. Sometimes urinary incontinence becomes a problem. Many women experience "stress incontinence," that is, the spontaneous loss of urine due to anything that causes increased pressure on the pelvis—laughing, running, coughing, sneezing, or lifting. Infections of both the vagina and urinary tract become more common, probably because the cells that line the genitourinary tract are thinner, easier to abrade, and less resistant to the bacteria that are always present in the region.

CHANGES IN MENTAL SHARPNESS

Women going through menopause often complain of becoming forgetful. Suddenly you have to make lists; you can't recall the lyrics to a song your children easily remember. Some of this forgetfulness can certainly be attributed to aging; clinical studies have proven that young men and women do better at recalling than do older men and women. These age-related changes in memory (a gradual loss in immediate and delayed memory) are practically inconsequential as long as you continue to exercise your brain by learning throughout life. Such recall delays are a different animal from the sudden though temporary loss of focus many women endure during menopause.

Although more definitive proof is on the way, I've seen enough to believe that this loss of memory is at least in part a real, physiological corollary to decreased estrogen levels during and after menopause. Estrogen bathes the brain throughout a woman's life and is critical to maintaining normal brain architecture; brain cells have specific estrogen receptors. Suddenly, during menopause, the amount of estrogen available to the brain plummets. This must have ramifications. Most convincingly, as we'll see, estrogen replacement therapy after menopause has been proven to better memory in postmenopausal women. Furthermore, neuroscientists have demonstrated that estrogen stimulates the production of a chemical messenger, acetylcholine, that is critical to message transmission throughout the complex brain networks.

EARLY SYMPTOM OR MYTH?

Hot flashes, genitourinary troubles, and even memory lapses are distinct physiologically based symptoms of menopause. But several other menopausal associations are far more suspect. These physiological and psychological "symptoms" may indeed accompany menopause in some form, but their severity has been so exaggerated that they are in fact more myth than truth.

MENOPAUSE, MADNESS, AND DEPRESSION

MYTH: *Menopause causes severe melancholia, clinical depression, and even insanity.* The belief that menopause goes hand in hand with melancholia or depression is deeply rooted in Freudian thinking. Dr. Helene Deutsch, an expert in women's mental health and author of *The Psychology of Women*, published in 1945, describes menopause in the most dismal of terms: "With the lapse of reproductive service, her beauty vanishes, and usually the warm, vital flow of feminine emotional life as well." Dr. Deutsch taught that this state was followed almost inevitably with either a short-lived "normal" depressive disorder or a long-term "morbid melancholia." A body of medical literature described this "involutional melancholia" as a depressive condition prevalent during a woman's midlife, related directly to menopause. Many women were hospitalized in mental institutions for years with this diagnosis. The myth of menopausal madness was well entrenched in mainstream medical thought and cast a dark shadow on virtually all women.

Even Simone de Beauvoir, one of the spiritual leaders of the women's movement when I was in college, described menopause in brutal terms: "Anguish is at the throat of the woman whose life is already done before death has taken her."

FACT: *Menopausal madness is a myth.* Contrary to the harmful medical and societal fantasy, menopause does not cause a major depression—an uncontrollable feeling of sadness and hopelessness, either without cause or way out of proportion to triggering events—or madness. I don't mean to imply that menopause isn't a time of mood swings and emotional tumult; it is. And women who see themselves only in terms of youth and femininity and who define femininity in terms of a Barbie-doll kind of sexuality are surely going to be set up for the blues when menopause hits. Others may face significant turmoil in their immediate environment with empty nest syndrome or a problem marriage that may aggravate mood changes or irritability associated with menopause. But many studies have shown that *women going through menopause have no greater chance of facing a severe depression than they do at other times in their lives.* Emotional shifts are not the same as a major depression, and you've no need to heap the worry that you're going crazy on top of what is naturally and understandably a *temporarily* difficult emotional time.

There are clear physical origins for the way you will feel. As I've explained, during menopause, women endure a major upheaval in their hormonal status: estrogen and progesterone levels drop, as do other circulating neurochemicals such as *endorphins* (the body's natural opiates), while relative levels of the male hormone testosterone increase. These complex fluctuations in the neurohormonal environment of a woman's body can create changes in mood (many women periodically feel sad or irritable), sleeping habits, outlook, and sense of well-being, or even in characteristics such as assertiveness or self-confidence.

In addition to these obvious physiological changes, menopause is a defining moment in a woman's life that engenders stress and anxiety, as do all major life passages. Menopause is a vivid biological marker of the end of one stage and the beginning of the next. Most women are likely to be struck by a certain sadness when confronted with the loss of the ability to have children—regardless of whether they have ever had any or wanted any. Because of menopause, women are forced to face squarely the turning point to the last half of adult life, to growing old, to no longer being young, however young they might look or feel. Men certainly are never hit with such a defining biological event; male midlife crises that are marked by slowing down, a weaker sex drive, or getting love handles just don't compare.

MENOPAUSE AND SEXUALITY

MYTH: *Most women lose interest in sex after menopause. The few who don't instead turn into sex-starved nymphomaniacs like Mrs. Robinson of the movie* The Graduate. This myth has clear origins in the point of view already noted in this chapter: a woman is only interesting sexually to a man if she can bear his children; after she cannot, she must therefore not be a sexual being. And if she is, she is violating the unspoken Victorian dictum that a woman engage in—and enjoy—sex only as a means of having a family. Fueling the myth of the "castrated woman" is the fact that sex *does* become difficult and painful for many women after menopause; before estrogen creams were available (see page 205), women with normal sexual desires were sometimes prevented by the idiosyncrasies of the body from enjoying intercourse.

FACT: *Sexuality, before and after menopause, is complex and individual, having far less to do with estrogen levels than with the way each woman feels about herself and her circumstances.* Some women report a loss of interest in sex as they go through menopause; others, albeit a smaller percentage, will tell you of increased sexual satisfaction and intimacy with their lifelong partner—almost a second honeymoon. A few claim to develop the voracious sexual appetite as depicted in *The Graduate*; I have observed a few women who went wild during menopause.

Biologically, while estrogen has a clear effect on the functioning of a woman's vaginal secretions and sexual organs and may play a role in ardor, it's testosterone that pretty much dominates the libido. So, if anything, as the ratio of testosterone to estrogen rises during and after menopause, a woman's sex drive could increase.

What is perfectly clear to me as a doctor and as a woman is that sexuality—especially at menopause—is an intricate mix of mind, body, and circumstances. Your mind allows you to love and feel the passion and desire for a mate; the circumstances grant you that mate. Your health has a clear impact on your sexuality. If you have a satisfying sex life before menopause, it should continue through and way beyond menopause, external circumstance permitting. Although no one can speak with authority for every woman, the most important perspective to hold is that the need for a loving and intimate relationship and the ability to enjoy it are affected by neither menopause nor age.

The pattern of sexual activity of both men and women is sure to change with age, but sexual satisfaction from a meaningful relationship will not.

MENOPAUSE AND AGING

MYTH: *A woman hits menopause like a car hits a brick wall: she suddenly and drastically ages, decaying mentally and physically overnight.* When I was in medical school, most people, doctors included, believed that after menopause a woman becomes instantly old in every respect. The fifty-year-old woman is old; the fifty-year-old man is in his prime. This sentiment is vividly stated by Dr. Robert Wilson, gynecologist and author of the 1966 bestseller *Feminine Forever*:

> Nature plays a trick on her. During her best years, she encounters menopause—the end of her womanhood. To be suddenly desexed is to her a staggering catastrophe. . . . The transformation, within a few years, of a formerly pleasant, energetic woman into a dull-minded but sharp-tongued caricature of her former self is one of the saddest of human spectacles. The suffering is not hers alone—it involves her entire family, her business associates, her neighborhood storekeepers, and all others with whom she comes into contact. Multiplied by millions, she is a focus of bitterness and discontent in the whole fabric of our civilization.

FACT: *Women age gradually after menopause.* It is true that hormones modulate the aging process, and that many of a woman's organs—without estrogen replacement after menopause—age more rapidly than they did before. However, "more rapidly" is a very relative term. First, estrogen, before or after menopause, is not a fountain of youth. Aging is a process that goes on relentlessly and inevitably, in women *and* men. Before menopause, the estrogen in a woman's body slows down the aging process of many key organs: specifically the heart, the bones, and probably the brain. In the ten or twenty years after menopause, the lack of estrogen causes those organs to catch up in age to where they would have been without its intervention (to where a man's organs, particularly of his cardiovascular system, already are).

This process is quite gradual; the myth that a woman is somehow older than a man at the same age is nonsense. In fact, protected by estrogen before menopause and likely to live longer than men, women are "younger" throughout their lifetimes.

Of course, we all age, and while genetics plays an undeniable role, so do our overall health and attentiveness to our bodies' needs throughout our lives.

LONG-TERM CONSEQUENCES OF MENOPAUSE

As women move through the years after menopause, their health and illnesses become as much related to age as to the physiologic consequence of the menopause. But for at least three major organ systems—the cardiovascular, the musculoskeletal, and the brain—menopause has a major impact.

Cardiovascular disease (see chapter 8) markedly accelerates after menopause. Before menopause, women virtually never develop atherosclerotic coronary disease (unless they have a major risk factor like juvenile—Type 1—insulin-dependent diabetes or a rare disorder of fat metabolism). After menopause, women become very much like men in their cardiovascular risk for disability and death. Stroke also increases in postmenopausal women. Protecting women of childbearing age against heart attacks and strokes seems to be nature's way of keeping women healthy as they rear their young, sparing them what has been one of the biggest killers of men in midlife. This protection is in part due to estrogen's effects on the composition of circulating blood lipids to decrease cardiovascular risk (see page 343); exactly how else estrogen does its good deeds for women's hearts and blood vessels, however, is still Mother Nature's secret.

Osteoporosis is clearly one of the major health challenges facing all women. A condition in which bones turn into eggshells susceptible to ready fractures, osteoporosis is a virtual epidemic among women after the age of menopause and a major cause of debility in the otherwise fit elderly. It is primarily a woman's disease—and one in which life choices can make a big difference. We'll look at osteoporosis in detail in chapter 10; for now, it is important that you recognize that decrease in bone mass accelerates during menopause and that there is a clear relationship between the level of estrogen in your body and the speed at which osteoporosis develops.

The link between *Alzheimer's disease* (see chapter 11) and estrogen depletion is by no means as well established as the connections of estrogen to heart and bone health, but I see enough evidence to suggest strongly that the relationship is one that bears watching. We know that Alzheimer's affects both women and men, but far more women get the disease than men. We've learned that men get the benefit of estrogen in their brains, too: some of a man's testosterone is converted to estrogen by the brain. Since testosterone levels do not fall significantly as men get older, their brains continue to have an estrogen benefit at a time when women are estrogen deprived. We also know that the incidence of Alzheimer's rises drastically after menopause. Part of the explanation may be a woman's greater longevity or the aging process, but that is not likely to be the whole story.

Some exciting studies currently under way are examining, at long last, the role of female hormones in maintaining the health of the human brain. A developmental biologist, Dr. C. Dominique Toran-Allerand, suggests that estrogen is instrumental in creating and maintaining the elaborate connections between nerve cells in the brain—cells that are linked to memory, learning, and thought processes of all kinds. This at least hints that there may be a critical link between loss of estrogen and a predisposition or vulnerability to Alzheimer's, one that is just beginning to be unraveled in this very young field of neuroscience (see page 474).

HYSTERECTOMIES AND SURGICAL MENOPAUSE

A *total hysterectomy,* where the ovaries as well as the uterus are removed, amounts to a sudden, surgically induced menopause. A process that naturally occurs over a ten-year period—almost the length of an entire childhood—is slashed into an overnight experience. The shock of surgical menopause on a woman's body is not to be taken lightly, contrary to the attitude espoused by some in the medical community and, unfortunately (and probably as a result), by many women.

I remember a common quip that I heard in medical school from the mouths of my esteemed professors; practices suggest not much has changed today: "There seems to be no testicle bad enough to come out and no ovary good enough to stay in!" Although said with a twinkle and a smile, it captures the mind-set that makes this major procedure so overperformed. And indeed, it may well underlie the view of both women and their doctors that a hysterectomy is somehow a trivial procedure rather than the serious medical encounter that it is.

Close to twenty million women in the United States have had a hysterectomy; it is among the most common operations performed in this country—by most accounts, far too common. It is estimated that almost 40 percent of women will have had such surgery by the age of sixty, and the high rate of hysterectomy in this country has not changed much over the past twenty-five years. Benign diseases such as uterine fibroids and endometriosis are the major reasons doctors perform this surgery. Cancer accounts for about 10 percent of these operations; some have estimated that as many as 10 percent are performed for sterilization alone in the face of very minor symptoms.

Almost always in women over forty, the ovaries as well as the uterus are removed. (When the ovaries are also removed, the formal medical term is *total hysterectomy with bilateral salpingo-oophorectomy*.) Hysterectomy does bring with it relief from menstruation and other "monthly" difficulties; it eliminates the risk of uterine and cervical cancer and, when a total hysterectomy is done, ovarian cancer as well.

But surgical menopause is not a benign procedure. It forces a "cold turkey" withdrawal from the many hormones that have been pouring out of the ovaries for decades. It is a wrenching change that brings with it the same symptoms as menopause, but with a far greater severity. Hot flashes, incontinence, vaginal dryness, and hormonally induced mood swings and memory loss are particularly harsh after a total hysterectomy. More crucially, hysterectomy in premenopausal women is associated with increased risk of both coronary disease and osteoporosis. (These afflictions are diminished—but not eliminated—if a premenopausal woman's ovaries are not removed. Retained ovaries continued to produce hormones, but not as effectively, and seem to fail sooner after a hysterectomy than they would otherwise.)

I question the sometimes cavalier attitude about performing hysterectomies (for uterine fibroids, endometriosis, heavy bleeding or mild uterine prolapse, and other benign diseases). I have seen women who have undergone hysterectomies for "convenience" and as a means of birth control; I question the judgment of a doctor who would perform a hysterectomy for such a reason. A hysterectomy should be taken very seriously and performed for life-threatening illnesses (such as cancer, uncontrollable bleeding, or infection) or when symptoms are clearly debilitating and interfere with quality of life (such as extensive endometriosis causing intractable pain and pelvic abnormalities, or severe uterine prolapse where the uterus is protruding out of the vagina).

After menopause, a hysterectomy should still be taken seriously, but it obviously won't have the same hormonal effect on a woman's overall health, since her ovaries have already ceased to function.

TREATMENTS FOR MENOPAUSE

As you read through this section, I'm sure you couldn't help but notice that most symptoms I mentioned have been shown to be related to the

GETTING INTO ESTROGEN

When we speak of estrogen, we are really speaking about a class of estrogenic compounds in the steroid family (just as testosterone is a steroid) that are naturally produced by your body (estradiol, estrone, or estriol) or ones that are synthetically made (such as ethinyl estradiol). When they occur naturally, they are produced from an important steroid building block, cholesterol (the grandmother of all hormones), which is converted by various tissues of the body—including the liver, ovaries, and adrenal glands—into estrogenic hormones.

Estradiol is the major and most potent of the naturally occurring ovarian hormones. It is poorly absorbed when given as an oral treatment and is rapidly converted to estrone by both the liver and the intestines. Less potent than estradiol, estrone is another ovarian hormone; its advantage is that it is more readily absorbed orally. Estradiol and estrone are the two major estrogenic compounds that our bodies produce, and in a modified form these two hormones alone or together are the primary component of HRT in the United States.

Estriol is a third and even less potent naturally occurring form of estrogen. (Although there is no proof, some believe it is associated with a lower risk of breast cancer; it also has little beneficial effect on lipids.) In our bodies, the liver makes estriol from estradiol and estrone. Most postmenopausal HRT in the United States uses naturally ocurring estradiol and/or estrone. Estriol is available along with the other forms for oral use in Europe and Asia, but not in the United States.

lowering of estrogen in a woman's body during and after menopause. The most obvious method through which to attempt to alleviate those symptoms is by replacing the missing estrogen, which is essentially the definition of *hormone replacement therapy* (HRT). HRT involves administration of estrogen or estrogen plus progesterone—the two major hormones produced by a working ovary—to restore hormonal balance to premenopausal levels and thus achieve the physiologic effects of naturally produced hormones. (In the body, estrogen has different forms—as it does when given in replacement—see sidebar, page 188.) Even symptoms not known to have been caused by lower estrogen levels have been lessened through estrogen therapy. Replacing the estrogen no longer produced by a menopausal woman's ovaries might seem a logical and simple solution, but, as I'll explain in this section, hormone replacement therapy has proven to be one of the most controversial medical treatments of this century.

There are actually two major treatment issues for women to consider as they approach and go through their menopause. One is whether or not to take hormone replacement therapy—if so, which preparation and for how long; if not, which other treatments are worth exploring. The second is more personal and internal: how you will develop your own outlook on menopause and plan the next half of your adult life. Menopause is a time of reckoning, a natural point to think about your health and your future. Any treatment decision must be made in the context of your total health, so I'll devote the second part of this treatment overview to your emotional and attitudinal experiences of menopause. But first, HRT.

HORMONE REPLACEMENT THERAPY

Hormone replacement therapy has been around almost fifty years; but lack of knowledge—coupled with blanket, unresearched prescriptions for high dosages—has at times almost driven this critical therapy for women off the market. Many doctors and many women today feel, in my opinion, unnecessarily fearful or skeptical of HRT as a result of yesterday's mistakes driven by yesterday's ignorance. As you'll see, HRT has had a very rocky history.

HISTORY OF HRT

In the 1940s and 1950s, estrogen first became available for the treatment of symptoms of menopause, mainly for hot flashes. Estrogen was prescribed in high doses, but generally for a short time to get through the "difficult" years.

In the mid-1960s, estrogen use took on a much broader role as the notion took hold that it could keep women feminine, attractive, and young. The aforementioned *Feminine Forever* made a big impact on American women. Estrogen was now seen not just as a way to navigate a few years of hot flashes, but as a means of holding on to youth and feminity. The myth of sudden aging and decay after menopause was firmly held at that time; frightened by this dreary mythology, women in droves started taking replacement estrogen. And for many, the estrogen was a godsend. Word of mouth among women and satisfaction with its effects led millions of women to take it.

Then, in the mid- to late 1970s came many reports of endometrial cancer associated with estrogen treatment. The continuous stimulation of the lining of the uterus by the estrogen prescribed to menopausal women seemed to be the culprit. Estrogen was suspected of having a link to breast cancer, as well. Women also reported that gallbladder problems increased manyfold, as did the number of blood clots forming in women's legs that sometimes traveled to the lungs and caused a lung embolus.

Even the seemingly airtight protective effect of estrogens against cardiovascular disease appeared to fall apart. A major NIH-sponsored trial of estrogen to protect against progression of heart disease had to be terminated because so many subjects instead experienced *worsened* heart and vascular disease. Of course, it was reported later that this study had been done in an exclusively male population, but not before most of the population heard that "estrogen causes heart attacks!" (The "in men" end to this sentence never seemed to make it into print.)

Estrogen clearly had a bad reputation by the late 1970s and early 1980s. The NIH issued a statement that estrogen's value was overinflated. In 1979 the National Institute on Aging sponsored a Consensus Development Conference pointing out the risks and questioning the benefits of estrogen use in postmenopausal women. It lamented the lack of carefully controlled studies of hormone use, particularly for women undergoing surgical menopause. The FDA issued warnings about the dangers of estrogen and approved only its limited use for hot flashes and other short-term problems of menopause. The FDA also counseled against its use in women with heart or vascular disease or with a history of breast cancer, liver disease, or blood-clotting disorders. Doctors became reluctant to prescribe estrogens, and women became scared to take them. Estrogen use plummeted.

Like any medication, estrogen is harmful in the wrong doses and in the wrong concentrations. In the mid-eighties the truth about the hormone began to emerge as more and more new studies demonstrated the protective effect of estrogen for a woman's heart and bones—in the proper dosage. Moreover, adding the hormone progesterone to the estrogen proved to eliminate the risk of uterine cancer posed by estrogen replacement alone (see page 197). Now, in the 1990s, hormone replacement therapy has become a truly viable option for women. Close to thirty-five million prescriptions for hormone replacement therapy are issued annually, making hormone replacement therapy one of the top ten prescription drugs prescribed. I know of no treatment or therapy that has been on such a roller coaster, and over so short a time period. And of course, women have been dragged along on the ride.

HRT now carries with it the burden of its past. Doctors of different ages and levels of awareness of current research have different ideas about HRT. Doctors who practiced through the 1960s and 1970s often still hesitate to prescribe estrogen, and not all doctors have a thorough understanding of proper dosages. At the same time, some prominent feminists, most notably Germaine Greer, take a hard philosophical stand against HRT, in a backlash against the myth that women must take estrogen solely to stay young and please men.

Your only means of finding your way through this maze is knowledge. Discuss information you read or hear about with your doctor— and, if necessary, with another doctor. Read this chapter closely and assess the risks and benefits for yourself. Fortunately, we now have gathered enough data that I feel comfortable making what I believe are sound recommendations.

Still, a word of caution: while I find the data convincing, I must note that most of the knowledge we have is based on laboratory work and observations of large populations of women who take estrogen. Estrogen users are apt to be more educated, informed, and health conscious—the so-called healthy user syndrome. Still lacking are the carefully controlled clinical trials in which similar matched groups are followed with and without treatment, trials that would provide certain proof of positive health outcomes and the specifics of health risks. These studies should have been done twenty or thirty years ago, in the wake of all the controversy; fortunately, they are finally under way (see sidebar, page 192).

BENEFITS OF HORMONE REPLACEMENT THERAPY

There are numerous benefits that come with hormone replacement therapy; for many women the benefits clearly outweigh the risks. (As we'll see on page 202, most currently prescribed HRT includes a combination of hormones, generally estrogen and progesterone together. The benefits listed below are largely the same whether the estrogen is taken alone or with progesterone.)

HRT and Early Symptoms of Menopause

Most women going through menopause report feeling better on hormone replacement therapy. Their hot flashes are eliminated or decreased, and vaginal dryness, pain on intercourse, and problems with urination are eased or even prevented. Even local application of estrogen with

STUDIES TO WATCH FOR

PEPI

In 1989, the NIH took a very important step in solidifying our knowledge of the short-term effect of HRT on postmenopausal women. It began the Postmenopausal Estrogen/Progestin Interventions (PEPI) trial, under the leadership of Drs. Elizabeth Barrett-Connor and Trudy Bush, to study in a controlled way how various forms and dosages of HRT in the short term (three years) impact cardiovascular risk factors (including blood cholesterol and blood-clotting factors), bone mass, general body metabolism, and overall quality of life. PEPI uses so-called surrogate markers, such as blood pressure or cholesterol levels, which would predict better health. It does not follow patients long enough, nor is PEPI large enough to determine treatment effect on disease development. In 1995 we heard some of the results of this study, which so far have confirmed the beneficial effects of HRT on cardiovascular risk factors, indicated no adverse effects on blood pressure or blood clotting, and reaffirmed the need for combination treatment using estrogen and progesterone in women with vaginal creams has been shown to be highly effective in dealing with the genital tissue atrophy and dryness that can impair sexual function.

Some women report that their skin "glows" with extended estrogen use. As we age, our skin becomes thinner and loses collagen. Estrogen improves skin texture, collagen content, and skin thickness. The feeling that estrogen keeps one young may well relate to the very visible effects on a woman's skin.

Many women claim that estrogen improves mood, sleep, memory, and interest in sex. (It's likely that the increased interest in sex has more to do with increased comfort during sex than it has to do with estrogen's impact on the libido.) Such behavioral benefits are more difficult to prove scientifically because the effects are hard to measure precisely. For example, some studies have found estrogen provides no documentable relief of the illnesses of major or minor depression; the FDA therefore denies the role of estrogens in fighting depression in

intact uteri. Other important findings from PEPI are sure to emerge over the next few years.

The Women's Health Initiative

What's obviously absent from the PEPI trial is the long-term impact of HRT on total health or prevention of disease and on specific outcomes (such as heart attacks or stroke) rather than only on the surrogate markers. The Women's Health Initiative (see page 10) will provide the missing pieces of our knowledge. Early, observational results of this decade-long WHI study, begun in 1993, will probably be available in about four or five years, and more conclusive results will follow well into the twenty-first century. In addition to its many other focuses, the WHI will study the long-term effects of HRT in a holistic and interconnected manner. Not only will we learn about the relationship of HRT to heart, brain, bones, and overall health, we will also learn how long it is safe to take HRT, how long a woman needs to take HRT in order to reap its benefits, how HRT needs may change over time, and how they may vary with the overall health, particularly nutritional health, of each woman. Long-awaited definitive answers are on the horizon!

women in their menopausal years (see chapter 7). But the beneficial effects of estrogens on a woman's mood and general outlook cannot be discounted in the wake of numerous anecdotal reports of improved sense of well-being, diminished anxiety, and decreased irritability.

My own impression from my patients is that most on HRT do feel less distracted, less moody, and more in command of their memories. It seems to me these are lucky side effects of the more concrete benefits, rather than necessarily direct results of the hormone on the brain. HRT definitely improves sleep (according to many studies, in both quality and quantity) and relieves hot flashes (and with them the anxious feeling that a hot flash may strike at any time). With better sleep and less anxiety, a woman will remember more and feel better on all fronts.

Long-Term Health Benefits of HRT on Osteoporosis, Stroke, and Alzheimer's Disease

Bones clearly benefit from estrogen replacement therapy during and after menopause. Estrogen increases calcium uptake by the gut, decreases excretion of calcium by the kidneys, slows bone breakdown, and may slightly increase bone buildup (see chapter 10). It is the most powerful intervention presently known to reduce the ravages of osteoporosis, clearly more beneficial than either calcium supplements or exercise. Estrogen is particularly effective in preventing osteoporosis when combined with calcium supplements and weight-bearing exercise. If you are planning to live to ninety, you should at least consider long-term hormone replacement therapy based upon this benefit alone.

The aforementioned male-only study of estrogen and *heart disease* (see page 190) has nothing to do with a woman's body, contrary to popular opinion. Men's bodies do not require large doses of estrogen to function; the men in this group were not given replacement hormones, but unnecessary toxins to their systems. Appropriate studies of women show, time and again, that women's heart and blood vessels benefit from long-term hormone replacement. In studies comparing women who take hormones with those who do not, the women on estrogen reduce their chance of getting coronary disease or having a heart attack by about 50 percent. Researchers believe that this risk reduction is related, at least in part, to favorable changes in blood cholesterol. Estrogen reduces LDL cholesterol—the so-called bad cholesterol—by 20 percent or more, and increases the levels of good HDL cholesterol in the bloodstream by as much as 10 percent. But estrogen has other beneficial effects on the heart and blood vessels that are not as well studied. It decreases certain blood-clotting factors, like *fibrinogen*, which decrease heart attack risk. It appears to dilate arteries mildly throughout the body, including the brain and possibly the heart.

There is also growing evidence that *stroke*, a deadly disease of the elderly, may be decreased through HRT, and that HRT does not raise blood pressure, as was once feared. Most strokes are caused by the same kind of arterial disease that causes heart attacks. A recent observational study from Sweden shows that estrogen replacement therapy decreases the incidence of stroke by 30 to 40 percent in postmenopausal women. While it is not sufficiently well documented for me to advise you to take HRT just for this benefit, I nonetheless find it quite convincing and eagerly await the results of future studies, including the Women's Health Initiative, that I believe will have the chance to verify this early finding.

We've discussed mood shifts and memory loss as short-term symptoms of menopause, which, at least by some claims, improve with HRT. There are also some potentially important long-term benefits of HRT for the *brain* that have just begun to be recognized and studied. The human brain, as we've seen, is built to employ estrogen, and estrogen is important to the building and maintenance of nerve networks from very early in life. Exactly how the brain uses the estrogen its receptors receive is still a matter being explored mostly in laboratories, but even these findings are provocative in light of other studies being conducted among the elderly. In his group's study of almost nine thousand postmenopausal women, Dr. Victor Henderson of the University of Southern California found that those on long-term estrogen lived significantly longer. In addition, by the time of their deaths, women who used estrogen had a 40 percent lower incidence of *Alzheimer's disease* than those not taking hormones. In a related study, not only was estrogen associated with a significantly decreased occurrence of Alzheimer's, but those who were afflicted suffered a milder impairment. These findings, if they hold up in the future, are truly extraordinary. Reducing the toll of Alzheimer's disease in the very group that carries an excess risk would be a major breakthrough on many fronts. Efforts toward that goal would encourage us to understand the mysterious role that estrogen plays in normal brain function, would tell us something about the underlying cause and progression of Alzheimer's disease, and, as a bonus, would help to relieve the economic burden of Alzheimer's disease with a relatively safe and low-cost treatment.

Considering our aging population, the expected leap in the incidence of Alzheimer's into the next century, and the devastating nature of this disease in both human and economic terms, we should vigorously pursue any lead we have, especially one so promising. Although we are spending some three hundred million dollars a year at the NIH on Alzheimer's research, I believe the estrogen/Alzheimer's connection merits highest priority.

THE RISKS AND CONTRAINDICATIONS OF HRT

Even properly prescribed HRT carries with it some real risks, which you should know before you make personal treatment decisions. As mentioned on page 191, an important fact to remember is that virtually all of the long-term studies showing the dramatic benefits of hormone replacement therapy suffer from the healthy user syndrome—that is, the women who use hormones are most apt to be the ones who take care of themselves, eat right, see their doctors, exercise, and lead generally healthier lives. So the studies themselves are skewed when it comes to getting a clear sense of the benefits or risks to women who are either ill or not healthy overall. Again, more definitive research is on the way; for now, here's what we do know about the risks and negative factors worth considering.

Quality-of-Life Issues and Life Outlook

Even though many women report an overall improvement in the way they feel, reaction to medicines can be highly individual and some women experience uncomfortable side effects from estrogen. Tenderness and swelling of the breasts, abdominal cramps, legs cramps, headaches, and water retention are not uncommon. Addition of progesterone tends to bring more complaints, such as fatigue, feeling irritable, a decrease in libido, and, for many women, the inconvenience of continued monthly bleeding (see page 202). Most often, though, all of these problems (including bleeding) can be eliminated by adjusting and tailoring the individual dosages of hormone, altering the mode of administration, or changing the particular preparation being used.

Some women hold a serious philosophical objection to the entire concept of HRT, believing that menopause is a natural state of being and that it is inappropriate—and perhaps sexist, perpetuating the male fantasy that a woman must be "forever young"—to disturb the natural state with hormones. Others believe on principle that normal, healthy women should not be given a lifelong prescription when they are aging according to nature's plan.

These are thoughtful and serious objections to HRT; as you assess the physical risks, you must also assess your feelings, and determine whether HRT is an acceptable compromise for you.

Endometrial Cancer

There is virtually no risk of an increase in cancer of the endometrium (the lining of the uterus) when HRT includes a combination of estrogen and progesterone. (The reason is that the progesterone causes the endometrium to shed each month, which means that women continue to have monthly bleeding. This is an unacceptable side effect for some women.) Women who take estrogen alone, without progesterone (called "unopposed" estrogen), do face an increased risk of endometrial cancer. This form of cancer is rare to start with but has been shown to increase as much as five- to tenfold in those women who take unopposed estrogen treatment, with this increased risk starting to show up after about one year of use. The ongoing PEPI study (page 192) showed that one-third of women on estrogen alone developed potentially precancerous abnormalities in their uterine lining cells within three years of use, although less than 2 percent developed endometrial cancer. Endometrial cancer is slow growing and is usually detected early (at which point it is fully curable by hysterectomy) when a woman reports abnormal bleeding or her physician notices enlargement of the uterus. If a woman chooses to take unopposed estrogen recognizing the risk, she must have annual gynecologic evaluations with periodic endometrial biopsies, which are performed in a gynecologist's office as a fairly routine outpatient procedure.

Breast Cancer

Higher doses of estrogen, with or without progesterone, have definitively been shown to increase risk of breast cancer. It is a low risk, but one that should not be discounted. Virtually all studies, though, show that an increased risk does not show until after about ten years of treatment. With hormone doses in the range of 1.25 mg per day or higher, taken for more than ten years, the risk increases by about 10 to 20 percent and grows to 25 to 30 percent in women who have taken these doses of HRT for fifteen years and at least doubles as twenty years is approached. Importantly, however, these observations were made in women taking about twice the dose of estrogen that is commonly prescribed today. A large analysis in which observations from many studies were pooled has shown that there is a lesser risk for breast cancer when the dose of estrogen is lower (0.625 mg per day). These observational studies are encouraging, but of course I'll be most sanguine when we obtain more definitive information by a clinical trial.

Other Risks

Women taking estrogen have reported a slightly higher incidence of gallbladder disease. Although today's low doses minimize the risks, discuss the matter with your doctor if you have a history of gallstones. I am less concerned about gallstones, though, than I am about the risk of estrogen in pill form for women with liver disease (although there is no proven relationship of liver disease to HRT). Estrogen taken orally is metabolized by the liver and becomes highly concentrated there. It seems intuitively clear to me that if you have liver disease, you would want to avoid any drug that stresses an already weakened organ and exposes it to high levels of a powerful hormone, especially when there are other preparations that bypass the liver. (For forms and doses of estrogen, see page 202.)

Higher doses of estrogen—at the levels used in birth control pills—have also been associated with blood clot formation in the veins of the legs. Although the lower doses of estrogen used at menopause have not been tied to this risk, prudence has led most physicians to at least warn women about the theoretical risk, especially if they have a history of clot formation in the veins of their legs, particularly during pregnancy or with the use of oral contraceptives. On a short-term basis the PEPI trial showed no significant increases in thromboembolic disease in women taking estrogen with or without progesterone.

A history of blood clots or gallstones may or may not be sufficient for your doctor to warn you away from HRT. I would make my recommendation based on each individual case. If you have liver disease, I would not suggest you take HRT orally, but a transdermal estrogen patch—where the hormone gets absorbed directly into the bloodstream, bypassing the liver—may be a viable alternative for you to discuss with your doctor.

Pregnancy Risk During Perimenopause

Some women start to have symptoms of perimenopause such as hot flashes long before their ovaries permanently fail. In this perimenopausal state, their FSH levels are mildly elevated (20 to 50), and they continue their periods, although irregularly. One way to alleviate symptoms and provide birth control simultaneously is to use birth control pills—but only if the woman is not a smoker. Birth control preparations provide continuous synthetic estrogen and progesterone for three weeks, followed by one week off the pills altogether. Transition to menopause will be signaled by absence of a period during the monthly withdrawal of the birth control pills and/or by determining that FSH levels have exceeded 100 International Units per milliliter. When this occurs, a doctor will switch the patient to HRT if she so chooses.

Who Should Definitely Not Take HRT?

Definite is never definite when it comes to current knowledge of women's health. As we've seen, exhaustive studies in key areas are finally under way, but at the time of this writing, I (and your doctor)

STUDIES TO WATCH FOR:
CAN WOMEN WITH HEART DISEASE TAKE HRT?

Although we have strong evidence that HRT is beneficial in preventing heart disease from occurring, there is concern that once heart disease hits, hormone treatment may then increase risk—mainly because of observations from years ago suggesting increased strokes or heart attacks in women on birth control pills. Consequently, the National Heart, Lung and Blood Institute has just initiated the Hormone Estrogen/Progestin Replacement Study (HERS) to see whether or not hormone replacement therapy can be shown to slow down the progress of already existing heart problems in women known to have cardiovascular disease. I predict there may well be a time when we prescribe HRT for every woman admitted to a coronary care unit with a heart attack!

must rely on data that will surely and quickly change. At least for now, most doctors and researchers agree that women who have had breast cancer or who have a strong family history of breast cancer should not take HRT. Nonetheless, some doctors are beginning to question this dictum, calling for a study of HRT in breast cancer survivors; a study is under review by the National Cancer Institute.

As this book is being written, an exciting discovery has just been announced: we have isolated and identified the breast cancer gene, and we should have a screening blood test within a year. Women carrying BRCA genes have an 85 percent chance of getting breast cancer in their lifetimes, and these women obviously should stay away from HRT for now. There is no hard evidence to support this view, but it makes common sense.

Although there are no definitive studies of HRT therapy in women who have had hysterectomies for early-stage uterine cancer, the American College of Obstetricians and Gynecologists advises that the vast majority of cancer specialists now approve the use of estrogen replacement in such women. But for more advanced tumor, HRT is to be avoided. Each woman faced with this choice must discuss with her doctor her personal risks and the benefits she wishes from HRT.

BENEFIT VS. RISK OF HRT: WHERE DO THE SCALES TIP?

The decision to take HRT can only be your own, made after serious thought and in close consultation with a trusted physician. I have outlined both risks and benefits as clearly as possible, using the latest studies available as of this book's writing. Here's my strongest recommendation: revisit any decision you make yearly, since the most conclusive research has yet to be finished. Understand also that each woman is different and that no one can make blanket recommendations for all women. Your decision to take HRT or not can be changed at any time; it is not a commitment for life.

I can tell you my personal position on HRT. When I hit menopause, I will begin HRT without a blink. The studies I've seen thus far, insufficient as they may be, nonetheless convince me that HRT presents no major risk to a healthy woman, and, to me, the benefits are nothing short of remarkable. Distilling all the reports, I conclude that long-term hormone replacement therapy may not make one feminine forever, but it clearly offers the chance for being healthier far longer. The benefits of hormone replacement therapy on individual diseases or specific organs are impressive. But when the benefits are looked at in aggregate, they are compelling. The total health of a woman as she gets older is largely what determines her quality of life, what allows her to view the last half of her adult life as a blessing and a second prime. All current evidence points to the fact that many of the major risks any woman faces as she ages—heart disease, stroke, osteoporosis, and Alzheimer's disease—are or may well be reduced by hormone replacement therapy. Even mood seems to improve with the right prescription. The risks of endometrial and breast cancer are of some concern to me, but they are in part controllable by tailoring the dose and preparation and consistent follow-up screening by your doctor.

My view may be altered in the future by new information; twenty years from now, my daughters reading this might say, "Mom, you were wrong." But a decision *not* to consider hormone replacement is a health decision too, just as is the decision not to take a flu shot or get a hepatitis vaccination. As I see it, women have a competitive health and survival edge before menopause. Women during their childbearing years are protected against many problems that affect men. I see no reason to relinquish that advantage after menopause—not if I can help it.

FORMS AND DOSES OF HRT

The decision to embark on hormone replacement therapy is only a first step. The next questions you must answer with the help of your doctor are

STUDIES TO WATCH FOR

Baltimore Longitudinal Study of Aging (BLSA) *is a longstanding project supported by the National Institute on Aging of the NIH, originally following men only. This study is now looking at differences between men and women as they age, including genetic, endocrinal, and lifestyle factors; transdermal estrogen combined with oral progestins in older postmenopausal women (short term); transdermal estrogen compared with other forms of estrogen administration; urinary incontinence in postmenopausal women (with various interventions such as behavioral training and exercises); and cognitive changes with aging, including short- and long-term recall and Alzheimer's. Results of this study will be out before the decades end.*

- Should I take estrogen alone or in combination with progesterone?
- Which chemical preparation should I take?
- In which form? A pill? A patch? A cream? A shot?
- What dose is appropriate?
- What schedule should I follow?
- How long should I take hormone replacement therapy?

Addressing these questions can seem a bit overwhelming, but they break down into some fairly straightforward choices. I'll go into them below. The more types of treatments available to you, the more likely you are to find the treatment that is perfect for you. Through trial and error—trying different preparations, different doses, different schedules—you should ultimately be able to work with your doctor to find a personalized prescription that provides the greatest benefits and fewest side effects.

• Should I take estrogen alone or in combination with progesterone?

For most women, the answer to this question should be quite clear: if you have your uterus and you take estrogen, you must take it in combination with progesterone. Progesterone, also known as *progestin* (the name used to describe an entire class of modified forms of natural progesterone, as well as synthetic progesterone and progesterone-like drugs), reduces the estrogen-increased risk of uterine cancer to next to nothing. Progesterone does not diminish the heart or bone benefit of estrogen, but with some preparations, progesterone lessens the beneficial rise in HDL cholesterol that comes with estrogen replacement alone.

When you cycle progestin with estrogen, you may have monthly bleeding, although there are now treatment schedules available that pretty much eliminate even the monthly bleeding after about six months (see page 206).

• Which chemical preparation should I take?

There are now more than fifteen different estrogen preparations used in HRT and more than five forms of estrogen/progesterone combinations—and that's just in the United States. There are more than one hundred in use in Europe. Some are naturally occurring; others are synthetic. As more studies are done, however, we are learning more about the different schedules and preparations. As noted above, one schedule eliminates monthly bleeding; another has a more favorable effect on

HDL cholesterol or a less certain effect on bone. Such differences will be factored in as you and your doctor decide what is best for you.

Estrogen Alone

Estrogen alone has been the most common hormone replacement given to women going through menopause over the past many decades. Today, estrogen alone is given only to those postmenopausal women who have had a hysterectomy—which, as we've seen, is a large number.

By far the most commonly prescribed form of estrogen alone is Premarin, an estrogen in pill form that is extracted from the urine of pregnant mares. It is a mixture of several forms of naturally occurring estrogenic compounds (called *conjugated estrogens*), most (50 to 60 percent) in the form of estrone. Relatively inexpensive and reliable, it has been in use now for more than fifty years. Other mixtures similar to Premarin and also given orally are called Estratab and Menest.

Combination: Estrogen plus Progesterone

Progesterone added to estrogen causes the uterine lining to slough away each month, mimicking the normal menstrual cycle and thereby eliminating the risk of endometrial cancer. The most commonly used progesterone is Provera (medroxyprogesterone acetate), a synthetic hormone also sold under the brand names of Amen, Curretab, and Cycrin. Another form, micronized oral progesterone, chemically identical to the natural human form of hormone, has a more favorable effect on HDL cholesterol when given in combination with estrogen. This finding was just confirmed by the PEPI trial, but the drug is not yet available for general use in the United States. (See page 192.)

Megace (megestrol acetate) is a progestin that is used as a remedy for hot flashes (in women who cannot take estrogen because of breast cancer risks and also in men who have hot flashes after removal of their testes—orchiectomy—for prostate cancer). Progesterone alone, however, does not provide relief for the other symptoms of menopause or the health protections of estrogen.

Another less commonly used progestin is norethindrone acetate, packaged under the names of Norlutate and Aygestin, the progestin commonly used in birth control pills. Your doctor will prescribe a chemical preparation of progesterone, depending upon his experiences and your own reaction to different brands.

Combination: Estrogen plus Testosterone

Although testosterone continues to be produced by a failing ovary, it too diminishes over time. Testosterone administration along with female hormones has been shown to improve libido, energy, mood, and sleep. But be careful. We have very little scientific backing for its use, and I personally wouldn't recommend its widespread use until we know more. The obvious concern is that too much testosterone would diminish the beneficial effects of estrogen's decreasing cardiovascular risk and also might lead to troublesome side effects such as facial hair and acne. Testosterone is available now and used in low doses, including Estratest (estrogen and methyltestosterone) and Deladumone (estradiol and testosterone), mainly to help boost the libido.

- **In which form?**

Most preparations of estrogen alone are now available in pill form, in shots, as a patch on the skin, and as a vaginal cream. Progestins are available in pills or shots. Each form has clear advantages and disadvantages, and you should discuss each thoroughly with your doctor based on your own particular needs.

Pills to be taken orally. Most HRT today is taken in pill form, with separate pills for estrogen and progestins. When taken as pills, though, the estrogen goes first to the liver, where it is converted into a form the body can best use. In the liver, as we've seen, it can provide more rapid cholesterol benefits (raises HDL, lowers LDL cholesterol). But it also can, occasionally and modestly, increase the chance of gallstones. Concerns that HRT in oral form raises blood pressure have not been substantiated. If for any reason you want to bypass the liver, another form (patch or cream) may be better for you; talk with your doctor about these issues.

A patch on the skin. A new form of estrogen is *transdermal* (by skin patch); placed almost anywhere convenient on the skin (the abdomen is typical), the patch provides a slow, steady absorption that actually mimics the body's natural production of estrogen more closely than does a pill. Usually applied twice a week, it can be used by women who take estrogen alone or along with a progesterone pill.

The estrogen released by this "transdermal" form may provide less long-term protection against osteoporosis and heart disease; we don't know for sure.

Vaginal creams. Estrogen also can be administered through a vaginal cream. In addition to giving local relief to menopausal symptoms of vaginal dryness, the hormones are absorbed into the bloodstream through the vaginal lining. Women employing combination therapy would use the cream in conjunction with a progesterone pill.

Again, when estrogen is absorbed through the vaginal lining, the liver is pretty much bypassed. However, the problem with creams is that dosages are harder to control than in any other form. The cream alone is preferred by women who are especially troubled with atrophic changes in the lining of the vagina. Be aware that estrogen in the form of a vaginal cream is basically as potent as estrogen taken any other way; all the risks and benefits apply. Indeed, it could be risky for women to apply this as freely as hand cream, not thinking it is really a medication!

Intramuscular administration (a shot). Estrogen, or estrogen with progesterone, can also be taken in the form of an injection, either a few times a week or once a week depending on the type of estrogen. Most women don't choose this method, though, because it is obviously inconvenient and uncomfortable. For the most part, intramuscular administration is used only for women who can't take medication orally for a short time, such as some hospitalized patients.

• **What dose is appropriate?**

The proper dosage is dependent on the form of HRT you choose and on your doctor's recommendation. Your main concern should be that you are taking the minimal amount possible to achieve heart and bone protection and still relieve symptoms. We've learned that this balance can be achieved by a dose equivalent to 0.625 mg of oral estrogen; commonly prescribed doses for estrogens range from 0.3 mg to 1.25 mg per day if taken orally, with doses sometimes modified on a trial-and-error basis depending upon a woman's symptoms. Provera (medroxyprogesterone acetate) is administered in doses of between 2.5 and 10 mg daily, and oral micronized progesterone at a dose of 200 mg daily, prescribed according to a set schedule with estrogen administration.

• **What schedule should I follow?**

If you are taking estrogen alone, your dosage will be simple and straightforward—a pill a day or patch with cream as advised. If you plan to take combination estrogen and progesterone, you and your doctor will have several options to discuss:

Mimicking the natural cycle. On this schedule, estrogen is taken either orally or in patch form for three weeks. In the second and third week progestin is added; during the fourth week, both hormones are stopped and withdrawal bleeding occurs.

Progestin every two weeks. Another approach is to give estrogen continuously and add progestin two weeks out of every month. With this approach, there are no symptoms of estrogen withdrawal, which some patients complain about.

Continuous administration. More recently, both hormones have been combined in constant levels, using a lower dose of progestin (2.5 mg). This approach has the advantage of being the most simple, since the regimen does not change from week to week. Such continuous use may be tolerated better because monthly bleeding is less and usually stops or is reduced to occasional spotting after about six months or so. At this point, we don't know whether one schedule is better than another in terms of long-term health risks and benefits; we'll learn over the next decade as the results from studies come in (see pages 192–93).

- **How long should I take hormone replacement therapy?**

The short answer is that we don't have an answer yet. If you are going to embark on a course of HRT for its long-term health benefits on your heart, your bones, and your brain, and you are not at high risk of breast cancer, then you should take them a decade or longer. The WHI study (see page 10) will provide us with a larger body of research with which to evaluate the safety of such a long-term approach.

ALTERNATIVE TREATMENTS TO HORMONE REPLACEMENT THERAPY

If you either cannot or choose not to take HRT, you do have options. That's the good news. The bad news, as you may expect, is that no option has proved to be as effective as HRT in either the short or the long run, and some are actually dangerous. You may consider either a variety of non-hormone drugs—none of which I find advisable—or alternative, natural treatments.

NON-HORMONE DRUGS

Some physicians prescribe blood pressure medications to relieve flushing and palpitations. This makes sense to me only if you have high blood pressure to begin with; otherwise, I don't recommend it and in fact strongly recommend against it. These medicines carry their own side effects and are not likely to bring benefits worth the risks.

For a very long time tranquilizers have been prescribed to menopausal women who feel anxious or restless, and sleeping pills given almost as a reflex to women who have insomnia. The one tranquilizer that has specifically been approved by the FDA for relief of menopausal symptoms is Bellergal; Bellergal is actually a mix of a tranquilizer, a sedative, and an agent that constricts blood vessels. My view is that all these medications are dangerous, not only because they can be addictive but because they somehow reinforce the myth that women going through menopause should be treated as if they are experiencing a serious anxiety disorder that requires psychotropic drug therapy.

None of these approaches remedy either the genitourinary problems or the long-term health consequences of menopause, namely, heart disease and osteoporosis, since they don't replace the body's own natural substances.

NATURAL REMEDIES

I wish I could give you substantive information on the many natural remedies that have become part of folklore for treatment of menopause; here, though, so little research has been done that I can tell you only which products have been used historically to combat menopausal symptoms. For example, some health practitioners believe that vitamin E provides relief from hot flashes and vaginal dryness and improves energy. Vitamin E is known to play a key role in estrogen metabolism, and while there is no evidence to support the benefit of vitamin E for menopausal symptoms, it has not been disproved either. I have enough respect for the growing importance of vitamins to our health to not dismiss this piece of folk wisdom out of hand without decent study.

Ginseng, a root used in Chinese herbal medicine, has been used in teas and syrups for generations to alleviate menopausal symptoms. Little or no research has been done on ginseng, and since it is a natural food product, it falls outside the normal category of drug treatment. Ginseng, available in health food stores, has been touted for a wide range of therapeutic values including improved mental performance, mood, awareness and memory, and even anticancer effects, but the fact is we don't have the facts.

There is growing interest in the class of naturally occurring plant hormones that are present in large amounts in certain diets. One family of compounds, in particular—the isoflavonoid phytoestrogens—are similar to naturally occurring human estrogens and bind to estrogen receptors. Soybeans and soy sprouts as well as peas and yams are a rich source of the isoflavonoid phytoestrogens and some suggest may account for the lower reported incidence of hot flashes among menopausal women in countries like Japan. The estrogenic isoflavonoids found in soy products (including the compounds genistein, daidzein, equol) are detected in high levels in the urine of Japanese women, about thirty times higher than levels measured in groups of American and European women. High dietary intake of these isoflavonoids has been linked not only to fewer menopausal symptoms but also to a lower noted incidence of breast (and prostate) cancer. This finding has led to the supposition that the weaker plant estrogens displace more potent ones (estrone, in particular) on breast tissue receptors, thereby causing less growth stimulation. No controlled studies have yet been done, however, on dietary modification to test these observations in menopausal women. (Perhaps we need a plant-PEPI study!)

There are many alternative treatments that have a following, but little or no proof of efficacy; these include garlic, assorted herbal teas, acupuncture, and megadoses of vitamins B and C. We need more studies of these natural products that often have a historical basis for use but have not been subjected to rigorous scrutiny. Such natural therapies could point the way to approaches not yet imagined. This kind of medical folklore is the very reason we established an Office of Alternative Medicine at the NIH. Sadly, it's an office that has had a hard time surviving in a world not used to the alternative paths.

THE TREATMENT-FREE TREATMENT: A NEW ATTITUDE

Menopause is not an easy time. Beyond its real and significant physiological and psychological symptoms, it can symbolize ominous things to many women:

- It signifies the loss of the ability to have children, which, for some women, means the loss of an identity, a place of value in the world.
- For many readers of this book, it evokes memories of whispered fears of madness and death.

- It is an unarguable marker of the passing of time.
- It can bring into question our desirability as sexual beings, both to ourselves and to many men.

Real as these issues are, the fact is that every woman who lives past fifty will go through menopause; some will have an easier time than others. The challenge is to find the commitment and inner strength to maintain equilibrium and a strong positive sense of self while our bodies and psyches are under such stress. Step one in finding a healthy attitude at this point is to recognize that these doubts and fears are not trivial; they give rise to normal and natural questions.

Obviously, the treatments suggested thus far can be a big help. But attitude can also be a powerful force for the good. Many women throughout history have seen both menopause and the years after it as the most exciting, most powerful, freest time of their lives. We have plenty of role models to turn to for inspiration, both past and present.

OTHER SOCIETIES

In those societies where the elder woman has a special, often elevated status, menopause can be seen in a positive context. In some Native American cultures, women beyond menopause take on an expanded role in the community, hold greater power, and can assume responsibilities of the shaman, a doctor-priest who uses magic powers to cure the sick and control happenings that affect the welfare of people. In some South American tribal cultures, menopause is seen as liberating, giving women more social freedoms and expanded authority.

MODELS FROM THE PAST

Despite the ingrained mythology of earlier times (women = womb), there were plenty of women who did just fine living beyond their ovaries. Looking back, you can build a pretty good case that through the ages women have handled menopause best when either they or others perceived that they had a role in society besides reproduction. It boils down to a woman's sense of her own personal worth in or outside the home.

Margaret Mead seemed to celebrate menopause. This great talent and pathfinder, student of cultures and societies, of human development and human interaction, described a state of "menopausal zest"—

a phase of creativity and energy. Mead worked into her late seventies, vibrant, productive, and—according to her interviewer Gail Sheehy— taking estrogen on the sly. In *Blackberry Winter*, her autobiography, Margaret Mead describes that something "very special" happens to women when they know that they can no longer have children: "Suddenly, their whole creativity is released—they paint or write as never before, or they throw themselves into academic work with enthusiasm."

The first hundred years of the women's movement were typically led by women midlife and beyond. Elizabeth Cady Stanton was in her mid- fifties when she and Susan B. Anthony, then age forty-nine, founded the National Woman Suffrage Association, and she served as its first president until she was seventy-five years old. These two women also published and lectured extensively late into their ninth decades. Lucretia Mott, another great leader of the early women's rights movement, was in her fifties when she began to travel widely, speaking out on both the abolition of slavery and women's rights. At age fifty-seven she wrote the book *Discourse on Woman*, in which she condemned the economic, educational, and political limitations women faced throughout the Western world. Emmeline Pankhurst, who fought long and hard to get women the vote in Britain, was the next-generation suffragette who lived long enough to see that happen. As a widow in her late forties, Pankhurst broke with some of the earlier suffragettes by taking more aggressive action, such as organizing marches on Parliament and breaking windows in Parliament Square. She and her followers (including under her mentorship her two adult daughters) staged hunger strikes and endured rough handling by police and even imprisonment on several occasions, all on behalf of their cause. And in her later years she wrote an important book about the effort, *My Own Story*.

These many women had a mission and the energy to pursue it. They transformed their society at a time when the average life expectancy of women was less than fifty and when women were still being defined by their youth. The lives they lived, even independent of their cause, defined a new perspective for women and for women's health.

In our time we can all look to great women who led their countries when they themselves were over the age of fifty—Golda Meir, Indira Gandhi, and Margaret Thatcher, for example. But to younger readers, I assure you, you won't have to look far for proof of the power of the postmenopausal woman. By the time you reach menopause, you'll have more women on your side of the passage than ever before in the history of the world. More than anything, the sheer numbers of visibly successful, sexy, and active menopausal baby boomers will render any menopausal myth so obviously false that much of this chapter, I'm glad to say, will be obsolete.

For other readers, women of my generation and older, I offer the following suggestions:

- View menopause not as an end, but as a beginning. You are at a uniquely exciting turning point in your life. You have the wisdom and identity gained from having spent a considerable amount of time on this planet, yet you have fully half of your adult life left to live. Put menopause in its proper place—as a natural state of being to pass through en route to a very meaningful and productive portion of your life.

- Assess your total physical health and take action. You are at an age when modifying lifestyle, focusing on health risks and disease prevention, and actively pursuing healthy behaviors will surely alter the next thirty or more years of your life. Pay attention to diet, weight control, exercise. Consider the health benefits of hormone replacement therapy.

- Assess your self-confidence. Is your sense of personal worth wrapped up in your role as a mother? You are a uniquely powerful being. There is much you can add to the world through your creativity, your ability to nurture, to manage, to give birth to ideas and actions as well as to children. Don't take this opportunity lightly. If you can't seem to shift your outlook, get outside help. There are women's groups and excellent therapists available in every community. Menopause is not a reason for your sense of fulfillment to end; if you feel it is, you are probably using menopause to cover up what's really bothering you. Get it out and get on with your long, wonderful life.

QUESTIONS FOR YOUR DOCTOR

As you approach menopause, you must feel certain that your physician is aware of and comfortable with all aspects of menopause and menopause treatment. The following questions will help you assess her familiarity with current medical findings and also give you the answers you need to make your own decisions.

- Does your doctor work with her HRT patients to find the best treatment? How frequently do her patients tend to change treatments? Does she have a regular method of ascertaining satisfaction with each treatment—a follow-up plan? What are your personal risks with HRT?
- What are the alternatives to HRT?
- Can you still get pregnant? What is the best kind of birth control for you? How will you know when you are no longer at risk?
- What general nutritional advice can your doctor give you?
- When does your doctor believe a hysterectomy is appropriate? What are the indications? Will she be removing your ovaries? Will she be recommending HRT? (And get a second opinion about hysterectomy advice.)
- What is the appropriate schedule for screening tests on HRT? How often should you have a mammography? Pap smears? An endometrial biopsy, if at all?

Questions to ask yourself:

- Are you comfortable discussing with your doctor such issues as your mood, your sexual activity, your sexual satisfaction?

Research on menopause has been in the Dark Ages for a long time. Thanks to the studies mentioned throughout this chapter, the answers we need are finally on the way. Be aware of this information as it emerges, especially as it relates to these questions:

- What's the latest on how long you should take HRT?
- What are the health benefits of each combination schedule short- and long-term?
- What is the role of testosterone and should it be replaced?
- What are viable alternatives to HRT? Have we learned more about diet? Phytoestrogens?
- What are the true risks of low-dose HRT and breast cancer? For women who have survived breast cancer? For women who have survived heart attacks or strokes?

- What are the proven long-term benefits of HRT?
- What are the risks and benefits of hormone-like alternatives to estrogen alone?
- If you have the breast cancer gene, should you avoid HRT?

WHAT WOMEN CAN DO PERSONALLY AND POLITICALLY

Medical schools must address the concerns of women at midlife in their curricula; primary care physicians and interns must be well trained in the intricacies of menopause. And we simply need solid information on the condition of menopause. Women from all walks of life must help make these things happen, keeping the pressure on the medical community, on industry, on their elected officials, and on the media. Menopause will affect every woman, and it is every woman's responsibility to make her voice heard.

That larger issue is also the easier one. You can show by your life and your actions that the old myths are only myths, and they must be discarded. Don't buy into anybody's preconception that you don't belong wherever you want to be—in the workforce, active and aggressive, on a mountaintop, or wearing sexy lingerie. The baby boomers in twenty years will shatter any final doubts, but your life is now, and quite possibly you are about to embark on your best times ever.

Any adult woman living today has been bombarded with information about menopause. Secrecy, mystery, and fears of decay have influenced clear thinking and plain speaking about menopause. "There is nothing good about turning fifty," a woman friend of mine lamented to me some twenty years ago. Fortunately, this perspective has changed for many women; it must change for all. Menopause marks entry into a woman's new prime.

SIX

CANCER

Hurry for a Cure

When I was little I used to lie in bed at night and think about how glad I was that I was a girl and not a boy 'cause boys had to go into the army. I never wanted to fight in a war; it seemed too scary. Now, here I was, deeply embroiled in the battle of my life—a war against cancer taking place inside my own body.

— GILDA RADNER,
   IT'S ALWAYS SOMETHING, *1989*

I have known many women who have fought their own cancer wars: friends and relatives, and patients who have shouldered the double burden of heart disease and cancer. As I sit here thinking of them all on this cold December day, I ache too, over the memory of my father's long, painful, and cruel struggle with lung cancer. But perhaps my keenest understanding of the distinct emotions this disease engenders comes from an encounter with a woman I barely knew.

I met her briefly in Washington, where she had come to lobby the Hill on behalf of women like herself. Tragically, this young woman, probably in her mid-thirties, with several young children, had metastatic breast cancer, which had spread throughout her body. She told me with hope that she was about to undergo what I knew would be an extremely difficult treatment to combat her cancer. Though her face was already devastated by the disease, her skin pale, her hair gone, she radiated strength and beauty. As we parted, she looked at me intensely but with a warm smile, took my hand, and said, "Dr. Healy, hurry!"

A diagnosis of cancer brings with it a sense of urgency as no other disease can. Early detection and immediate action may well make a life-or-death difference. Movies may have overplayed the question

"How long do I have, Doctor?" but it is nonetheless a devastating one to have to ask. As a group, cancer patients have engraved the need for haste into each of our perspectives, by being more active than any other group in lobbying for public awareness and government funding for research. Cancer advocacy groups mix energy and visibility; their compelling vibrancy stems from a sense of precious time passing.

As a nation, we all associate cancer with the ticking of the clock, possibly because the cure seems so close—even within our grasp, if we could only reach out that extra inch. Since World War II, explosive change in cancer treatment has given us great optimism; cancers that once meant nothing but death can and are being beaten back, every day. We are steadily learning new things about the origins of cancer through the exploration of our own genes, possible only because of technological breakthroughs undreamed of twenty years ago. And yet, every day, people are dying. Women are dying, sometimes needlessly, of cancers that can be prevented.

The exigency of cancer takes on special significance for a woman. For one thing, the number of female sufferers is formidable: cancer is fast gaining on heart disease as the biggest killer of women; all told, in 1995 cancer will claim the lives of more than a quarter-million U.S. women, while more than a half-million others will be newly diagnosed. What these shocking figures do not reveal is the scope and depth of anguish that accompanies cancer for a woman. For a man, cancer is a life-threatening, terrifying disease. For a woman, cancer often threatens not only her life but her essence, her identity, her woman's soul. Why? Half of all the cancers that attack women are unique to women. Cancer for a woman can mean the permanent loss of fertility, the loss or disfigurement of her breasts, her ovaries, her uterus.

Women are, as we'll see throughout this chapter, made more or less vulnerable to cancer through our sexual and reproductive choices, and even through our societal conditioning. A woman's own sexuality can turn on her and become her enemy from within. There is no evidence in this lopsided world that the procreative decisions men make throughout their lives—choosing many or few sexual partners, fathering one or twenty children, getting vasectomies—influence their getting cancer.

Yet it is also in the cancer fight that we women can find our greatest model of achievement in women's advocacy. We have wielded our power to achieve funding, attention, and medical advances in breast cancer that have saved thousands of lives.

For all these reasons, I focus the bulk of this chapter on the crucial forms of cancer to which women are particularly exposed. "Hurry" for a woman must signify more than the urgency prompted by the disease's clear progression with time, or the loud voices of advocacy groups, or the optimism of the cure around the corner. "Hurry" for us must mean a rush to understand our own cancer profiles: to find hope in what we've already accomplished, to acknowledge our unique risks, to be less afraid, and to take more control over what we do.

WHAT IS CANCER?

Cancer is not one disease, but a variety of diseases that share one key property: uncontrolled and invasive growth of an alien form of a normal tissue. (Cancers can actually be "solid" and tumor- or mass-forming, or liquid and floating in the blood or lymph system, such as leukemia. We will be looking at the more common "solid" cancers in this chapter.) Some combination of factors—inherited, environmental, or simply inexplicable—induce our own cells to mutate and suddenly attack the very body they were created to preserve. All it takes is one tiny cell to turn; once it does, it will divide and reproduce itself constantly, like the water buckets in Disney's *Sorcerer's Apprentice*. Initially, the cells produced will cluster into a clump or mass of visible tissue, called a *tumor*. The tumor grows larger and larger; its size doesn't get in its way, for the malevolent cells that constitute it know how to provide their own blood supplies. They sprout their own capillaries and vessels, which siphon off nutrients from our bloodstream.

Cancer cells seem eventually to grow impatient at being in one place. When a tumor is unchecked, cells ultimately break off and show off their unnatural mobility as they spread throughout the body, or metastasize. They secrete enzymes that destroy the membranous barriers that enclose them, and penetrate the walls of normally impervious tissue; they wander like vagabond thieves through the circulatory system of the body—through both the blood vessels and the lymph system—and invade parts of the body where they have no business being, attaching themselves to a remote vessel wall or a distant, unrelated tissue. A nest of cancerous breast cells may take hold in the brain or the liver, for example, or ovarian cancer may invade the bowel.

This progression—from one sick cell, to the microscopic nest of cells, to a visible growing tumor, to a metastasized cancer—can develop over as many as ten or twenty years, or as quickly as a few months. The treatment and prognosis depend in large part upon how far the cancer has spread, and on the type of cancer cell (some grow faster than others). Physicians find it useful to pinpoint the progress of most types of cancer by using the label of "stages." Not all cancers conform precisely to a neat staging scheme, but the concept of stages remains key to any cancer treatment, and you'll find it throughout this chapter.

WHERE CANCER COMES FROM

What is the factor that causes that one wild cell to mutate and initiate the horrible cancer chain reaction? As with so many other illnesses, the causes of cancer are complex and often intertwined. But cancer, we've recently learned, always boils down to the deepest molecular level—cancer occurs when the masterminds within an individual cell, the genes, tell it to divide into an abnormal variation or fail to provide a check or balance on growth.

Every one of the millions of cells in our bodies (except the egg and sperm cells, which carry twenty-three single chromosomes) carries twenty-three chromosome pairs; each chromosome carries thousands of genes. Most of the genes in each cell lie dormant, but those genes that are "expressed," or active, regulate the entire cell—its growth, its traits, how frequently it divides, and so forth.

Cancer is never the result of just one gene's perverse instructions. For the cell to turn, it needs to be the target of several (some estimate from three to seven) genetic "hits." Genes are constantly dividing and reproducing themselves—billions of times through the course of a lifetime. In the course of the division, there can be a spontaneous error, an unhappy accident—one hit. Some cancers can be traced directly to an inherited faulty gene that multiplies itself billions of times—another hit. External and often controllable environmental factors can prompt a gene to mutate—yet another hit. As we'll see later, some of the genes we carry have a counterbalancing role, causing an abnormal cell to self-destruct, or correcting errors of cell division. If one of these counterbalancing genes malfunctions, and its protective job becomes perverted, that may mean another hit, the one that triggers the start of cancer.

Obtaining a fundamental understanding of what makes a cancer cell a cancer cell is the greatest hope we have for working out a cure. And we are very close—we are in the midst of an explosion of knowledge about the molecular basis of cancer. This understanding of the

GENES, THE GENOME, AND THE MOLECULE OF THE YEAR

Researchers have discovered that the genes present in cancerous tumors are in fact mutations—not strange external creatures, but related in some way to normal cell growth. We have now been able to identify more than a hundred gene mutations that in some way contribute to the multifarious interactions that allow a cancer to take off, and take over.

CANCER-RELATED GENES

Many cancer-related genes identified, mostly through the support of the National Cancer Institute's "War on Cancer," fit into several categories:

• ONCOGENES *are genes that are critical to normal growth but for some reason appear at the wrong place at the wrong time, contributing to the transformation of a normal cell into a cancer cell.*

• SPELL-CHECKER OR EDITING GENES *double-check the genetic code every time it duplicates itself in a cell division. When the spell-checker gene is not functioning properly or is not present, there is nothing to stop an error from continuing to replicate itself.*

• GENES THAT REGULATE THE SURFACE APPEARANCE OF CELLS *may lead us to identify tumor cells.*

• TUMOR-SUPPRESSOR GENES *are supposed to stop cells from forming tumors. When they break down, cancer can result.*

One important cancer-related gene was named "molecule of the year" by Science *magazine. This gene, eloquently called by the code name p53, is a tumor-suppressor gene, normally programed to keep us from getting cancer by slowing down cell growth (or even bringing it to a brief halt) so that natural repair mechanisms can get to work. The p53 gene is also a* so-called defending angel that brings cell death when damage is too extensive to be repaired. A mutation in the gene is associated with tumors that spread throughout the body very quickly, and a lower chance of survival. By the close of 1993, researchers had identified more than fifty types of tumors containing p53 mutations. That means that p53 isn't limited to one type of cancer, but that cancers of different types may be related. This astounding fact affords great optimism to all searching for a cancer cure. If a recurrent mutation exists that prompts many types of cancers, there may be a generally applicable way of supporting this gene so that it doesn't transform, and perhaps halting the progress of many types of cancer.

THE HUMAN GENOME PROJECT

Many disease-causing genes are being identified under the auspices of one of the most important new programs of the National Institutes of Health, the Human Genome Project. Its goal is to map and sequence the entire "human genome"—that is, every human gene present on each of the forty-six chromosomes. Remember—even though the form differs from person to person, each kind of gene is present in all humans, carrying out a certain kind of function. Also remember, however, that not all the genes in the genome are "expressed." In the process of identifying the fifty thousand to a hundred thousand total genes, the NIH hopes to target the five thousand or more expressed genes, the ones that determine our traits and when abnormal, can explain the development of human disease. This project has an especially critical role to play in our war against cancer. Being able to link a gene on a specific chromosome with cancer allows us to describe precisely how the cancer is initiated. (Of course, identifying genetic flaws that might lead to cancer can be treacherous, and is not without its controversial implications, several of which we'll be exploring.)

complex genetic underpinnings of the disease is probably the most exciting, ongoing discovery of this century. Now that we've learned it takes many factors to trigger cancer, we can probably block the development of the cancer by getting in the way of just one of those factors. We may be able to put up a barricade by actually altering our genes (see sidebars, pages 218–19), and in the meantime, whether or not we are genetically predisposed to cancer, we can be foot soldiers in our own anticancer wars all our lives. We can weaken the enemy by eliminating or lessening the risk factors we can see in our own environments, as I will discuss throughout the chapter.

GENERAL CANCER RISK FACTORS

Any graph of the path cancer cuts across our nation would show odd and wandering shifts in its incidence. The erratic jogs and jags of this path reflect the changing character of our society, and its good and bad habits and differing environmental hazards. We'll examine the actions and environments that put women at risk for specific forms of cancers later in this chapter; here are the risk factors that apply to all.

AGE

Every decade an adult woman lives brings with it a doubling of her chances of getting some type of cancer. Most cancers occur in midlife, or later, with a sharp increase at age fifty. This means that, as we get older, we must all get wiser about cancer risk, prevention, and early detection.

DIET

Though at this point no sound scientific studies have been made, I'm convinced we'll soon find a strong link between diet and many types of cancers. There are hints everywhere we turn: we can't ignore the large population studies showing clear relationships between the diets of entire cultures or subgroups of individuals and the prevalence of cancer, and I suspect in time we'll also learn more about the very specific factors in certain foods that affect the overall tendency of cells to mutate. Specifically, a high-fat diet among certain population groups has repeatedly been linked to many of the cancers we'll discuss in this chapter, as has a diet low in fiber. Oriental diets high in tofu or other soy products have been linked to less incidence of breast and prostate cancer, regular consumption of garlic to less colon cancer. Many cancers have been tied to heavy consumption of salt-cured, pickled, or smoked foods, and alcohol in excess.

EXERCISE

A sedentary lifestyle is suspected to increase the risk of many types of cancer, although a definitive controlled trial has yet to be done. Certainly exercise promotes the health of the immune system, our natural cancer fighter.

ENVIRONMENTAL HAZARDS

You may find it surprising to learn that environmental chemicals are not major cancer risk factors. Yes, they are often linked to cancer in laboratory animals, but circumstantial evidence, at least, suggests there is not a strong or obvious connection in humans. Though the number of industrial chemicals present in our environment over the past fifty or so years has increased, the incidence of most cancers—after one corrects the statistics for tobacco and age—has not.

Radiation is the one environmental hazard known to be clearly linked to cancer—not only the radiation from radioactive substances and X rays, but also and especially the ultraviolet radiation emanating from the sun. (Electromagnetic radiation from power lines, computers, and a host of other devices has recently been labeled a cancer cause, but years of epidemiological studies have failed to establish a definite relationship; this suggests that if such a relationship exists it is at the most very slight.)

TOBACCO

Tobacco is a well-known carcinogen, linked to many cancers. It's an insidious enemy; though cigarettes trigger cancer early, most cancers do not show up for perhaps twenty or thirty years after the first exposure to the toxin. Women did not start to smoke in any great numbers until the 1950s—and we are just now seeing the impact. The picture is not pretty, as we'll explore beginning on page 259.

VIRUSES

For years scientists have pursued the theory that cancer is itself a virus, but have been unable to prove this in any large-scale way. A few viruses have been shown to be clear risk factors for specific types of cancers. Epstein-Barr, hepatitis B, and HIV all directly or indirectly contribute to cancer causation, and as we'll see on page 246, the human papilloma virus (which sometimes causes genital warts) is a critical precursor to cervical cancer. Curiously, where viruses may end up having the most relevance to cancer is in cancer treatment, through the new science of gene therapy: we may be able to use viruses to carry into the cancerous cells therapeutic genes that manufacture cancer-fighting molecules—in effect, using the infecting properties of the virus to contaminate the cancerous cells with the "disease" of a cure.

DETECTING CANCER

What all cancers have in common, no matter the cause or the type, is that no single medical intervention saves more lives than early detection. Early detection can mean a cure rate of 80 to 90 percent; late detection can mean a life will end within a year.

THE EARLIEST DETECTION: FINDING CANCER IN YOUR GENES

As we've seen, we are on the verge of being able to ascertain each individual's genetic risks for cancer long before any symptoms appear. You could take a blood test right now, and discover the likelihood that you will be stricken with certain types of cancer—such as some endocrine gland cancers and a rare eye tumor called retinoblastoma. There are now tests for abnormalities in the p53 gene, and tests for the genes for colon and breast cancer are being developed; these indicate an increased risk for cancer with sometimes uncanny precision, as we will see later. Again, such abnormalities do not mean you have cancer, only that you have one hit against you and are at greater risk.

The implications are enormous, of course. Peering into a genetic crystal ball to learn of a risk that is not a certainty, when a cancer cure is still unknown, leads to bewildering and unanswerable questions, such as "Do I want to know?" A clear genetic risk can be an obvious incentive to screen aggressively and take powerful precautions to minimize other, controllable risk factors. But even larger medical, ethical, economic, and legal issues accompany such knowledge—issues we as a society have yet to address.

For some women, such as Gilda Radner, detecting the genetic risk doesn't require a test tube. Her dad died of a malignant brain tumor; her grandmother succumbed to stomach cancer; her mother, Henrietta, had breast cancer; and her mother's sister, Elsie, died of stomach cancer. Gilda's cousins battled breast cancer and cancer of the ovary. Many women who would test for a cancer gene come from similar backgrounds. These women know we cannot escape our genes—but we may be able to control them, and it is likely that such diagnostic genetic testing will lead us to a clear understanding of just how such genes and their products work within a given cell to cause a cancer. Knowing the enemy is good. Knowing what the enemy will do is better. This knowledge puts us on the road to cures.

DOCTOR VISITS AND SELF-AWARENESS

We are not at that futuristic point where we can get a blood test and screen for all cancers (perhaps some would say, "Thank goodness"). Currently, the best means of detecting cancer early is through regular visits to your primary care physician or gynecologist so she can monitor any changes in your body and perform routine screening tests. The screening tests that a good doctor insists upon can expose a problem before it begins to show itself to you. Even so, you are probably the best analyst of your own body. Know your body, and keep in mind the early warning signs:

THE AMERICAN CANCER SOCIETY'S SEVEN
EARLY WARNING SIGNS OF CANCER

- A change in bowel or bladder habits.
- A sore that does not heal.
- Unusual bleeding or discharge from the vagina or rectum.
- A thickening or lump in the breast or elsewhere.
- Indigestion and/or difficulty swallowing.
- An obvious change in a wart or mole.
- A nagging cough or hoarseness.

Women need to be aware of their bodies. Many are not as familiar with their bodies as they might think. When you notice a mole or lump or funny discharge, you shouldn't have to struggle to remember if it is new or something that you have had for years. Such signs or symptoms are prompts, and mean that you should see your doctor—without procrastination.

If your physician suspects cancer, and early screening tests support his concern, you have now at your fingertips a number of incredibly sophisticated and accurate tools through which to identify and describe the nature and scope of the cancer very early on. Which of the tests your doctor recommends depends upon the type of cancer and your symptoms. A cancer specialist, called an *oncologist,* is trained to help you with these decisions and to manage cancer treatments.

COMPUTED TOMOGRAPHY (CT OR CAT) SCANS

These use X rays to create images of an organ in "slices" a millimeter wide or less. Newly developed computer programs then take the images and turn them into a three-dimensional reproduction of the organ and/or the tumor in the organ. That image can be rotated and studied from any angle at the punch of a few computer keys.

MAGNETIC RESONANCE IMAGING (MRI)

This new and even more advanced technology uses electromagnetic fields and computer analysis to create very accurate three-dimensional images that can pinpoint virtually any organ in the body. The evolving technology is getting better all the time; for example, a new method of processing the image allows an image to be taken in less than twenty seconds. MRI can also measure certain biochemical functions in tissues.

ULTRASOUND IMAGING

A less costly technology involving no X rays, ultrasound can be performed in a physician's office. An ultrasound machine directs short pulses of sound toward the tissue; the sound waves bounce back, providing two-dimensional images of internal organs.

RADIONUCLIDE SCANS

Various compounds that have been tagged with minute quantities of nontoxic radioactive isotopes are injected into the bloodstream and concentrate in various organs, such as the brain, bone, and liver. A camera or computer registers the radioactive emissions externally and creates an image. The sensors that detect the radiation are extremely sensitive, and getting more so. New combinations of isotopes and proteins that bind to specific cells are also under continual development, to make these tests even more specific for a given cancer.

POSITRON EMISSION TOMOGRAPHY (PET SCAN)

Positron emission tomography is a method of scanning specific organs with radioactively charged elements—including carbon, hydrogen, nitrogen, and oxygen—that take part in the cell's biochemical processes. Computer techniques then construct three-dimensional images of the scanned tissue. Tumors tend to have more active metabolism than normal tissue, and PET scanning has been valuable in detecting tumors, particularly in the brain, by picking up this more rapid or distinctive biochemical function. The technology is expensive, however, and not available in most medical centers.

ENDOSCOPY

The most powerful and least invasive way to identify a tumor without actual surgery, endoscopy has been around more than thirty years, but has been turned into a lifesaver by recent technology incorporating fiberoptic cables, computers, and video cameras. In any type of endoscopy, a tube is inserted into your body, generally through a body cavity (through the mouth and throat in bronchoscopy, to examine the lungs; through the mouth and esophagus in gastroscopy, to examine the stomach; through the anus in colonoscopy, to examine the colon). Through the tube, a myriad of functions can be performed. It can be used as a camera; tiny surgical blades and lasers can be fed through it to gather suspicious tissue or actually perform minor surgery.

Sometimes the endoscopy does require an incision through the skin. With a laparoscopy (an outpatient procedure), a specially fitted fiberoptic tube is inserted into the abdominal cavity through a tiny incision in the belly button. That tube can be snaked around the inside of the abdominal and pelvic cavity to obtain images of the ovaries, the surface of the uterus, and nearby structures such as the wall of the pelvis and the outer surface of the intestines.

TUMOR SAMPLES OR BIOPSIES

Though the tests above can be used both before a definitive diagnosis (to determine the likelihood of a tumor) or after (to determine the position and extent of the tumor), almost the only way to know for sure whether you have cancer is if a sample of the tumor itself is studied under the microscope by an expert, usually a cancer pathologist. The tissue can be obtained by biopsy, the cutting out of a small piece of suspicious tissue, which can sometimes be performed through endoscopy. Or sample cells can be captured by taking body fluid that bathes a suspicious area (such as bronchial washings, or fluid from an ovarian cyst), or by taking a scraping of the tissue to get surface cells (as is done with a Pap smear).

TREATMENT

We may not yet have found the secret in our genes that can irreversibly rid our bodies of cancerous cells, but we have learned to fight the good fight in the meantime. There are three established approaches to cancer treatment—surgery, radiation therapy, and chemotherapy—and one emerging approach, immunotherapy. All are designed to remove or destroy the cancer cells while doing as little damage to healthy tissue as possible.

SURGERY

Physically removing the tumor through surgery is usually the primary treatment. Tumors have been removed by surgery for more than thirty-five hundred years. For cancer in an early stage, it is still the most effective and often the most curative therapy. Of course, techniques have changed over time. The technological imaging devices described above that are used to detect cancer also allow surgeons to pinpoint and remove tumors with greater accuracy and confidence than ever before. New tools are being developed as well, ranging from "electrosurgery" (used thus far to treat epidermal cancers of the skin and rectum through electric current) to "cryosurgery" (which employs liquid nitrogen to freeze tumors, particularly superficial skin cancers) to laser surgery (using a high-intensity light beam that destroys cells it touches but leaves adjacent cells healthy; this is applied to cancers of the larynx and esophagus, and used for benign conditions such as endometriosis, ovarian cysts, and fibroids).

The basic philosophies behind cancer surgery have also recently undergone substantial change. For most of this century, there was but one surgical approach—a radical one. The belief was that, the more adjacent (and healthy) tissue, bone, skin, and muscle you could cut out, the more successful you would be at preventing the spread of the cancer cells. We now know that in most cases such drastic measures are not necessary: less radical approaches may bring equal benefit and produce far less disability.

For thousands of years, surgery was employed as the only method of cancer therapy. Not anymore. To stop the spread of cells invisible to any surgeon's eye, surgical procedures are combined with chemical and radiation treatment before and/or after the operation (see below). Although this practice, called *adjuvant* therapy, reduces the risk of recurrent cancer and death in most patients, its effectiveness will vary with the tumor type.

RADIATION THERAPY

It is a bit ironic that a risk factor for cancer is also one of its most established methods of treatment, but radiation therapy is a powerful and effective means of shrinking or even destroying cancerous tumors. Radiation kills cells, especially when they are in the process of dividing—and cancer cells divide incessantly. It also destroys normal cells, and must therefore be used only in a rigidly controlled and targeted manner. The therapy appeared on the scene early in this century, and was first given in one or two giant doses—not, we have found, the safest thing to do. During the past thirty years or more, we have seen radiation therapy change from an anticancer weapon resembling a cannon to one more like a high-powered rifle. Treatments now consist of a few minutes' exposure to the radiation beam on a more or less daily basis for several weeks, depending on the size and nature of the cancer being treated. It penetrates more deeply and strikes tumors with greater accuracy than ever before. (Doctors who prescribe and administer radiation therapy are called *radiation oncologists*.)

For some well-defined tumors, radiation may even supplant surgery as the primary approach, but it is usually used as an adjuvant therapy, applied before surgery to shrink a tumor or after therapy to destroy cells and cell masses the scalpel may have missed or been unable to reach. Sometimes short-term radiation treatments are given to increase the comfort of a dying cancer victim by shrinking a painful tumor that is too large to remove. This is called *palliative* treatment.

Radiation is painless, but its side effects can range from fatigue to skin changes, including dryness, itching, and sometimes redness and irritation, like a sunburn. Nausea, vomiting, and diarrhea may also occur. Most of these effects can be minimized by targeting the radiation exposure.

Both surgery and radiation therapy are effective in fighting the primary tumor and its local extension. What they cannot fight are the small clumps of cancer cells that get into the circulatory system and hide in distant sites. Most often, it is this metastasis, or distant-spreading, that destroys the body and a life. Chemotherapy is the tool used to battle it.

CHEMOTHERAPY

From an ugly agent of death used in World War I in Europe was born a chance for life for today's cancer victims. This nefarious chemical weapon, nitrogen mustard gas, damaged cells' ability to divide. When troops were exposed to it, their lymph nodes shrunk dramatically; researchers noted this fact, tested nitrogen mustard on advanced lymph node cancers, and found breakthrough success. Based upon that experience, another cell growth inhibitor, methotrexate, was tested in advanced cancers in the late 1940s, again with extraordinary results. Methotrexate was first successful in young women, causing choriocarcinoma, a rare cancer of the placenta, to regress and in some cases to disappear entirely. And so chemotherapy was begun.

The term *chemotherapy* was derived from these deadly cell-killing agents, but now has been expanded to include any drug therapy used in the treatment of cancer. During the past fifty or so years, numerous chemotherapeutic agents have arisen that work in much the same way as those first noxious drugs: by infusing the body with a toxin that interferes with the fundamental machinery of gene replication, thereby destroying rapidly reproducing cells—namely, cancer.

Depending on the tumor type, your oncologist will choose the drugs that research has shown are best suited to your illness. In many cases, several different chemotherapeutic drugs are used at once, in an effort to overcome the resistance tumors can develop to one agent alone. Many chemotherapy drugs are naturally occurring substances: doxorubicin (Adriamycin) and mitomycin (Mutamycin) are antibiotic-like substances produced by bacteria and used to fight cancers such as breast, lung, cervix, and bladder; platinum, a naturally occurring element in nature, is the core component of cisplatin, used to fight tumors of the testes and ovary; arabinosyl-cytosine, found in ocean sponges, has been of great value in treating leukemia; and vincristine and vinblastine are found in the periwinkle plant. The bark of the yew tree gave us one of the newest anticancer drugs, Taxol, which interferes with the cancer cell's internal architecture and has produced some dramatic responses against advanced cancers with distant spread, such as those of the ovary, and holds promise for other cancers.

Many naturally occurring hormones or drugs that block them, including estrogens, progestins, and androgens, are effective chemotherapeutic drugs for hormone-sensitive tumors. Often making a direct impact on the growth and development of certain cells, these can have a significant effect on cells that are dividing out of control.

These powerful and toxic anti-cancer drugs do inevitably affect normal cells as well as the rapidly dividing cancer cells, causing side effects (which vary from drug to drug) including nausea and vomiting, loss of appetite, hair loss, general weakness, kidney or temporary nerve damage, and interference with the functioning of the bone marrow. The bone marrow is the center where the most rapid dividing of our healthy cells takes place, including new red blood cells, which carry vital oxygen through our bloodstream to all our organs; new white cells, critical to our immune system; and platelets, which help with blood clotting. When the bone marrow is damaged, we become vulnerable to anemia, infections, and bleeding. Most of these effects, including the suppression of the bone marrow, are transient, but some other serious effects may linger, such as loss of fertility, weakness of the heart muscle, and, rarely—but it happens—an increased risk of getting a second cancer.

IMMUNOTHERAPY

The newest strategy in combating cancer, immunotherapy, encourages the body to start its own sort of chemotherapy—one that lacks many of standard chemotherapy's side effects. Such therapy would have been impossible to imagine without the progress we have made in understanding the molecular basis of cancer, in identifying particular genes, and in understanding the complex mix of cells and proteins the body produces in its own natural defense against invading organisms or alien cells. With immunotherapy, the body's own army of cancer-fighting agents is marshaled, strengthened, and sometimes augmented in a wide variety of ways.

In one approach to immunotherapy, drugs or the patient's own killed tumor cells are administered to prompt tumor cells to produce inordinate amounts of tumor-specific markers. These markers act as a clear bull's-eye, encouraging the body's own immune system to speed antibody bullets to destroy the tumor. It is as if the tumor cells are made to taunt, "I am a cancer, come and get me." Certain drugs

STUDIES TO WATCH FOR: BONE MARROW TRANSPLANTS FOR CANCER TREATMENT

Bone marrow transplants have been used to treat certain cancers of the circulatory system, such as lymphoma and leukemia, for more than twenty years. More recently, the procedure has been modified to treat very advanced solid tumors in other parts of the body. Though the new use of this treatment has obvious relevance for women, it is controversial and unproven over the long term.

In this experimental therapy used to treat very advanced cases of cancer, samples of a cancer patient's own bone marrow (autologous bone marrow) are removed and stored. In more recent approaches, the patient's blood system is stimulated by special growth factors to produce more bone marrow stem cells (stem cells are the precursors from which the circulating red and white blood cells originate). Then, some of these cells are obtained from the bloodstream, obviating the need to take marrow. The patient is next given very high levels of chemotherapy and/or radiation, basically killing off all rapidly dividing cells in the body (tumor cells and also bone marrow cells). After that, the patient's own preserved bone marrow cells are restored.

The theory behind this therapy is that, when a portion of the bone

(BCG and levamisole) stimulate the immune system and enhance the body's ability to destroy tumor cells actively. This approach to cancer treatment is even now being applied to cancers that are unresponsive to conventional chemotherapy, such as colon cancer and malignant melanoma.

In another approach, the patient's tumor is removed at surgery, antibodies are developed from it in a laboratory, and then, through a chemical bonding process, radioactive molecules or chemotherapy toxins are actually attached to the antibody. The antibodies are then injected back into the body; they zero in on the specific tumor antigens from which they were created and deliver toxic payloads of radiation

marrow is removed and held in reserve, you can give exceedingly high doses of cancer-fighting drugs, knowing that, even if the existing bone marrow is destroyed, it will be replaced. Generally, the higher the drug dose, the more effective it is in killing the tumor—and the greater its toxicity, especially to the bone marrow. If we can hold on to our healthy marrow and kill off the tumor, the replaced marrow will produce only healthy blood cells, and ultimately the body will be rid of the cancer.

Autologous bone marrow transplantation has been used for breast and ovarian cancer patients. Researchers have shown lengthened survival in those with breast cancer who have ten or more lymph nodes positive for cancer but no other spread; a study is now looking at those with five to nine positive nodes. But the practice has as many detractors as it does advocates. ABMT is a toxic treatment (a patient is without any reliable immune system for a period of weeks), as well as an expensive one; we do not know the full consequences of highly toxic levels of chemotherapeutics on other parts of the body; some women have found the treatment unendurable and the results negligible.

A randomized clinical trial of this treatment involving medical centers throughout the country is being conducted by the National Cancer Institute (NCI) under the leadership of researchers at Duke University. Since many years of follow-up are needed to see if cancer recurs, the final results are not likely to be available before the end of the decade.

or toxins, like the biologic equivalent of smart bombs. This approach, still under investigation, holds the promise that high doses of drugs can be used without causing the usual great damage to normal cells; but its long-term effect on survival is by no means established, and has in fact been disappointing in some patients.

An even more recent form of immunotherapy, called *biological response modifiers,* exposes the tumor to high levels of purified molecules, *cytokines,* which naturally augment the human immune system. For many of these natural molecules, genes have been isolated, making it possible to produce them in large quantities and then administer them to patients just like a drug. The interferons, molecules produced in small quantities normally by white blood cells in response to viral infections, in higher concentrations will inhibit tumor cell growth, destroy some tumor cells, and attract and activate powerful white blood cells called *macrophages* and *killer lymphocytes* to attack the tumor. The interferons have shown promising results with certain advanced cancers including those of the lymph system and the kidney. Interleukin-2, another cytokine, marshals several different kinds of lymphocytes to attack tumor, and has been shown, by Dr. Steven Rosenberg and his colleagues at the NIH, to be effective against some advanced forms of the skin cancer malignant melanoma. Other biological response modifiers include *tumor necrosis factor* and certain "colony"-stimulating factors that cause the body's own tumor-fighting cells to multiply rapidly.

Dr. Rosenberg and others in the field are now combining immunotherapy with gene therapy. Since the genes for most of these naturally occurring biological response modifiers are known, cells from the patient's own tumor can be genetically engineered to manufacture very high levels of these tumor killing compounds selectively, locally at the tumor site. The tumor in essence takes up a poison pill that is otherwise a normal part of the body's immune system. The power of tumor-specific gene therapy to carry in natural killer molecules to the tumor, wherever it has spread, may allow us to develop vaccines for cancer, able to work even when the cancer is advanced.

WHEN THERAPY FAILS: HOSPICE CARE AND PALLIATION

The late Elizabeth Gee captured the spiritual dimension of dying in her book *The Light Around the Dark,* in which she recounted her struggle as a young wife, mother, and educator afflicted with a highly aggressive form of breast cancer in her mid-thirties. "Before I had cancer, I would spend time in seemingly mundane activities: reading a newspaper, outlining a research project, loading the dishwasher. Now I can't go a day without reflection. . . . Is this my dying time? I must learn to die. What is death's lesson? Is it to inform one of life, to throw light on the moment? Without death, would we ponder the mystery of being?"

Advanced forms of cancer that have defied our medical miracles force us to face with our loved ones a "dying time," a period of weeks to months when we prepare together for the end. Though there has been in our society a growing awareness of the needs of the terminally ill, far too few hospice facilities or palliative care providers are available to ensure the type of individualized care that is needed. In an ideal hospice, the emphasis shifts from medical combat, to relief of pain and suffering and the providing of companionship, spiritual comfort, overall physical and emotional support, and help with the basic functions of the body. Specialist nurses and other health care workers are present around the clock, administering music therapy, massage, beauty treatments, and spiritual counseling, along with conventional medicine. Alternatively, for those who wish to die at home, the best of palliative caregivers would help the family care for the terminally ill patients, assisting them with home health services and periodic visits.

Hospices exist and flourish out of a core respect for the dignity of the dying and for the struggles of the family. In many ways, the hospice transcends medicine; it is a reflection of the values of a community.

THE CANCERS OF WOMEN

When I was sixteen, my mother suggested that I visit a family friend in her late thirties who was in the hospital just a few blocks away from my high school. I didn't know why she was there, only that she had a mysterious "problem" that needed surgery. I was intimidated by the huge hospital, and a bit frightened to see her—she looked so fragile and pale in her sterile, narrow hospital bed. Marilyn whispered to me that she had breast cancer; tearfully she showed me the mass of white bandages encasing her chest and her abdomen, the result of radical breast surgery and another surgery to remove her ovaries. I tried to comfort her, chatter about school, take her mind off the coldness around her. Finally, I sat up straight and, in my best rendition of what I thought a doctor should be, said very directly and firmly that I knew she would get through this because she was such a strong woman. She gazed at me for a moment and said, "But, Bernie, that's the problem. I don't think I am a woman anymore."

Physicians don't treat breast cancer in this way today, but the cancers that strike only women still involve such intimate and personal dimensions of our lives and our bodies that our womanhood cannot be separated from any discussion. Cancers of the breasts and reproductive organs are obviously unwelcome potential consequences of being a woman (although you may be surprised how much the choices you make as a woman influence your risks); lung cancer, colon cancer, and skin cancer have long been viewed as "men's diseases," but the changing world around us has made these cancers women's diseases as well, and dramatically so. I hope through this chapter to demystify these diseases, to help put them in their appropriate place as illnesses that, though women are vulnerable to them, do not have to rob them of their womanhood, or in many cases of their lives.

BREAST CANCER

Twenty years ago, breast cancer was a disease spoken of only in whispers. For one thing, it was generally not spotted until it had progressed beyond the point of successful treatment. It also served as a horrifying symbol of how women viewed themselves, and how much of society viewed women—women were objects with little or no ability to decide their fate; they were put to sleep on operating tables with no idea of whether they would wake up with or without their breasts, depending on what the surgeon did or did not find; doctors did not talk to women about choices, and women did not complain.

None of this is true now. The transformation is almost beyond belief. Breast cancer has come to embody the standard on which all women's health efforts can be modeled. Women began asking questions individually, participating in research that led to less radical treatment. Women began to become partners in their own health care. In groups, we insisted that women become educated, and breast cancer self-examination became part of the vocabulary (and habit) of most women. Breast cancer entered the political arena, empowered by First Lady Betty Ford's great gift of coming forward to publicly speak about her struggle with breast cancer, opening the way for many others to tell their stories. Today the research budget exceeds four hundred million dollars.

Such advances are not without their flip side. Be aware that breast cancer has taken on another symbolic meaning, becoming a code word for *women's health* in the mouths of many politicians and government agencies. A candidate will often say, "I support breast cancer research," and do so, in the hopes of getting the female vote—and at the expense of most other critical areas in women's health and an understanding of the importance of attention to the larger issue of women as whole humans.

The battle against breast cancer is not yet won. As inspiring as this battle is as a model of advocacy, the disease remains a devastating issue for any woman who contracts it. Breast cancer generates about a third of all cancer death in women; it's the leading cause of death in women between the ages of forty and fifty-five. This year alone, more than 200,000 American women will be diagnosed with breast cancer, and 46,000 will die of the disease. Each of us individually faces a one-in-eight chance of getting breast cancer in her lifetime. Despite our many advances in treatment, the incidence of breast cancer keeps rising, and no one knows exactly why. It may be that the population is aging and the illness correlates with age, or perhaps it has to do with unproven and poorly defined environmental factors. We may well simply be better at diagnosing the disease and correctly labeling cases we would have missed in the past. The good news is that the mortality rate has gone down by 5 percent over the past twenty years—although a modest gain, it is a testament to earlier detection.

RISK FACTORS FOR BREAST CANCER

All adult women, particularly as they move beyond their fourth decade, must see themselves as being at high risk for breast cancer. White women have more breast cancer than African-American and Asian women; but no woman is immune because of her race. There are factors for the illness that make some women more vulnerable, but only about 20 percent of all women who are afflicted can be shown to have experienced either inherited or other recognizable risks that set them apart from other women.

Family History and Inherited Genes

The most powerful risk factor for breast cancer is heredity—but even heredity accounts for only 5 to 10 percent of all breast cancer. Heredity is a more powerful determinant of breast cancer at a young age; a quarter of all women who have breast cancer under the age of fifty also have first-degree relatives—mothers or aunts or sisters—who have experienced it.

One of the most exciting health discoveries of the nineties will surely prove to be the recent identification of the specific family genes associated with breast cancer. The research has been part of a highly targeted, nationwide gene-hunt. In late 1994, mutations in BRCA-1, an unusually large gene making up part of chromosome 17, were isolated in women with strong family histories of breast and ovarian cancer, by a group from Utah headed by Dr. Mark Skolnick. BRCA-1, which may also be linked to cancer of the colon and prostate, appears to be a tumor-suppressor gene; about half of all families in which there is a recurrent history of breast cancer are now believed to have a mutation in this gene, and four out of five families with strong histories of both breast and ovarian cancer at a young age carry abnormal BRCA-1. If an individual woman is found to have a faulty copy of BRCA-1, she has more than an 85 percent chance of getting breast cancer in her lifetime.

No sooner had BRCA-1 been reported than the race shifted to a second, equally important breast cancer gene, called BRCA-2, which is located on chromosome 13. Flawed BRCA-2 is associated only with breast cancer, and in men as well as women. (Yes, men do get breast cancer, but very rarely.) These two genes together are thought to account for almost all hereditary cancers of the breast.

Hormones and Reproductive History

The tie between our reproductive hormones and breast cancer is complicated and still a bit perplexing. It appears that women's choices as to when to have babies, and whether or not to have abortions, may have an impact on their ultimate risk of breast cancer. Also, the hormones women produce naturally or as therapy seem to affect their risk.

The primary female hormone we produce naturally, estrogen, works as a woman's strong health ally, by protecting her from heart disease, stroke, perhaps Alzheimer's, and certainly the many symptoms of menopause. But estrogen is no defender against breast cancer. It actually induces breast cell proliferation; progesterone, another important female hormone, which works hand in hand with estrogen, only enhances the effect. The more the cells proliferate, the greater the chance that a replication will go awry, producing a cancerous cell. The longer a woman is fertile, the more her body is exposed to estrogen, so the finding that an early menarche followed by late menopause is associated with increased breast cancer seems to be common sense. Early menarche or not, women who have their menopause after age fifty-five have been shown to run nearly twice the risk of breast cancer that women who reach menopause by age forty-five do.

Our bodies don't always behave as expected. Since both estrogen and progesterone levels rise during pregnancy, one might think that the risk of breast cancer would also rise for each pregnancy. The opposite is true—delayed childbearing and no childbearing have been linked to an increased likelihood of breast cancer. (Remember that there are three forms of estrogen in our bodies—estradiol, estrone, and estriol—as discussed on page 188. Though estradiol and estrone have been clearly implicated in breast cancer risk, estriol, which has not been connected to the cancer and may even decrease risk, is produced in huge quantities by the placenta during pregnancy.)

A 1994 study conducted by the Fred Hutchinson Cancer Research Center and the University of Washington School of Public Health— new evidence of just how complicated the tie between reproductive hormones and breast cancer may be—showed that induced abortions, not miscarriages or spontaneous abortions, pose a significant risk for breast cancer. This study, supported by the National Cancer Institute, showed that an induced abortion more than doubles a woman's breast cancer risk, which becomes greater the younger the woman and the later the stage of pregnancy at the time of the abortion. The breast cancer appeared an average of ten to fourteen years after the abortion. The possible explanation is that the sudden pregnancy termination interrupts hormonally driven changes occurring in the lining cells of the glands and ducts in the breast at a time when they are vulnerable to cancerous transformation. These observations must be pursued to see if the link bears out. Some 1.5 million women undergo abortion in this country each year; if the breast cancer connection is valid, we will be seeing a continuous rise in breast cancer in this country for many years into the future.

A woman must also consider the risk of breast cancer in her choice to take the various types of hormone therapy available. Birth control pills contain estrogen, but the vast majority of studies have failed to find a connection to breast cancer—possibly because the doses of hormones in oral contraceptives are low relative to normal estrogen exposure in childbearing-age women. For women after menopause, the majority of observational studies performed around the world show that estrogen replacement therapy slightly increases the risk of breast cancer, but only if the hormone has been taken for more than ten years. Risk is increased by 20 or 30 percent after more than a decade of use, and by fifteen to twenty years of use, the risk may as much as double. Most studies, however, have been of women using the higher doses of estrogen—1.25 mg of Premarin per day or higher, rather than the 0.625 mg used most commonly today. The Women's Health Initiative will provide controlled information about the breast cancer risk, but not for a decade or more.

Lifestyle and Education

A number of lifestyle issues may bear on breast cancer risk, but we know very little with certainty. Fat in the diet (see page 37) and obesity are the two dietary factors that recurrently match with breast cancer in large population studies, but we've no definitive proof. Studies have recently come out that link exercise in young women to less breast cancer under the age of fifty, but, again, women who exercise are also likely to be leaner and have healthier overall lifestyles. Smoking does not appear to be a risk factor for breast cancer—probably one of the few major diseases for which it is not.

For most illnesses, from heart disease to Alzheimer's, lower educational achievement increases the risk. The opposite is true for breast cancer. Women who have reached higher educational levels and are in higher socioeconomic groups and from urban rather than rural communities have more incidence of breast cancer—perhaps because more educated women also tend to detect breast cancer earlier, through self-exams and the other methods described below.

DETECTING BREAST CANCER

More than 90 percent of women who find breast cancer in its earliest stage will be cured—even though we have no known definitive cure for breast cancer and do not fully understand its causes. The surest cure for breast cancer is *early* detection, and this is well within your power to control.

Breast Examination

You can detect a lump in your own breast at a very early stage in its development—and thereby save your own life. In fact, most cancers are found first by the patient. Something new, a lump in the breast or discharge from the nipple, prompts a woman to seek medical advice; most of the time, the findings do not turn out not to be cancer.

Mammography

Monthly self-examination for early breast cancer is not enough as women move into the high-risk breast cancer years. Mammograms, which can pick up breast cancer at its very earliest stage, when a lump is too small to be felt, have now become routine. And with good reason: I've noted that nine out of ten women with breast cancer detected early will be cured, and that some 80 percent of new breast cancer occurs in women with no known family history or other risk factor. So,

EXAMINING YOUR BREASTS

Thanks to the incredible campaign for national awareness of breast cancer, most women have learned how to examine their own breasts. Here's a refresher course.

Every woman should develop a lifelong habit of monthly breast self-examination. The procedure is simple, and done in no particular order. While in the bath or shower, run your fingers over your breasts, feeling for lumps or bumps. Out of the shower, look at your breasts in the mirror with your arms at your side and over your head. Look for changes in shape or skin color, or changes in your nipples. Lying in bed, systematically and gently feel each part of your breast, sweeping first at the outer part of the breast and then in concentric circles inching toward the nipple. Finally, squeeze both nipples, looking for any kind of discharge.

Your primary care doctor or gynecologist will routinely examine your breasts. This is a good time to go over how well you are performing self-examination.

although we don't know who is going to get breast cancer, we do know how to discover it and get rid of it. Mammography, which uses low-level X ray to provide an image of both breasts taken at different angles, saves thousands of lives each year. The technology is continually improving; it can now detect smaller and smaller cancers, with less and less radiation exposure. Paired with the injection of dye or other newer technology in development, such as heat sensors, screening mammography can be made more precise in distinguishing a malignancy from a noncancerous lump, obviating the performance of a biopsy in some cases.

The benefits of using mammography to screen for early breast cancer have been solidly proven in women over fifty, the age range in which most breast cancer develops. There is less certainty—and suddenly some controversy—about using screening mammography on women between the ages of forty and fifty. Testing every two to three years for women over forty (and every one to two years after age fifty) had become part of the catechism of women's health care, endorsed by the American Cancer Society, the National Cancer Institute, and most other involved medical groups. The controversy centers on the overall economic cost if all women over forty get screened, and the fact that in younger women, with denser breasts, there is a higher false-positive rate. We don't have definitive studies of the effectiveness of mammography in women over forty to fight these contentions—but that's because most studies have yet to focus on younger women.

The issue became especially heated when the Clinton Health Security Act removed mammography screening of women in their forties from their comprehensive benefits plan, and then the National Cancer Institute, in a turnabout from its own long-standing position, withdrew any official recommendations for women on this matter. This NCI action was opposed by the organization's own outside standing advisory council, and was disputed by the American Cancer Society and most other independent medical professional groups.

My own opinion is clear: stick with the existing recommendations until we have certain information for women in their forties. Breast cancer developing in women under fifty tends to be more aggressive and fast-moving, and there is growing evidence that modern and better mammography can cut the under-fifty death rate from breast cancer by more than 20 percent. My belief is that, for the twenty-nine thousand or so American women under age fifty who develop breast cancer each year, we need better mammography, not no mammography; we may even need more frequent mammography, not less; and we surely need better treatment, not later treatment. And, finally, I've personally seen too many patients who have developed breast cancer in their forties to be willing to buy into any change in existing recommendations until we have solid scientific evidence otherwise.

Other Noninvasive Detection Methods

A number of other techniques are in use or being developed to screen for cancer, but none of them have proven to be superior to mammography. One of these is thermography, which looks for hot spots—cancers are hotter, since they grow faster. Ultrasound will tell us if a lump is a cyst, sometimes ruling out a tumor, but it is not accurate enough for routine screening. MRI and CAT scans are very expensive alternatives. Your doctor might recommend them if the mammogram is unclear, as sometimes happens with very dense small breasts.

Biopsies

If your doctor suspects cancer, from either examination or mammography, the next step is a biopsy. Usually this is a simple outpatient procedure, sometimes using a needle inserted into the lump to pull out tissue. Biopsies will tell us whether or not the lump is cancer, and what cancer type it is.

TREATMENT

Treatment of breast cancer involves either surgery alone, or surgery plus chemotherapy. The success of the treatment hinges on "hurry"; when the tumor is past the early stage and larger than about an inch, or has spread to one of the lymph nodes under the arm, treatment will help 60 to 80 percent of women to survive five years beyond the therapy. When the cancer has progressed deep into the lymph nodes, or out of the lymph nodes and into the chest, about 40 to 50 percent of stricken women will survive long term with treatment. If the cancer has metastasized into distant sites, the outlook is quite grim, even with surgery: a five-year survival rate of about 10 percent.

Surgical Treatment for Breast Cancer

For most of this century, there was but one surgical approach to treating breast cancer—the *Halsted radical mastectomy,* in which the entire breast was removed, along with chest muscles and all lymph nodes under the arm. This method was more than disfiguring; it could also be disabling, the removed muscle making it difficult for a woman to raise her arm, for example.

The procedure was first called into question by Dr. R. McWhirter after conducting studies in Canada and Europe in the late sixties, and a few years later in the United States, notably by Dr. George (Barney) Crile, Jr., of the Cleveland Clinic. Dr. Crile proposed less radical cancer surgery in general, including local tumor excision or lumpectomy for breast cancer. This assaulted all the proper surgical tenets of the day— and led to Dr. Crile's being vilified and labeled as a dangerous kook. Years later, the less radical approach was proven to have an equal or better outcome in a large-scale study conducted by the National Cancer Institute under the leadership of Dr. Bernard Fisher of the University of Pittsburgh. (Serious problems in one center contributing to this study led to a recent recheck and rereview of all the data. According to the NCI, the conclusion that less extensive surgery is as effective as radical surgery stands firmly from these and other studies.)

The surgical approach today is conservative and conserving wherever possible, and far more respectful of the desires of the patient. Women are now involved in the treatment plan from the very beginning, having biopsy results in hand well before surgery so that they can review alternatives, and prepare and participate in the choice of their treatment. The simplest procedure for breast cancer is *lumpectomy,* the removal of the tumor and lymph nodes under the arm as necessary. If the cancer has spread somewhat, a *segmental mastectomy* is performed, removing additional nearby breast tissue along with the tumor. A *total mastectomy* removes the entire breast and sometimes all the lymph nodes under the arm. A *modified radical mastectomy* removes the breast and underlying tissue and some lymph nodes but preserves the chest muscles.

Adjuvant Therapy

Although they have been practiced for years, we have only recently confirmed that both radiation therapy and chemotherapy can be lifesaving additions to surgery. Radiation therapy is most effective after surgery of early-stage cancer: after a lumpectomy, it can catch and destroy any discrete microscopic tumors that the surgery itself might have missed. And for virtually all breast cancer patients, chemotherapy after surgery reduces the risk of recurrent cancer and death.

One noteworthy drug employed in breast cancer chemotherapy is the synthetic hormone *tamoxifen*. Tamoxifen blocks estrogen receptors in the breast tissue, and therefore prevents the prolific breast cell divisions that estrogen normally prompts. In postmenopausal women, especially those whose cancer cells are shown to be estrogen-sensitive as measured by the presence of estrogen receptors on the tumor cells, the drug as part of a regimen of chemotherapy has been shown to reduce recurrence by 45 percent. (We are far less certain of tamoxifen's benefits to premenopausal women. Scientists are concerned that it might paradoxically induce the ovaries to produce more estrogen to counter the agent's hormone-blocking effects. Research is under way.)

A Note on Breast Reconstruction

Any disfiguring surgery can be followed by reconstruction, but not quite as easily as in our very recent past. Most women are by now well aware that breast implants containing silicone gel, which cosmetically are superior prostheses, were banned by the FDA following the unproven and now discredited claim that they triggered immune diseases. So, safe though it may be, silicone is no longer an option for you. Saline-filled implants remain available, but they don't have the same natural feel as silicone, and do occasionally (and harmlessly) rupture. (Other fillers using natural fats are in development.) Many women are turning to the alternative of having their own abdominal tissue used to reconstruct the breast, with excellent results.

Silicone or no silicone, do not dismiss the benefits of a good cosmetic repair after breast surgery. Beyond your personal preference, there is no reason for you to face daily the physical evidence of your bout with cancer; cosmetic surgery to repair damage done by a car accident, for example, is common and unquestioned. It is not vanity to wish to repair visible disfigurement, and for some women such surgery may well speed up rehabilitation, given its positive impact on their emotional well-being and self-esteem—a symbol of facing and conquering an illness in the past and looking clear-eyed into a long future. In any event, it is a woman's choice.

PREVENTION OF BREAST CANCER

The simple fact is that we have no certain way of preventing breast cancer. The best prevention, again, is early detection and continued investment in research. We are not without possibilities, however, that offer considerable promise as we look ahead.

Lifestyle Issues

Although the effect may not be great, I would not ignore the potential that a diet low in fat and rich in fruits and vegetables may somewhat decrease your risk (besides being a healthy choice overall). Also—and without scientific verification—some chemicals found in certain foods have been promoted by practitioners of alternative medicines as having anti-breast-cancer qualities. One such chemical, indole-3-carbinol, which occurs naturally in certain vegetables—including broccoli, cabbage, and cauliflower—does interfere with the action of the more potent forms of estrogen, estradiol and particularly estrone, on breast tissue.

And if induced abortion is indeed a risk factor for breast cancer, young women can protect themselves through responsible sexual behavior and the avoidance of unwanted pregnancies. If you or your daughter chooses an abortion, however, remember—the earlier in the pregnancy it is performed, the less the breast cancer risk.

Precancer Surgery or Drugs

Some women at very high risk for breast cancer have opted for prophylactic treatment, removing part or all of their breasts before any actual cancer is found. Surgery to prevent breast cancer has actually been with us for a long time; when I was in my residency, I saw several women undergo prophylactic mastectomies because they dreaded facing repeated biopsies of their lumpy but cancer-free breasts. This issue will become more acute as we develop tests for the cancer gene. Women will know they carry a risk—but is that risk worth such a radical remedy? We have to focus on this issue and find a way to determine risks and benefits on a case-by-case basis.

High-risk women today also have the option of taking drugs in the hopes of minimizing their risks. Although already used by some women under the guidance of their physicians, such *chemoprevention* has not yet been proven effective in any form. (See sidebar, page 245.)

STUDIES TO WATCH FOR IN CHEMOPREVENTION

Obviously, finding a drug that can painlessly reduce breast cancer risk is a very exciting and popular area of research. Some of the more promising possibilities:

- *Low-dose aspirin, recently noted for its anticancer properties, is the subject of a major clinical study supported by the National Institutes of Health that is looking at its protective effect in both heart disease and breast cancer in women.*
- *Retinoids are a family of substances that are part of the vitamin A family, including beta-carotene. They specifically regulate the kinds of cells that line the breast ducts, and experimental studies at least suggest that they may suppress the development of breast cancer formation in its earliest stage. Retinoids are currently being studied by several groups for their general cancer-fighting qualities.*
- *Tamoxifen, which until recently has been viewed as a treatment only, is now being examined in large clinical trials in many countries— including the United States, under the aegis of the National Cancer Institute—as a possible preventive agent. The drug has some serious side effects, including a small but real increased chance of getting cancer of the uterus. Tamoxifen also brings on some symptoms of menopause.*

CANCER OF THE CERVIX

Cancer of the cervix is increasing in epidemic proportions in this country. Even though it is not among the deadliest of cancers, I believe that, if we're not very careful in all our life choices, it could quickly become a needlessly common killer of women. Currently, about seventy thousand women each year contract this illness, and cervical cancer, unlike most other cancers, hits women when they're young. The earliest and more easily treated form of cervical cancer tends to show up when a woman is in her mid- to late thirties; the more advanced forms in her mid-forties.

Even though more women get cervical cancer each year, the number dying from the disease—about forty-four hundred each year—is continually decreasing. I say that's still forty-four hundred too many. Cervical cancer is well within our grasp to stop before it gets started— or at least before it gets started growing. Knowledge of cervical cancer is an easy lifesaver.

The cervix is the round, knoblike opening of the uterus; it protrudes into the vaginal canal and can be easily touched and examined. Its small opening, called the *os,* is plugged with mucus secretions, which serve as a shield to keep bacteria and other foreign invaders from getting into the uterus. The inner edge of the os (called the *squamocolumnar junction*) is the place where most cervical cancers start, growing slowly as they spread from the os and into the uterus or out to the vagina.

RISK FACTORS FOR CERVICAL CANCER

Cervical cancer demonstrates one of nature's great inequities. Sexual choices put women at risk in a way no man must face. But at least in this disease the risk factors are clear, and generally avoidable.

Sexual History

The major risk factor for this cancer is an active sex life. Having multiple sex partners, having a first sexual encounter before age eighteen, having had more than five pregnancies, and having a history of virtually any sexually transmitted disease, ranging from gonorrhea to syphilis to herpes, markedly increases the likelihood of developing cancer of the cervix. Not surprisingly, cervical cancer is almost never seen in nuns—and is exceedingly common among prostitutes. In all likelihood, one primary reason an active and varied sex life is such a major risk is that the odds are high that a diaphragm or condom is not used with each and every new encounter.

Human Papilloma Virus

There are in America today an estimated 250,000 to 300,000 women with a smoldering precancerous infection in their cervixes—the incurable venereal disease known as *human papilloma virus* or *HPV.* (See chapter 4.) About 90 percent of all cervical cancers contain this virus (although only about a third of the many types of HPV affect the cervix). Simply having the virus doesn't mean you'll get cancer, but it does mean you are at increased risk; you're at the highest risk if the strain of HPV you develop is numbered 16 or 18.

You contract HPV from a sexual partner who has the disease; you're made more vulnerable if your cervix is already injured or contains abrasions, as can happen from sexual intercourse, or ulcerated from other infections, such as herpes.

Cigarettes

Smoking increases your chance of getting cervical cancer fourfold—no matter how safe the sex you practice. It's possible, though, that the smoking itself is not what causes the disease but that it correlates with some other behavioral risk factors.

DETECTING CERVICAL CANCER

Fewer women are dying of cervical cancer because more women are taking responsibility for their own health, at least in the doctor's office. Women are exposing themselves to more risks—multiple partner sexual activity and smoking have both been on the rise—but are detecting and waylaying the resulting slow-growing disease early through the simplest of tools, the Papanicolaou test, or Pap smear. Most of the time, cervical cancer is picked up through a Pap smear before a woman experiences its symptoms of abnormal vaginal bleeding or bleeding after sexual intercourse.

To get the Pap smear, the physician gently uses a small spatula to scrape off cervical cells, which are then smeared on a glass slide, processed, and looked at under the microscope. A newer test, called a *Virapap,* also detects the presence and particular strain of any HPV infection present.

The slide is generally sent to a lab for analysis. You may have heard reports over the past few years that the resulting lab reports are unreliable. I believe most labs are trustworthy and professional, and see these reports only as reminders that you are in control of your own health, in partnership with your physician. Ask your doctor about the lab's track record, and whether it is accredited. Note too that some flawed Pap smears are not the fault of the lab, but of the sampling process. The gynecologist must carefully scrape the cells from the squamo-columnar junction for the most accurate results. Pick your physician carefully. And regular Pap smears can pretty much eliminate any risk of error—the more tests you have, the less likely it is that any mistakes will be made. If the cells in the Pap smear suggest cancer, the next diagnostic step is a closer examination of the lining of the vagina and cervix with a special magnifying instrument called a *colposcope,* and a biopsy.

TREATMENT

Treatment of cervical cancer usually involves some type of surgery, as long as there is any hope of positive results. The adjuvant therapy that is most effective with this disease is radiation.

Cervical cancer in its earliest stage, when it is a microscopic invasion (called "in situ") involving only the cells lining the cervix, is easily halted. The cancer has not broken out of the superficial layer of cells in which it started, has not invaded other, normal cells, and has done no damage. The abnormal tissue is removed in a simple outpatient operation using local anesthetic, the uterus and cervix remain intact, and, as long as the diagnosis was accurate, the recovery rate is 100 percent.

When the cancer has spread out of its original site but is still present only in the cervix, a total hysterectomy (see page 186) is necessary, but the chance of a complete cure is still excellent, in the range of 90 to 98 percent. Cancer that has spread beyond the cervix into the upper part of the vagina but not into the pelvis requires a radical hysterectomy with removal of pelvic lymph nodes, plus radiation treatments. Five-year survival now falls to 60 to 80 percent. If the cancer grows to involve the internal pelvic cavity or the lower part of the vagina, it requires removal of all of the above, plus as much of the tumor as possible. Surgery is followed by radiation, and survival at this stage falls to below 50 percent. And, as in all cancers, cancer of the cervix can progress beyond the point of surgical removal. When the tumor has metastasized beyond the pelvic wall into the nearby organs, including the rectum or the bladder, or into distant organs like the lung, it is inoperable (except for "debulking" surgery, which, for the comfort of the sufferer, removes as much of the tumor mass as possible), and radiation therapy is the only available treatment. Few patients survive a year, and fewer than 15 percent make it to five years.

PREVENTION

With such blatant risk factors, and such positive results from early detection, I suppose the means through which you can prevent cervical cancer are fairly obvious. Don't let this detract from their value—you can prevent this disease, and you can educate your daughters to take care as well.

I'm certainly not going to tell you not to have sex, or not to have sex often. But do understand the importance of common sense. If you aren't absolutely sure about your partner's sexual history, use a condom and a diaphragm. Knowing your partner is AIDS-free isn't enough to save your life; all types of sexually transmitted diseases are still out there, including herpes, gonorrhea, HPV, and syphilis; protecting yourself against them also means protecting yourself against cancer.

Diaphragms have been definitively shown to help prevent cervical cancer; women who use diaphragms with spermicides have an even lower incidence of the disease.

And if you do contract cervical cancer, you can easily conquer it. Any woman who is sexually active, or over the age of eighteen, should see her gynecologist yearly and have a Pap smear. If after three years the Pap smears have been completely normal, the exams can be every two to three years, depending on your risk factors, your own concerns, and the advice of your doctor. Catch this cancer early. It makes all the difference to your quality of life, your ability to have children, your happiness, and your survival. And it's mostly up to you.

And, of course, stop smoking.

CANCER OF THE ENDOMETRIUM

Cancer of the lining of the uterus, the endometrium, affects about thirty-three thousand women each year, about one-sixth the number that get breast cancer; each year, about fifty-five hundred women die of endometrial cancer. More common among white women than any other ethnic group, endometrial cancer almost always attacks post-menopausal women, with the average age at detection being close to sixty. Any woman with a uterus is at risk for endometrial cancer, but the risk is controllable.

RISK FACTORS FOR ENDOMETRIAL CANCER

Virtually the only risk factor for cancer of the lining of the uterus is im-balanced exposure of the uterus to the hormone estrogen—not estrogen in excess, but estrogen without its natural partner, the hormone proges-terone. In the natural cycles of our bodies, estrogen prompts endome-trial cells to keep dividing, and progesterone causes the endometrial cells to mature. When the progesterone is withdrawn each month, the cells slough off. We learned a very hard lesson about the risks of "un-opposed" estrogen in the early seventies, when thousands of women who were taking high doses of estrogen alone as a part of postmenopausal hormone replacement therapy were stricken with this disease.

Endometrial cancer has been steadily declining, probably in large part because hormone replacement therapy now includes carefully bal-anced amounts of both estrogen and progesterone (see page 197). There are other circumstances, however, in which a woman can be ex-posed to estrogen out of balance. Certain estrogen-producing tumors and menstrual abnormalities are linked to increased occurrence of this cancer, and women who are infertile or who have never had children are also at an increased risk, possibly because both conditions are of-ten caused by hormonal imbalances. Obese women are at risk too, probably because fat cells convert a hormone secreted by the adrenal gland into the estrogenic compound, estrone.

DETECTION OF ENDOMETRIAL CANCER

For most premenopausal women, a routine gynecological exam should be a sufficient early screen for endometrial cancer. Your doctor will regularly check the size and firmness of your uterus for any abnormal-ities. In younger women, the signs of endometrial cancer are nonspe-cific, but include the sudden development of heavy or irregular periods or bleeding after intercourse.

After menopause, many women detect this cancer themselves, by recognizing the warning sign of the sudden development of a watery, bloody vaginal discharge. With or without these warning signs, if your doctor finds an enlarged uterus, he will perform a uterine biopsy. This procedure, done in your gynecologist's office, involves dilating the cervical canal, inserting an instrument into the uterine cavity, and taking a sample of the lining cells for examination under the micro-scope. If the biopsy is normal, but suspicious signs or symptoms continue, your doctor may recommend a full D&C (dilatation and curettage), in which all the lining cells are evacuated and studied under the microscope.

Another means of examining the uterine cavity involves the use of ultrasound to measure the thickness of the lining cells of the uterus. With endometrial cancer, the lining cells of the uterus become thick; if the lining cells are very thin and atrophic, there may be no need to biopsy; if they are thick, however, a biopsy is necessary, since you cannot tell whether the thickness is cancer or a noncancerous change without looking at the cells under the microscope.

TREATMENT

Enodmetrial cancer is treated with surgery and chemotherapy, the outcome of which is affected by the extent to which the cancer has spread and the relative aggression of the cells making up the tumor. In its earliest stage, when the tumor is limited to the lining of the uterus (or has only minimally penetrated to the inner muscular wall of the uterus), treatment is a complete hysterectomy with removal of the ovaries and fallopian tubes and nearby pelvic lymph nodes, and in certain cases chemotherapy or radiation treatment. The chance of surviving for five years is in the range of 80 to 90 percent with early treatment. With each subsequent stage, as the cancer spreads first into the cervix and then to the vaginal wall or into the pelvis, the treatment becomes less effective and the survival rate plummets. When the cancer has spread into the bladder or rectum or into distant organs usually within the abdomen, debulking surgery plus radiation and or chemotherapy is tried, but the outlook is poor, with an estimated 7 percent chance of surviving more than five years.

PREVENTION

You cannot eliminate your risk of getting endometrial cancer as long as you have a uterus. What you can do is be alert to your risk, based upon your own hormonal history, and when contemplating any kind of hormone replacement therapy. As with most cancers, the best prevention is the earliest possible detection, and that means regular visits to your gynecologist, and, depending on your personal medical history, more intense screening tests after menopause.

Also, having lots of babies—or being on oral contraceptives with lots of progestins, which make your body mimic a pregnant state—may reduce your risk of endometrial cancer by about half.

CANCER OF THE OVARY

Ovarian cancer is among the most dangerous of cancers. Although only about 15 percent of all cancers involving the reproductive tract occur in the ovaries, this cancer is responsible for more than half of all deaths related to cancer of a woman's reproductive tract. It is so dire for one reason: early detection is the key to defeating any cancer today, and ovarian cancer is hardly ever detected early. It is a quiet cancer that initially grows without symptoms, and we have no reliable test for it in its first stages.

This insidious cancer tends to strike women over age sixty, but not always. A woman faces a 1 to 2 percent chance of getting ovarian cancer in her lifetime; as she gets older, her chances increase.

As we've seen, the more frequently a cell divides, the more susceptible it is to mutating into cancer. The cells lining the surface of the ovaries, the epithelial cells, must replicate after ovulation each month so as to re-cover the exposed surface of the ovary, where the egg has broken loose from its follicle, and 85 percent of the time these epithelial cells are the origin of ovarian cancer. (Epithelial, or covering, cells also line the surface of body cavities, enclose different organs, and form the outer layer of the skin, or epidermis.)

RISK FACTORS

Cancer of the ovaries can be provoked through inherited susceptibilities or spontaneous gene mutation, far out of the control of any woman. But a growing body of evidence suggests that it may also be triggered by choices within a woman's control, choices to enhance or reduce fertility that can in themselves be instigated by heartbreaking circumstances. Must we, for example, choose between fertility drugs and ovarian cancer?

Genes

Although only 10 percent of ovarian cancers run in families, it is likely that a woman under sixty stricken with ovarian cancer has inherited it. An individual woman who has an immediate family member with the cancer has a 50 percent chance of contracting the disease in her lifetime.

Some of the same genes that are tied to breast cancer may also play a role in predisposing a woman to ovarian cancer—such as the recently discovered BRCA-1 gene, which serves as a tumor supressor. Gene abnormalities implicated in colon cancer have also been shown to play a role in ovarian cancer; for example, defects in the spell-checker gene MSH-2 give women a risk for ovarian cancer that is ten times higher than normal. This genetic information confirms what we have known for years—that a family or personal history of breast or colon cancer increases ovarian cancer risk substantially.

Reproductive History

Life is never easy for a woman. The choice whether or not to have children shouldn't, it seems, rationally bear an impact on a woman's risk of cancer; but it does. Cancer of the ovary is tied to any condition that leads to "incessant ovulation"—that is, never giving the ovaries a rest. So choosing not to have a child can place a woman at an increased risk for ovarian cancer.

On the other hand, for a woman struggling with infertility who wants desperately to have a child and cannot, the choice to stimulate the ovaries artificially to produce multiple eggs at once, with drugs such as clomiphene (see chapter 3), may also increase her risk of ovarian cancer years later. The reports, which include several from the NIH-supported Collaborative Ovarian Cancer Group and, more recently, one from the University of Washington, Seattle, are fairly convincing, but longer-term studies are needed. New reproductive technologies have exploded over the past decade, but the fact that it often takes a decade or more for such cancer to develop means we cannot yet accurately assess the risk of these new therapies, and the answers are still far off. My view is to respect the risk, study it vigilantly, and advise any woman of the hazard to her own life that undergoing these treatments may pose. I am concerned about the sometimes cavalier and too-quick dispensing of fertility drugs, and suggest we all be very cautious, never casually using such powerful agents until all other recourses have been exhausted.

Talc

The use of talcum powder is an easily controlled but unfortunately little-known risk factor for ovarian cancer. Women who use talcum powder on their external genitalia after bathing, or on their sanitary pads, run a greater risk for ovarian cancer. It is presumed that the talc is carried into the vagina and works its way up into the pelvic cavity to the ovaries. I'd even caution against the use of talc on diaper rash.

Diet

In many studies from all over the world, a diet high in saturated fats has been linked to cancer of the ovary (and also the prostate). Why, we do not know. In any case, as I've said again and again, it is always healthy to eat a diet low in fat.

DETECTION

Cancer of the ovaries cannot be seen and often cannot be felt until it has broken out of its bounds within the ovary and seeded the pelvic cavity. Since the ovaries move rather freely within the pelvic cavity, a tumor-enlarged ovary doesn't press or tug on adjacent structures and cause pain or dysfunction, as tumors in most other locations would. Accordingly, symptoms all too often do not develop until the tumor is large and has produced problems like fluid accumulation in the abdomen, abdominal bloating, or vague abdominal distress, nonspecific bowel discomfort, or uterine bleeding. Because the symptoms are so general, most women wait almost a year to consult their doctors. And because most women have no idea they have this cancer until it has advanced beyond the ovary, the overall survival rate of ovarian cancer is less than 40 percent. A doctor first suspects ovarian cancer when she feels an enlarged ovary on pelvic examination in a woman over the age of fifty. (Palpable or enlarged ovaries in premenopausal women are common, and therefore don't by themselves lead to suspicion of cancer.) Although only about one in ten enlarged ovaries in postmenopausal women turns out to be cancer, the finding must be pursued.

The discovery of an enlarged ovary prompts several steps.

One is getting a blood test for elevated levels of carbohydrate antigen 125 (CA-125), a protein from the surface of epithelial tumor cells. (Unfortunately, CA-125 often looks normal in early stages of ovarian cancers and therefore cannot be used as a routine screening tool. Also, it can be misleading, for it may be elevated in the blood of women with breast cancer or inflammatory diseases of the abdomen and pelvis as well.)

The second step is a pelvic ultrasound. With the ultrasound probe inserted into the vagina, the ovaries can be seen on a monitor, and tumors or other innocent forms of enlargement can be detected. Ultrasound can reveal ovarian cancer earlier than all other tests, but an ultrasound cannot always distinguish a tumor from a benign growth. Therefore, ultrasound in ovarian cancer has a very high rate of false-positive readings. Studies of several thousand women have shown that, for each instance of ovarian cancer signaled by an ultrasound, there were as many as fifty women labeled with the suspicion of cancer who were in fact perfectly healthy. (For this reason, unless you're high-risk, vaginal ultrasound is discouraged as a routine screening device.)

The next step in evaluating an enlarged ovary is more invasive, involving a direct look at the ovary through a laparoscopy, and a biopsy or other means of extracting cells for examination under the microscope. In cases where an ultrasound does provide unmistakable evidence of an advanced tumor, speed is of the essence. Your physician will then choose to dispense with any further exploratory techniques and undertake a full-scale abdominal operation (called a *laparotomy*) to detect, diagnose, and, if necessary, remove the tumor and surrounding tissue as necessary.

Clearly, we must find some way of identifying ovarian cancer early and without invasive surgery. One promising method is the use of more sophisticated forms of ultrasound with color-flow Doppler (a special form of ultrasound that can measure blood flow and use color to define tissue better), which may provide more precise information than current ultrasound and enable physicians to separate benign enlargement from early ovarian cancer. Stay tuned.

TREATMENT

Treatment of ovarian cancer involves surgery as long as it can be effective, and often adjunctive treatment through chemotherapy. (The chemotherapeutic drug most recently associated with ovarian cancer is Taxol, which has been shown to be somewhat more effective than standard anticancer drugs. Taxol comes from the bark of the yew tree, the home of the rare spotted owl, and has therefore sparked many heated arguments between environmentalists and cancer research advocates. The controversy is being resolved by discovering alternative drug sources.) Radiation isn't generally useful, except as a means of alleviating pain by shrinking obstructions after all other options have failed.

When ovarian cancer is found before it has visibly spread beyond a tumor in the ovary, the survival rate is actually quite high: 90 to 95 percent of women live more than five years. But only 20 percent of ovarian cancer is picked up this early. The surgery even at this stage is extensive: it calls for total hysterectomy, removal of the ovaries and fallopian tubes, removal of nearby lymph nodes, and the taking of tissue samples from surrounding organs and samples of fluids to determine both the type of cancer cell and whether microscopic pieces of the tumor have spread outside the ovary. If the cancer has spread, or if the type is an aggressive one, additional treatment with chemotherapy will also be given. If the cancer type is lower-risk, and the cancer confined to one ovary in a younger woman who wants to have children, sometimes only the cancerous ovary is removed. A woman must carefully weigh the risks and benefits to this approach.

When the cancer has spread outside the ovaries into other parts of the pelvis—such as the uterus or fallopian tubes—the five-year mortality rate sinks to 30 to 40 percent, and the surgical philosophy is simply to take out as much as you possibly can. When the cancer progresses to the next stage—beyond the pelvis into the abdominal surfaces, including the surface of the liver—the philosophy remains the same, and rate of survival falls to below 30 percent; when ovarian cancer has metastasized to distant organs, such as the lung, survival falls to below 10 percent. These more advanced stages all require adjunct chemotherapy.

PREVENTION

Preventing such an unpredictable and uncommon disease is not really something I can advise most women to concentrate on in their day-to-day lives. When you are under sixty and do not face a high risk by virtue of heredity, until we have a reliable screening measure I can only advise you to be aware of ovarian cancer risks in all of your choices concerning reproduction, and weigh them, in consultation with your physician, against the other risks and benefits each decision brings. If you are at high risk, however, you can take a drastic measure to protect yourself from this dread cancer: prophylactic surgery.

Preventive Surgery

Women with a strong family history of ovarian cancer face a one-in-two chance of getting the disease, and for these women prophylactic removal of the ovaries (oophorectomy) is a realistic preventive option. Extreme as this approach may seem, it has recently been endorsed by the NIH, which in late 1994 recommended that women with this type of hereditary risk have annual pelvic exams, CA-125 measurements, and transvaginal ultrasound visualization of the ovaries until the age of thirty-five, and that after age thirty-five they should seriously consider a prophylactic bilateral oophorectomy.

I agree with this new approach, which, in the absence of good screening technology for the cancer's early stages, and given the fifty-

A NEBRASKA WOMAN'S STORY

The October 13, 1994, issue of the Journal of the American Medical Association *reported on the economic and legal battle between a woman and her insurance company. The woman's mother and aunt had died from ovarian cancer in their late forties, and she therefore faced a clear one-in-two chance of encountering ovarian or breast cancer. She decided to have prophylactic surgery, but her insurance company refused to pay for it because, since she did not actually have cancer, they deemed it was not "medically necessary." The case wound its way through the courts of Nebraska; judgments went both ways. Finally, on appeal, the woman won. This is one of the first such cases, but it won't be the last. As we continue to move forward, as we must, in identifying specific genes that are cancer risks, we will be facing manifold questions like these, which transcend economics to become an ethical, medical, legal, and social dilemma as well. Will insurance cover preventive medical or surgical treatment? Where should the lines be drawn? How should health care plans account for these cases? Such tough decisions will have a direct impact on the health care of tomorrow's women, and demonstrate the need for individuals to stay aware of health policy matters.*

fifty risk, can be a difficult but lifesaving option. It is your choice, and you must be fully informed of the risks of inducing a surgical menopause at a young age and the likely need to take long-term estrogen replacement therapy (see page 189).

There is an added caveat. Even with prophylactic oophorectomy, there is a 5 percent risk that the cancer will occur after the ovaries have been removed. Cancerous cells can remain, hidden in the lining cells of the abdomen. Nonetheless, a 5 percent risk is far more palatable to many women than a 50 percent probability.

Interventions in Ovulation

As might be expected, events such as one or more full-term pregnancies, which reduce the frequency of ovulation, also reduce the risk of ovarian cancer. Oral contraceptives reduce the risk of ovarian cancer too, since they suppress ovulation, although the lower doses of today may well be less effective against the disease than the otherwise unnecessarily high doses of yesteryear. Ovarian cancer has in fact decreased by about 10 percent over the past twenty or so years; many physicians, including me, directly attribute the decrease to a coinciding increase in the use of oral contraceptives.

I will go even further out on my limb. If I had chosen not to have children, or were periodically on fertility drugs, I would take birth control pills for an extended period of time in order to give my ovaries a rest and, possibly, reduce my chances of encountering ovarian cancer.

The Nurses' Health Study (see page 46) demonstrated that tubal ligation decreases a woman's risk of getting ovarian cancer by more than 70 percent, and hysterectomy, particularly if done early in a woman's adult life, can reduce the risk by as much as 30 percent. There is no good explanation for the effects. I'm certainly not advocating that any healthy woman run out and get either operation for this reason alone, but the findings are provocative, and perhaps comforting to women who have undergone these serious procedures.

VAGINAL CANCER LINKED TO DES

Vaginal clear cell adenocarcinoma, a very rare cancer, occurs in one of every hundred daughters of mothers who used diethylstilbestrol (DES) during pregnancy. (DES, from the late 1940s through the early 1970s, was prescribed to prevent miscarriages.) The cancer strikes women in their twenties or thirties, and sometimes even younger. It is often misdiagnosed, for as many as 50 percent of DES offspring also have had other reproductive tract abnormalities, including benign changes in the cells lining the vagina and part of the cervix.

Fortunately, vaginal cancer can be detected on routine exam with a Pap smear. Its treatment and outcome are very similar to those of cervical cancer—if it is found early, the five-year survival rate is 90 percent or more.

LUNG CANCER

Whereas women were celebrating triumphs in many other fields throughout the 1970s and 1980s, 1986 must be marked as one of our more dismal setbacks. In that year, lung cancer surpassed breast cancer as the leading cause of cancer death in women, a record that will stand for at least the next decade. And this tragedy was preventable.

If you look at any charts of cancer-related death in women over the past fifty years, you will see that rates for virtually all cancers have stayed steady or falling. Lung cancer is the dramatic exception to this, for the figures have risen relentlessly and steeply. Since the mid-1950s, the lung cancer rate in women has risen by more than 400 percent and is still rising; in men, it has increased by about 130 percent but is now falling.

Incidence of lung cancer is soaring in women today undoubtedly because smoking somehow became a sign of women's liberation back in the 1960s: smoking like a man somehow would enable women to be given the salary, credibility, and prerogatives of a man. Sadly, lung cancer will continue to skyrocket in our daughters' futures, because, although our generation may have stopped smoking, our daughters are smoking in ever-increasing numbers.

Lung cancer is a killer. Seventy thousand women lose their lives to it each year—and each year seventy thousand new cases in women are diagnosed. Although early detection lengthens survival time for those with most cancers, the patient diagnosed with lung cancer rarely survives for five years, regardless of when it is found. And this doesn't have to happen.

RISK FACTORS

Smoking

The more and the longer you smoke, the more likely you are to get lung cancer. Eighty to 85 percent of all lung cancers can be traced directly to tobacco (with the minor exception of those related to scars caused by tuberculosis). In 1995, just as many women as men will be smoking. And just as many will be dying—not only of lung cancer but of heart disease, stroke, chronic obstructive pulmonary disease, and cancers of the mouth, esophagus, larynx, pancreas, bladder, and kidney.

Industrial Exposure

Certain industrial hazards have been linked to lung cancer; in virtually all cases, the risk is increased manyfold if the exposed person also smokes. Most of these dangers are no longer risk factors for women, though. Asbestos, for example, is a well-known menace that is rarely used today, and the industries using asbestos dangerously in the past did not tend to employ many women. Radiation exposure at one time increased the likelihood of lung cancer, but that risk is now tightly monitored. Any environmental risk pales in comparison with that posed by smoking.

DETECTION OF LUNG CANCER

We have no way of detecting lung cancer at an early stage, or screening for it. Early lung cancer simply doesn't show up in chest X rays, and clear symptoms don't manifest themselves until the disease is far advanced as a persistent cough, bloodstained sputum, or chronic chest pain; occasionally a woman will be hoarse, or have peculiar facial swelling. Sometimes an advanced mass in the lung is inadvertently picked up during a chest X ray done to diagnose some other problem.

A definitive diagnosis of lung cancer is made by analyzing cells in the sputum—much like a Pap smear—or through a biopsy of the lining tissue of the windpipes, taken in a bronchoscopy.

TREATMENT

All lung cancer is treated in much the same way: surgical removal of any visible tumor if possible, followed by either radiation or chemotherapy or both. But often surgery cannot remedy the problem.

When lung cancer is diagnosed, the physician must determine whether the type of cancer cell present is a "small cell" or a "nonsmall cell" (describing what the cancer cells look like under the microscope relative to one another) before predicting the outcome of treatment. The progression of both small cell cancers and nonsmall cell cancers is identified in stages, much the same as for other cancers. Early lung cancer tends to be localized to one identifiable tumor; the next stage is called *regional* if the cancer has spread to an adjacent lung or to the lining of the lung; finally, *distant* lung cancer has metastasized to the bone, the brain, or other remote organs.

But small cell cancers are very much more aggressive than the nonsmall cell type. Because they metastasize early in their development, when a small cell tumor looks localized the odds are that microscopic cells have already seeded distant sites. Only 10 percent of small cell cancers can be treated with surgery. When a nonsmall cell cancer is at the early, localized stage (a stage at which it is diagnosed only 20 percent of the time), the five-year survival rate after surgery plus adjuvant therapy is about 40 percent. When the cancer has metastasized at the time of diagnosis, no matter what treatments are given, the rate of survival for five years remains less than 1 percent.

PREVENTION

Don't smoke. If you do smoke, stop. We can make lung cancer the rare disease it was in our grandmothers' day.

A few dietary factors may somewhat reduce the risk of lung cancer in women smokers. Consuming a variety of fruits and vegetables (or taking vitamin pill supplements), particularly those rich in the vitamin A family (see page 45) and vitamin C, has been shown in several different populations to decrease a woman smoker's chance of getting lung cancer. Taking vitamins or eating well, however, is not the whole answer. Throwing away your cigarettes is. Since risk of cancer is directly linked to cumulative lifetime exposure, anytime you stop will decrease your risk.

COLON CANCER

Colon (*colorectal*) cancer is on the rise, especially in American women. It trails only lung and breast cancer as our biggest cancer killer. I strongly suspect that one trigger of this rise lies well within our control: our diet. As we'll see, though heredity certainly plays a large role, and always will, the dominant cultural change that has accompanied the rise in colon cancer is the increasing amount of fats and easily digested food we now consume. Again, in the guise of making women's lives easier and more "liberated" in the late fifties and early sixties, high-fat, no-fiber convenience foods were perhaps innocently thrust upon us all. TV dinners, processed cheese, white breads and rolls—all gave us more time in each day, but perhaps, in the long run, less time to live.

Colon cancers develop within the lining cells of the large bowel almost anywhere in its tortuous course through the abdomen, but primarily in the left side near or in the rectum. This type of cancer lies dormant for a long period: it may take three to four decades for small harmless growths on the bowel's interior surface to grow into larger ones, and then, finally, to progress to cancerous tumors called *adenocarcinomas*. The growths take either the form of polyps, which are tumors that develop on stalks and may be completely benign or may contain precancerous cells, or benign tumors called *adenomas*, which have no stalks. Because the disease lies idle so long, its incidence increases as we get older; it mostly appears in those over the age of fifty.

It was through studying colon cancer that we first learned (through the work of Dr. Bert Vogelstein) that cancer is a disease of many "hits," a complex molecular disease created by a number of genetic aberrations, both inherited and acquired, as well as external toxins.

RISK FACTORS

Family History and Genes

Your family history is a strong risk factor in colon cancer; the susceptibility takes many forms. Generally, families carry the genes for precursor diseases, diseases through which members first develop polyps or adenomas that can eventually grow into the cancer.

Some of the rarer inherited vulnerabilities to colon cancer cause the disease to strike those younger than the norm. In familial adenomatous polyposis, offspring of afflicted parents have a 50 percent chance of getting colon cancer by age forty. Another, less common inherited polyp-forming disease is called *Gardner's disease*. Yet another type of inherited colon cancer, the *family cancer syndrome*, which usually hits before a woman reaches her early forties, doesn't involve early polyps at all, and often forms in the right side of the colon;

women in these families also have a markedly increased incidence of cancer of the ovary, uterus, and breast.

Whether inherited or spontaneously mutated, several of the specific gene abnormalities that play a role in colon cancer have now been identified. Dr. Vogelstein and his colleagues at Johns Hopkins discovered that mutations in the tumor-suppressor gene (APC) found on our chromosome 5 is associated with inherited colon cancer. Abnormalities in this same APC were also present in a large number of tumors from cases of colon cancer that occurred without a family history of the tumor (so-called sporadic cases). Researchers found another colon cancer tumor-suppressor gene, called DCC, on chromosome 18; presumably, if DCC is flawed, another rung on the ladder to cancer has been climbed. More recently, studies in patients with strong family histories of colon cancer uncovered another gene, called MSH-2, which is a repair or spell-checker gene; defects in this gene have been clearly tied to colon cancer.

Isolated Colon Polyps

Whether or not colon cancer runs in your family, having a single adenomatous polyp increases your chance of developing it. This fact places a large portion of our population at risk, especially among people over fifty. The very small polyps rarely go on to become cancerous, but if a polyp is more than 2 cm across (about 0.8 of an inch), the risk that it will turn into an adenocarcinoma is better than 50 percent.

Ulcerative Colitis

This uncommon inflammatory disease of the bowel leads to chronic inflammation of the lining of the large bowel and the rectum and is associated with bloody diarrhea and abdominal pain. The body's own immune system is thought to be the major culprit in the process by attacking the body's own cells—in this case, cells in the colon. Ulcerative colitis tends to run in families and attacks women in their twenties and thirties; it is associated with a tenfold or greater risk for colon cancer.

Smoking

Smoking once again rears its ugly head. A 1994 report from the Nurses' Health Study showed an increased risk of rectal and colon cancer among women who smoked. The risk more than doubled among women who had smoked a pack a day for more than ten years.

Diet and Exercise

Time and time again, studies in populations that eat a high-fiber diet both here and around the world show a very low colon cancer rate. Our high-fat, low-fiber diets are, I'm convinced, contributing to our deaths from colon cancer, although we cannot yet point to a controlled scientific study to back me up. We know that the large amounts of fat we eat are turned by large-bowel bacteria into chemicals that can irritate bowel cells and, after years of constant exposure, sometimes induce cancerous transformation in these cells. A high-fiber diet can decrease the exposure of the bowel lining cells to these toxic fat derivatives, both by diluting them and also by speeding up transit time through the bowel. (See chapter 2.) Although studies vary, several in different populations worldwide have linked colorectal cancer to diets lower in calcium and vitamin D. The Women's Health Initiative will also explore the effect of calcium and vitamin D supplements on the development of this cancer, providing a needed, definitive answer.

Sedentary Lifestyle

Being sedentary has been tied to colon cancer. It is surmised that exercise improves the tone of the gastrointestinal tract and may, like fiber, decrease the bowel's exposure to the carcinogens in food.

DETECTION

Colon cancer is fortunately a cancer for which we can easily screen. I urge you to make sure that your physician or gynecologist annually examines your stool for blood (this is generally a part of a routine gynecological exam). If you are over the age of fifty, the American Cancer Society recommends that your doctor perform a sigmoidoscopy, which looks at the rectum and the lower portion of the left side of the colon, every three to five years. Increasingly, however, doctors are recommending that the more extensive colonoscopy test, which looks at the inside of the entire colon, not just the lower portion, be administered every three to five years.

Warning signs that should alert you to colon cancer, particularly as you get older, are unexplained changes in bowel habits, blood in the stool, or rectal bleeding. Discuss any one of these signs with your doctor.

TREATMENT

The first stage of colon cancer (called *Dukes A*) is a localized but clearly cancerous tumor. Only about 15 percent of colon tumors are picked up at this stage, but if you can catch it, the five- to ten-year survival rate is 90 percent or better. Treatment, as you may guess, is surgery. Unlike many other cancers, though, colon cancer has not been shown to respond well to either radiation therapy or to chemotherapy, although these adjuvant treatments are used with some success for more advanced disease with lymph node involvement.

Once the cancer has grown through the bowel wall and involves the fat that covers the outer surface of the colon (called the *Dukes B* stage), survival with surgery falls to about 70 to 80 percent. Surgery at this stage means removing much of the colon. When the cancer has spread to nearby lymph nodes (*Dukes C*), the surgery is even more extensive, but the survival rate for five years after surgery is still about 40 to 60 percent. (Most of the time, removing the tumor does *not* require a colostomy, an opening in the abdominal wall through which wastes are eliminated into a bag.) At *Dukes D,* in which the tumor has spread to nearby organs or to distant sites like the lung or the brain, surgeons remove what they can through surgery, but the chance of survival beyond five years is less than 10 percent.

PREVENTION

If you are not at high risk for colon cancer through inherited factors, look first to your diet as a means of preventing this disease. Diets rich in fruits, vegetables, complex carbohydrates, and fiber, and low in red meat and saturated fats, seem to decrease your chance of getting colon cancer. The Women's Health Initiative is now looking at this very issue among a large group of women and should come up with definitive information. But don't wait. (See page 10.)

Early screening is a must, and any early polyps must be removed before they can grow into cancer. If colon cancer runs in your family, these screenings become crucial, as does a regular colonoscopy on a schedule you should set with your doctor. For those who have the familial polyposis syndrome, prophylactic removal of most of the colon is usually recommended fairly early in adult life. This was, in fact, probably the first cancer for which prophylactic organ removal became routine practice.

CANCERS OF THE SKIN

Cancers of the skin may not be unique to women, but they are a common and growing problem for women. Skin cancers are increasing worldwide, and we are not sure why. They are caused, in virtually all cases, by overexposure to ultraviolet light, which reaches us from the sun. People who live at high altitudes, or are exposed to the sun more frequently throughout their lifetimes, get more skin cancer. It seems logical to assume that, since being tan became a symbol of beauty in our culture, our sun-basking for vanity's sake before we had a clue about the sun's dangers may well be a contributing factor. We all did it, and we didn't know. But we know now—and, again, this is a type of cancer whose risk we can easily diminish.

Cancers of the skin come in three general categories, depending on the specific cell type within the skin that becomes malignant: *basal cell cancers, squamous cell cancers,* and *malignant melanomas.* All of them have the sun at their origins.

BASAL CELL CARCINOMA

The most common of all skin cancers are the basal cell carcinomas. These look like little craters or crusty sores on the skin, developing most often on the head or neck, particularly around the eyes or on the nose, and involve the deepest layer of the skin. This cancer grows slowly and locally and almost never spreads.

Risk Factors

The major risk factors for basal cell carcinoma are being a fair-skinned person and being exposed to the sun. Another is the existence of small, roughened, and discolored patches that appear mostly on the face, called *actinic keratoses.* These spots don't lead to basal skin cancer, but they are caused by overexposure to the sun, and serve as a reminder that your lifetime openness to the sun has put you in danger.

Detection and Treatment

Basal cell cancers are in ready sight in the mirror, and usually seen first by the patient. Treatment is by local excision with a scalpel, by freezing through cryosurgery, or through local radiotherapy. Treatment brings a cure, but your sun-exposed skin is likely to keep getting these cancers. You must stay alert for the development of new sores, so they can be treated early with a good cosmetic result.

Prevention

Avoid the sun. When you do go out in the sun, wear a sunscreen, especially if you are fair—and no tanning parlors!

SQUAMOUS CELL CANCER

Squamous cell carcinoma involves the most superficial part of the skin, the outermost cell layer, called the *squamous epithelium*. Like basal cell cancer, this tumor grows very slowly, but it can be more invasive and can ultimately spread distantly, although only about 2 percent of these cancers do. Squamous cell cancers first appear as a painless, firm round lump on your lip or ear; the lump may eventually turn into an ulcer.

Risk Factors

The major risk factor for squamous cell cancer is, of course, long-standing sun exposure, but there are other important risks to note. Though not a direct risk for basal cell cancer, the skin abnormalities mentioned on page 266, actinic keratoses, can turn into squamous cancer. Age is another risk factor for this type of cancer: most of the time, it turns up after the age of sixty. Scars from burns or chronic skin ulcers make a woman more susceptible to this cancer, and squamous cell cancers developing in burn scars have a chance of spreading ten times greater than do those developed from sun exposure. (Long-term skin exposure to certain industrial chemicals—such as tar, coal, or paraffin—is also a risk factor, but uncommon for women.) If you have had one squamous cell cancer, you are at risk for another.

Detection and Treatment

Squamous cell cancers are also easily spotted, by feel and in the mirror. When they become large enough to see, they are generally still small enough to cure without major surgery.

When the tumor is spotted early, it is generally removed through surgery, radiotherapy, or by freezing. On those rare occasions when it has spread distantly, or appears to have, anticancer drugs are given. When found locally, it is completely curable; overall, it has a 90 percent five-year survival rate.

Prevention

Avoid the sun. Protect yourself in the workplace from direct chemical exposure to your skin. If you have burn scars, keep attentive to any abnormalities in or around them. And bring any unusual or enlarging skin lesions to the attention of your doctor.

MALIGNANT MELANOMA

Malignant melanoma is the most dangerous of all the skin cancers. It develops in the melanocytes, the cells in the skin that produce skin pigment. These cancers too are increasing worldwide for no good reason beyond excessive exposure to the sun. In the United States we have seen a steady increase in their incidence—sixfold in the past four decades—and a death rate growing at 3 percent per year over that time. Although this cancer is more common in the elderly, its occurrence is increasing among all age groups, even among those in their twenties and thirties.

Gender differences favor women in the occurrence of this cancer: women have about half as many melanomas as do men, and a lower mortality rate. Melanomas also tend to appear in different spots on women than they do on men, first showing themselves in women somewhere on their lower limbs, including the soles of the feet (whereas in men they typically first show up on the trunk). Melanomas appear mainly in whites with fair, easily sunburned skin, and rarely occur in dark-skinned individuals or Asians.

Risk Factors

The relationship between malignant melanoma and the ultraviolet radiation in sunlight, and particularly a history of blistering sunburns early in life, is now well established. But, unlike the other skin cancers, sun exposure is by no means the whole story. Our inherited genes affect our melanoma risk. There appears to be a gene or genes on chromosome 9 tied to at least one form of malignant melanoma.

Detection

Melanomas often develop on parts of the skin that have had major sun exposure in the past—but unlike squamous and basal cell cancers, they can occur almost anywhere, even in the eye. About a third of the time, they develop in a preexisting mole. (Our body has numerous moles, but only rarely does one become malignant—literally about one in a million.) Women themselves are the ones most likely to pick up a malignant melanoma, by noticing a change in a mole's size or color or the development of an irregular border—or pain, itching, or bleeding in a new or existing mole.

Treatment

A suspicious mole must be biopsied; if it is cancerous, the treatment always involves removing the mole. Other forms of treatment, however, are very limited. These tumors tend to be resistant to radiotherapy, and only a small group of people have any response to chemotherapy.

If the malignant mole does not penetrate into the skin by more than 0.75 mm, removing the mole plus a margin of about 1 to 2 cm of skin around it will cure the disease in nearly 100 percent of instances. As the tumor grows deeper, the cure rate falls: penetration to 1.5 mm correlates with a five-year survival of about 90 percent; between 2 and 3 mm, survival falls to around 70 percent; and if the tumor is more than 3 mm thick, five-year survival falls to 40 to 50 percent. Once the cancer has spread to distant sites, such as the liver, the outlook is very poor, with less than 20 percent survival to five years.

Prevention

Avoid the sun, and particularly avoid blistering sunburns early in life. This means parents must be atuned to the sunburn risk in their children. After that, the best prevention is early detection—the only way to ensure a cure.

STUDIES TO WATCH FOR

We have yet to win the war against cancer. We have got to learn to cure it—to find it in its earliest and sneakiest state and to take it out without doing damage. I don't believe, though, that we will ever stop cancer from developing in the first place. Our bodies are filled with billions of cells, most dividing and reproducing in such a myriad of ways and times that monitoring and controlling all of them would simply be impossible. We cannot stop the occasional gene from mutating dangerously. But we can, I'm convinced, find ways to strengthen our immune system from within, to teach our own cells to demolish those devastating, aberrant cells, before they can destroy us. Curing cancer depends on expanding our base of knowledge in molecular biology, molecular immunology, human genetics, and genetic therapy. Here are a few specific areas to watch for:

• FINDING A CANCER VACCINE. *Fulfillment of one of the greatest dreams would be the discovery of a cancer vaccine. This would immunize us against the spread of a small tumor that has been identified and removed, marshaling the forces of the body's own immune system to identify and destroy the alien cells invading our bodies from within, much as vaccines for small pox or diphtheria already do.*

QUESTIONS FOR YOUR DOCTOR

- You should ask your primary care doctor to review your early detection plan for cancer. Include on such a plan your diet, other lifestyle issues, and a schedule of regular medical visits for routine screening. Ask about your own personal risk, including a review of your family history of cancer.
- What is your doctor's opinion on and experience with prophylactic medications or surgery for high-risk ovarian, breast, or colon cancer?

- FINDING NEW ANTICANCER DRUGS THAT CHOKE OFF BLOOD SUPPLY TO TUMORS. *One of the more malevolent aspects of cancer cells is their ability to set up their own life-sustaining blood supply. If we can block this ability, called* angiogenesis, *tumors would starve to death instead of spreading. Researchers are currently investigating several naturally occurring agents that may well turn out to serve this function. One such protein, called* tissue inhibitor proteinase 2 (TIMP-2), *prevents the formation of new capillaries and vessels in and around tumors. Other substances,* angiostatin *and* interleukin-12, *also inhibit tumor blood vessel growth. We must continue research efforts into this promising area. Given cancer's proclivity to consume its host, its death by starvation would be a most fitting end.*

- GENE THERAPY. *The importance of the genetic basis of cancer has been a consistent theme in this chapter. Gene therapy, which includes the immunotherapies discussed on page 229, is a whole new approach to human disease which involves focusing on the fundamental genetic error or errors that are causing the problem. The strategies vary. Some researchers are trying to replace or correct genes found to be missing or dangerously mutated. Others are inserting genes into cancer cells, to induce the cells to produce powerful factors called* cytokines, *which attract and stimulate immune cells to the tumor site. Still others are inserting into tumor cells genes that should make the tumor more susceptible to existing drugs and radiation. These and other gene therapies will change the face of medicine in the twenty-first century.*

- If you are told you have HPV infection in your cervix, ask which strain. Is it a strain that is especially risky for cervical cancer, and if so, what should be done? If you are planning to have children, does the problem affect the timing of that decision?

- Does your skin type place you at risk for skin cancer? What type of protection does your doctor recommend?

- From time to time, ask about any new diagnostic tests that have been released. Are they appropriate for you? What's new in genetic screening tests?

- What about the laboratory support system that your doctor uses? What laboratory does she use to examine Pap smears? Is it accredited? What can she tell you about its records? What about the radiology lab she's sending you to? How long has it been operating? Why does she recommend it? How did she determine that it would be the most accurate and skillful?

- If you are told you have cancer, do not hesitate to ask for a second opinion. Be sure to consult an oncologist; that is, a doctor specializing in cancer. Find out about that doctor's experience with the kind of cancer you might have.

- Is the biopsy of your tumor being reviewed by another cancer pathologist, to see if there is any question whether it is cancer or what kind? This is especially important before embarking on any major course of therapy.

- Always ask if there are alternative approaches to the treatment plan your doctor suggests. Why does she recommend this approach over others? Are there different forms of surgery? Radiation? Chemotherapy? Immunotherapy?

- How extensive will the surgery your doctor proposes be? What degree of deformity or disability can you expect? Are there less radical approaches? Is reconstruction an option? Can it be done at the same time as the surgery?

- If reconstructive surgery is being proposed after breast cancer, who will perform the reconstructive surgery? Why does your doctor recommend this person? Can you see photographs of his work, and speak to other people who have consulted him?

- If you have had endometrial cancer or breast cancer, ask about hormone replacement therapy.

- Ask about cancer support groups in your community that might be helpful to you or your family. What about home health services? Hospices?

WHAT WOMEN CAN DO
PERSONALLY AND POLITICALLY

"Hurry" is the prescription for the war against cancer; public activism has been the energizer. We know that the passionate actions of individuals can make a difference in finding medical cures—we know that primarily because of the enormous difference such actions have already made in combating cancer. Use the steps we have made in cancer as an inspiration never to give up, on cancer or on any other disease that seems incurable. And don't tire of the cancer war, now that we have come so far.

Some twenty years ago, Ann Landers, aka Eppie Lederer, wrote a column about the War on Cancer that led to the appearance of millions of letters in record time at the White House and the Congress. The public outpouring was instrumental in the passing of the National Cancer Act (which vastly increased funding for cancer research education and prevention and created a presidentially appointed national cancer board, among other achievements), a testament to the fact that letter writing can make a difference. One thing politicians do well is count!

Cancer research advocates have been effective at the grass roots as well as the federal level. The National Breast Cancer Coalition, cofounded by Fran Vesco and Dr. Susan Love, has exerted pressure on virtually all federal activities that affect breast cancer patients, and its representatives have been vocal at congressional hearings and served on advisory boards and initiated meetings at agencies like the NIH and the CDC. Numerous cities across the country have instituted "The Race for the Cure," a breast cancer marathon sponsored by the Susan B. Komen Foundation. This group, which now has branches in cities all over the country, was founded by one woman, Nancy Brinker, a breast cancer survivor, in the name of her sister who died from it.

For more inspiration, we can look to the American Cancer Society itself. It is among the largest of the volunteer health agencies, active in communities everywhere in America. ACS and local hospitals are often embarking on cancer screening efforts aimed at the public. Other cancers striking women now cry out for this same type of effort and education, particularly lung cancer, cervical cancer, and ovarian cancer.

Finally, the creation of humane hospices and hospice services has often been the domain of community activists who pull together to bring this service to a neighborhood or city. In my own Cleveland, a group of women led by Pat Modell energized the business community, the sports world, hospitals, and the general public to rally behind the cause of providing expanded hospice services for all patients dying of cancer regardless of their means—with the simple message that these patients should be free from pain and never be alone. Consider initiating or joining such a movement in your own community.

At a personal level, there is much you can do for yourself. Once again, knowledge is power. Learn as much as you can about the risks you can control, and especially about risks you face simply because you're a woman and your body is made vulnerable by your lifestyle in a way that a man's isn't. These risks might not be too well reported in the news; they are not all common knowledge. If you suspect a problem, get to the doctor without hesitation.

When cancer is the topic, you will have an almost endless number of questions facing you at every point, from simple risk factors through detection techniques through treatment choices and choice of oncologist and surgeon, and about emotional issues as well. Ask your questions, no matter how uncomfortable they might be.

I don't know the fate of the woman who told me to hurry on those Capitol steps. She was about to undergo a bone marrow transplant—something that ten years ago would not have been a possibility, and perhaps twenty years from now will not be a necessity. I do know there is a chance she survived, and I know that if we continue to hurry there is an even greater chance that, despite the risk of inherited breast cancer, none of her children will fight the same enemy. The battlefront against cancer is in constant motion, but the final and definitive contest will take place on the tiniest possible field—within our own cells. If we heed this young woman's advice, and hurry to support the research that will provide the weaponry, we will win this war.

SEVEN

DEPRESSION AND ANXIETY
Living Without Joy

Sorrow like a ceaseless rain
Beats upon my heart.
People twist and scream in pain, —
Dawn will find them still again;
This has neither wax nor wane,
Neither stop nor start.

People dress and go to town;
I sit in my chair.
All my thoughts are slow and brown;
Standing up or sitting down
Little matters, or what gown
Or what shoes I wear.

—EDNA ST. VINCENT MILLAY,
"SORROW," 1917

My slow and brown year began just before the Christmas of 1980. In the course of about twelve months, my father died an anguished death from cancer, and I was separated and divorced, finding myself a single mother with a very little girl and an oversized mortgage. That same year my pipes froze in one of the worst winters in Baltimore history, my furnace broke down, and my house was ransacked and robbed. I was in a funk I couldn't shake. I was anxious. I couldn't sleep. For a while I saw doom and gloom everywhere.

As it most often does for everyone, my cloud gradually passed. I clung to my work in medicine and my daughter and muddled my way into obtaining the support I needed—but not because I ever admitted to myself I needed it. That experience left me knowing that I, who had prided myself from my earliest recollections for being strong and sturdy, the one with true grit, was human and vulnerable to a dark period of the soul. It left me with greater insight into the depressive reactions I saw in many of my own heart patients. Maybe, as some psychiatrists say, being depressed is the common cold of psychiatry, but as a persistent state of mind interfering with life's function, it becomes the devil's grippe.

It's likely that any woman reading this chapter can identify to a greater or lesser degree with what I endured in that year. Most women would not hesitate to label my reaction as a depressive reaction and empathize with me. Intuitively, women seem to understand depression; this is not a sexist statement but a truism because there is less of a stigma for women to identify and express their emotions. Female gender and depression seem linked: the ratio of women to men who report symptoms of depression is more than two to one. Almost seven million American women are afflicted at any one time; anxiety disorders and/or depression will strike somewhere between 10 and 25 percent of all women in their lifetime.

DEFINING MOOD DISORDERS

Many researchers have found that depression can affect the immune system, making you susceptible to other illnesses (or contributing to the length of an existing illness); at the very least, it interferes with your ability to experience joy or to function as you should socially, at work or in relationships. But depression hasn't always been viewed as a serious illness. In part, that's an understandable result of the slippery nature of the beast; in part, as we'll see later in this chapter, it's a result of not so understandable historical and societal views about women.

For those who do recognize the impact of depression, analyzing it and treating it are no simple tasks. Although we now have some very good guesses, no one knows with certainty what, biologically, causes depression or anxiety. Diagnoses are therefore based solely on symptoms: not blood tests, not X rays, neither CAT scans nor MRIs. If we had to diagnose other illnesses this way, we'd be treating the symptom of chest pain as a heart attack in an intensive care unit, when the chest pain could have been caused in reality by a hiatus hernia—and treated with Tums.

Nature and nurture come together in depression and anxiety disorders as they do in perhaps no other. Psychological or environmental stresses work their damage on a human mind that is very much the product of its genetic and biochemical makeup and biological development. In the millions of women hit by depression, a trigger somehow is pulled, the brain chemistry shifts, and a depressive illness results. What may cause a depression in one person may not even affect another.

A further complexity: psychiatrists and researchers have been locked into constant redefinition of depression for most of this century. If you can't consistently identify the diseases, how can you begin to ascertain causes or prescribe treatments? The terminology has become more precise, but the field is still very much in flux. Before detailing the precise diagnostic criteria and treatment approaches in use today, I will start with a general discussion of this sometimes elusive condition called depression.

Depression is a tortured state of mind, which persists from weeks to months and sometimes longer, in which your predominant symptom is sadness and dejection. It occurs most often in the context of loss—loss of a loved one, job, home, or health. What begins, however, as a natural reaction of grief or loneliness veers out of control; the mood turns into an illness when self-esteem crumbles; feelings of self-reproach and powerlessness incite fears that there is no lightness ahead. You feel dependent, and feel unable to achieve mastery of your state of mind, your problems, or the outside world. The overriding feeling for most people in a depression is a sense of helplessness.

The key to this definition of a clinically significant disorder is the veering out of control. There is a critical moment when something "clicks" in your brain, and your despondent mood shifts into a true depression you cannot shake off. Freud had an even simpler but more powerful means of identifying a serious depression that demanded his intervention. He asked: Can you love and can you work? If you can't, something has "clicked."

Affect describes mood or emotion as seen by another person. The common forms of clinically significant mood disorders discussed in this chapter are lumped under the umbrella category of *affective disorders,* describing illnesses in which the most prominent symptom is a persistent or recurrent disturbance of mood—either up (*manic*) or down (*depressed*). Examples of psychological malaise that don't fit this category are simple mood swings or even short-term, severe emotional reactions to disturbing life events, and are referred to as adjustment disorders.

While the bulk of this chapter concerns depression, we'll also explore anxiety, which is a separate, distinct, and common emotion that sometimes accompanies depression and sometimes appears alone, but it may intensify to a debilitating fear or panic that is inappropriate to whatever has triggered it. Although we don't have the wealth of history and research on anxiety that we do on depression, anxiety does not carry depression's heavy historical baggage.

When we look at the definition above and study the symptoms, which we will do later in the chapter, it will be clear why women have experienced more depression than men throughout history. Women are, as a rule, still an underclass everywhere in the world, regardless of socioeconomic status. Social structures have made women emotionally and economically dependent; women have not routinely been allowed to feel the sense of mastery over their environment that men commonly do. Nor have women's accomplishments outside the home been encouraged—or even sometimes permitted. In such a social climate, it's no wonder that depression more often strikes.

Edna St. Vincent Millay, who penned the lines introducing this chapter, has always been one of my favorite poets. The first woman to win a Pulitzer prize for poetry, she celebrated the individual spirit and wrote personally and piercingly about love, emotion, conflict, and nature, always with the eye of a woman. She also battled depression on and off during her life. In Jean Gould's biography, *The Poet and Her Book*, Millay speaks of her "chronic moodiness and quixotic behavior" and of how she sought understanding and forgiveness for her "silly moods." "How silly I am!—and I know how silly I am! . . . Just Heaven consign and damn / To tedious Hell this body with its muddy feet in my mind!"

Perhaps her "moods" sprang in part from the conflict between her creative genius and a society that forced her to view her mood as "silly." For many women, the world can be and often has been a pretty depressing place.

WE CANNOT IGNORE OUR HISTORY

The evolution of our thinking about depression has been deeply rooted in our views of society and our views of women in particular.

COUNTERPOINT

Depression is a woman's disease . . . maybe. Certainly, the numbers of women who experience depression's classic symptoms—feelings of dependency, hopelessness, helplessness—far outdistance the numbers of men reporting the same symptoms. But symptoms are not causes. It's exceedingly possible that men may have the same "disease" of depression and entirely different symptoms (such as violent behavior, alcoholism, and suicide—all more prevalent in men). Until we have a concrete biochemical or physiological test to pinpoint depression, we simply won't know.

Additionally, the more severe the depression, the more likely it is to have originated in a biological or genetic problem, not necessarily to be triggered by an exterior life experience. Women more often report suffering the common, milder, more socially influenced kind of depression; men and women experience in more equal numbers the less common, more severe, biologically based varieties. In a different world it's certainly conceivable that women would no longer hold the numbers edge on depression.

In ancient times, Hippocrates contended that unexplainable illnesses such as depression and madness were based on emotions and originated in the uterus. Hence, the linguistic connection between hysteria, hysterectomy, and the Greek word *hysterikos*, which means "pertaining to the womb."

Two thousand years later the theory still held strong. In the Victorian era—much of the nineteenth century—in which psychoanalytic theory was born, hysterectomies were performed expressly to treat the emotional disorders of women. In 1850 Dr. Edward Jarvis wrote in the *American Journal of Insanity* that all of the "various and manifold derangements of the reproductive system, peculiar to females, add to the causes of insanity." Another prominent physician of the time, Dr. Horatio Robinson Storer, contended that a woman's health, character, and charms of body, mind, and soul were all due to her womb alone.

Throughout the Western world, until this century, women were chattel. They had no control over their lives; were owned by father, husband, or brother; had no property or rights of their own; had no political voice or vote; and served the sole and exclusive role of motherhood. They were expected to relish their dependency. The nineteenth century was a time of great restlessness for women, in which rebels such as Lucretia Mott, Elizabeth Cady Stanton, Elizabeth Blackwell, Emmeline Pankhurst, and others organized to define for the first time the concept of women's rights: economic independence, the right to vote, and maternal and child health, to begin with.

From this atmosphere came Sigmund Freud, who ushered in modern psychiatry. Freud was brilliant and insightful—and an inescapable product of his own environment. He lived in a milieu in which women were viewed as inherently inferior, and all too often repressed and depressed.

Freud put these components together in his study of the psychological dynamics of men and women and came up with the infamous notion of penis envy, which holds that women forever feel inadequate because they learn in childhood that they don't have penises; they can become psychologically whole and healthy as adults only by channeling any envy (or aggression or competitiveness) derived from the lack they feel into the wholesome craving for a husband or by bearing a child (preferably a son). Women, to Freud, have an innately passive nature that is perverted through "loss" of a penis; to find peace and satisfaction, a woman must recover her natural passivity. This view has permeated and colored both the field of psychology and the world's view of women throughout this century. In it, any woman striving for equality is simply expressing some kind of neurotic yearning to have a penis.

FREUD: FRIEND OR FOE TO WOMEN?

I "grew up" on Freud in college; in fact, inspired by his work, I thought for a while that I would be a psychiatrist. My interest and respect for the field continued despite the jocund taunts of "penis envy" I heard occasionally from some of my male colleagues when I noted the sex-bias irritants of my early medical training—like distinctively male bathrooms labeled PHYSICIANS ONLY or the fact that the salaries of married women interns were 10 percent less than those of the married males.

I could reconcile the conflict easily, for Freud, in my opinion, did as much for women and the world as he inadvertently did against them. Before Freud, mood disorders were seen as some kind of possession by demons. Freud recognized them as illnesses rooted in environment, heredity, biology, and early experience; he thereby was instrumental in bringing them respect and, more important, disciplined diagnosis and treatment. Because of the focus of Freud's work, women were finally seen as separate from the mental illness that afflicted them.

Freud gave us one of the earliest descriptions of affective disorders. He saw depression as a severe form of melancholia, in which the patient loses the ability to work or to love, and he likened it to mourning. He was the first to stress that loss of self-esteem was central to depressive illness.

Freud was highly respectful of women (even if, to him, they were inferior in social and psychoanalytic terms); he was way ahead of his time in his research into and analysis of women's mental health, and he fervently trained an entire generation of women disciples (including his daughter Anna) who became prominent psychoanalysts—prominent enough to challenge him in his own day.

Thanks, finally, to Freud's concentration on sex and gender as the cornerstone of psychoanalytic theory (and obviously in part to the sheer numbers of women evincing mood disorders), psychology is one of the few medical disciplines that has not neglected women in either research or practice. Yes, much of the resulting findings have been filtered through a man's eye (hence, penis envy), but women are still far more and better represented in studies here than in other crucial health areas, such as cardiovascular research.

Freud's students and disciples included two women, in particular, with influential and opposing interpretations. Helene Deutsch espoused a very literal interpretation of the concept of penis envy. Despite her own "liberated" life as a physician, writer, and teacher, she wholeheartedly believed that women struggle all their lives with an inferior organ (female genitals), destined for passivity and doomed to masochism.

Karen Horney, a German-born American psychoanalyst and student of Freud, brilliantly and generously challenged both Freud and Deutsch. In her classic work, *Feminine Psychology*, she noted Freud was constrained by both his own sex and by society, his limitations clear but understandable: "Almost all of those who have developed his ideas have been men. It is only right and reasonable that they should evolve more easily a masculine psychology and understand more of the development of men than of women." Horney saw male and female as complementary, not at odds. She introduced what to me was a highly creative way to expose the fallacies of penis envy: "motherhood envy." "Now, if we try to free our minds from this masculine mode of thought, nearly all the problems of feminine psychology take on a different appearance. . . . At this point I, as a woman, ask in amazement, and what about (. . . the ineffable happiness of . . .) motherhood? . . . from the biological point of view woman has in motherhood, or in the capacity for motherhood, a quite indisputable and by no means negligible physiological superiority."

The battle over these concepts of women's mental health raged mainly in the psychoanalytic field in the 1930s as Horney and others took on the views of the strict Freudians. In the 1970s it erupted more broadly as the woman's movement targeted the misogyny of Freud and Deutsch: their theories became symbolic of the oppressed and sure to be depressed woman.

CURRENT PICTURE OF MENTAL ILLNESS

Today, most professionals are able to separate Freud the man from his crucial insights. I see several other positive developments in the complex field of mental illness. First, a somewhat symbolic event: in 1992, after twenty years of separation, the National Institute of Mental Health was brought back under the umbrella of the NIH. This seemingly inconsequential reorganization was actually proof of a major shift in perspective: a recognition that severe mental illnesses have a strong biological basis and that the so-called physical illnesses like cancer and heart disease have a behavioral component.

In addition to the moves at the NIH, I note two important shifts that began with Freud but are only now well established in the medical world's understanding and treatment of affective disorders. First, these disorders are finally being characterized in precise detail as illnesses. This means they can be demystified and approached as any other medical illness would be. Second, we've seen electrifying advances in our knowledge of the biochemistry of behavior and the genetics of mental illness, which are pointing the way toward more precise classification and specific drug treatments.

All this greatly encourages me, as do the slow but steady societal changes empowering women and thereby lessening the psychological burdens that can lead to depression. But we have much to learn and far to go; many studies still show that the symptoms of depression and anxiety are taken less seriously in women than the same symptoms in men.

THE ORIGINS AND RISK FACTORS FOR AFFECTIVE DISORDERS

Our goal in dealing with any illness is treating it and making it go away. But accurate treatment relies first on a thorough understanding of cause—something we're still trying to achieve with affective disorders, which as we've noted have their origins in a complex mix of biology and circumstance. There is generally no overriding cause or common pathway to the disorder; rather, each instance of depression reveals a three-dimensional personal portrait of mind, body, and spirit. Here is what researchers have learned might precipitate the leap from health to illness of the mind.

BIOLOGICAL CAUSES OF AFFECTIVE DISORDERS

Intellectual battles have raged from the beginning of medical history regarding the causes of these disorders. The ancient Greeks, founders of medicine, felt that most illnesses, including those of the mind, were caused by an imbalance of internal, physical "humors." Later scholars insisted that mental illnesses were caused by external events such as childhood trauma. Medicine now appears to have completed a two-millennium circle. We have discovered that, in addition to the environmental factors, there are indeed entities in the body and brain that can have profound effects on mental balance. The ancient Greeks called them humors; we call them genes and hormones, neurotransmitters and neuropeptides.

YOUR GENES

Many studies have shown that both depression and anxiety clearly run in families at a significantly higher rate than many other illnesses, including breast cancer or heart disease. Heredity is just one risk factor of many, and a genetic predisposition does not mean you'll automatically have an affective disorder, but it's a critical one. Your genes influence both your biological and to some extent your psychological degree of risk (the latter through your inherited temperament, discussed on page 291). Your brain structure is genetically predetermined, as is much of the brain chemistry discussed below. In fact, in 1992 the American Psychological Association identified genetics as one of the themes that represents "the present and future of psychology."

In the following sections, we'll discuss many determinants of affective disorders, but most will ultimately come back to the genes. Our genes are the framework through which we interact with external events, since they establish the chemical systems and biological components of our bodies and then in turn are regulated by them.

HORMONES

Hormones are the vehicles of brain-body interaction, chemicals circulating throughout our bodies that are secreted into the bloodstream by specific glands. Several hormones appear to play an important role in mood and behavior and are tied in to the development of depression. The implications of such connections are enormous. If some types of affective disorders are caused by a pattern of excess or insufficient hormones that we can identify, then we can envision a next step: curing depression by selectively regulating hormones.

CRH, ACTH, and Cortisol—the Stress Connection

Cortisol—better known as cortisone (a manufactured version of our bodies' natural creation)—is a stress-sensitive hormone released by the adrenal gland (a little gland sitting on top of the kidney) in response to two other triggering hormones, CRH and ACTH. CRH (corticotropin-releasing hormone) comes from the hypothalamus in the brain; it flows through the entire nervous system and thereby stimulates the pituitary gland to release the hormone ACTH (corticotropin). The ACTH regulates the release of cortisol, causing more to be released when we are under stress. For healthy people, after the stress is relieved, the levels of CRH, ACTH, and cortisol fall to normal. People who are depressed, however, continue to pour out high levels of these elements twenty-four hours a day. We know specifically that CRH, the "master molecule," has been shown to be elevated in depressed patients—but we haven't yet figured out a reliable way to use the knowledge to make a specific diagnosis, or to pin down a certain cause.

Thyroid Hormone

Thyroid hormone produced by the thyroid gland regulates how cells use energy and perform chemical functions. Thyroid hormone has been tied to some depressive disorders: a small number of depressed people have low levels of this hormone, and people with a thyroid deficiency disease called myxedema often have depression that can be cured with thyroid replacement.

Sex Hormones

Sex hormones such as estrogen and testosterone are well known to affect mood. A number of affective disorders may relate to abrupt changes of estrogen, in particular. For example, postpartum depression and severe premenstrual syndrome have been linked to fluctuations in estrogen levels (see pages 315 and 317). Much needs to be learned about the role of female sex hormones in affective disorders and about their possible role in the gender differences between the way men and women suffer (or at least report) depression.

NEUROTRANSMITTER SYSTEMS

Neurotransmitters, chemicals washing through our brains, are the vehicles of brain-mind interaction, that is, they are the means whereby the complex structures of the brain are turned into the conscious and unconscious workings of the mind. (Sometimes the same chemical element is both a hormone and a neurotransmitter, depending on whether it circulates in the blood or stays solely in the brain.) But the chemicals themselves tell only part of a story, for the specific neurotransmitter holds little meaning outside of each complex system of nerves and chemicals that form a pathway within a specific anatomic site of the brain. The neurotransmitter systems create momentary signals through which our mind functions; each system is anchored, defined, or identified by a specific neurotransmitter.

Neurotransmitters are the means through which the estimated four billion nerve cells in the brain "touch" and influence one another. They flow through tubes called axons and dendrites, between nerve cells, and find other nerve cells to bind to and to excite. For every class of neurotransmitter there is a specific type and class of receptor, like the key to a lock. This whole interactive network comprises a neuro-transmitter system. There is no way to estimate the number of lock-and-key connections in the human brain; suffice it to say that there are more keyholes in the brain than there are stars in our galaxy. It is not that difficult, therefore, to see how the brain can produce the Sistine Chapel ceiling and great oatmeal cookies, nor is it difficult to see how the entire process might be disrupted by an imbalance of neurotransmitters.

Several neurotransmitters have been tied to mood and depression, but the most important of these are norepinephrine and serotonin. Dopamine and acetylcholine also seem to have an impact on depression, but to a lesser degree. How do we know? Mostly, accidentally.

Norepinephrine

Serendipity had characterized many important breakthroughs in medicine, from stumbling upon penicillin to the unexpected discovery of the hepatitis B virus, but it's hard to find a better example of a less expected yet more crucial discovery than that of the tie between mood swings and the brain's neurotransmitter systems. The breakthrough discovery: norepinephrine affects the state of mind.

Researchers noticed, in the 1950s, that the blood-pressure-lowering drug reserpine depleted norepinephrine levels in the brain and at the same time induced depressive symptoms. Other research has supported the connection: deficiency of norepinephrine coincides with depression, and an increase coincides with mania, a state of inappropriate elation and hyperactivity. Furthermore, an antituberculosis medicine, iproniazid, which as a side effect allows norepinephrine (and serotonin) to build up, was discovered to be a big mood uplifter in the tuberculosis patients who took it. These unexpected discoveries clearly positioned mental illnesses as having a biological—as well as psychological—dimension and initiated the era of psychopharmacology and drug therapy, revolutionizing psychiatry.

Serotonin

Serotonin was discovered inadvertently some thirty years ago by Dr. Irvine Page at the Cleveland Clinic Foundation, in the course of his research on high blood pressure. Serotonin did not turn out to be very important to most forms of hypertension, but later work identified serotonin as one of the most powerful and important of brain chemicals.

The serotonin system in the brain is linked to a wide range of functions including appetite, sleep, sexual behavior, and pain perception. When serotonin has been reduced in otherwise normal individuals, a variety of mood disorders has surfaced, including depression, anxiety, and lethargic behavior. Other studies have tied dysfunction in serotonin release to low self-esteem and lack of assertiveness. Low serotonin may also set the degree of anxiety or impulsivity, and increased levels of serotonin appear to enhance self-esteem, courage, assertiveness, calmness, flexibility, security, and resilience.

Melatonin (a derivative of serotonin) is linked to circadian rhythms—the normal glandular, metabolic, and sleep cycles that connect to the twenty-four-hour rotation of the earth, setting the body's biological rhythms. Melatonin normally increases at night (it has become a treatment sold in health food stores for insomnia), and depressed people have been shown to have a melatonin secretory pattern that is abnormally low. In other words, the notorious connection of sleeplessness to depression is not without its specific biological explanations. We swim in a complicated chemical soup, after all.

Dopamine and Acetylcholine

Although less well studied and more controversial, dopamine and acetylcholine may also be influential in causing some types of affective disorders. Much of the brain's dopamine is located in a region called the caudate nucleus. In studies conducted by Dr. Michael Phelps of UCLA and by others using special brain scanning techniques, depressed patients showed less brain activity in that region. Similarly, some symptoms of depression develop when stroke damages part of the caudate nucleus.

Acetylcholine plays a special role in our higher brain functioning, including memory. It is a powerful neurotransmitter that provides all nerve-to-muscle signals throughout the body, and it exerts a suppressive effect on many automatic body functions; for example, it slows the heart rate and lowers blood pressure. I'm afraid we know little about its role in mood and depression, but there are many hints that it may have an impact. A few studies have shown that large doses of choline, a building block of acetylcholine, decrease symptoms of mania in sufferers of manic depression (see page 318).

Other Noteworthy Brain Chemicals

Over the past few decades, we have uncovered a host of other brain chemicals that may modulate behavior, all lumped under the general chemical name of neuropeptides. (The name *peptides* merely refers to the molecular structure; many of these chemicals are too new to us to define by function. Technically, some of the hormones and neurotransmitters previously mentioned can also be classified as peptides.) The newly discovered peptides are often released at nerve terminals along with neurotransmitters, causing many researchers to suspect that they in some way modulate neurotransmitter activity. Like the major neurotransmitters, these peptides are particularly interesting because they are "site specific"; that is, they are localized to individual regions of the brain.

One peptide, GABA (gamma-amino-butyric acid), a generalized inhibitor of brain function, has a receptor in the limbic system of the brain—which is the fear and anxiety center. Certain tranquilizers that can quell anxiety states and produce sedation bind to the GABA receptor. Other neuropeptides include the opioids, oxytocin, galanin, neuropeptide Y, and substance P. Decreases or increases in these regulatory compounds have been connected to depression, but as yet not clearly or definitively. Research on this entire area is hot and will surely expand and modify our current thinking about the function of our minds in both health and disease.

WHO'S AT RISK?
NONBIOLOGICAL VULNERABILITIES

Depression is a vulnerability that comes with being human. Affective disorders are seen in virtually all societies and cultures worldwide. In the United States the prevalence of depression is reportedly lower than in most other developed parts of the world, including Canada, New Zealand, Britain, Scandinavia, Spain, Italy, or Greece.

The following risk factors are both psychological and environmental, derived from factors outside your physiological makeup. Each alone does not cause an affective disorder, but can make you more susceptible by increasing your experiences of some of the symptoms I mentioned at the opening of this chapter: *a continuing sense of loss; low self-esteem or insecurity; dependency; helplessness and lack of control.* In a continuing depression, the symptom also becomes the cause.

THE BIGGEST RISK FACTOR: A SECOND X CHROMOSOME

Being a woman means you're twice as likely to experience a mood disorder. Does this mean that we women truly are the weaker sex? I don't think so. Women may experience more depression, but we also seem to tolerate it better.

Biologically, the estrogen fluctuations women endure—monthly, with pregnancy, with menopause—do affect their mood. Estrogen is produced in the ovaries and plays a key role in all reproductive functions, but it washes over the brain as well, and affects thinking and feeling. An estrogen-born mood shift is not a depression; the illness of depression involves more than feeling temporarily blue or irritable. But women may well be set up, through their biological makeup, to be vulnerable should other causal factors come into play.

Psychologically, women are more openly emotional than men. Women cry more often, display more emotions, exhibit more dependency and often insecurity. All of these traits also have been shown to place a person at risk.

It is the social factors, though, that cannot be ignored as exposing women to risks of affective disorders. We've talked about Victorian society; today, the lip service given to equality in the face of the reality of glass ceilings, fragile or nonexistent support systems, unequal household burdens in two-career families, economic dependence in one-career families, and hundreds of mixed messages about what a woman is "supposed" to be—all contribute as social stressors that drastically raise a woman's susceptibility to this disease. Working mothers face loss day after day as both family and work must be balanced; few women I know feel a comfortable sense of control or mastery in today's conflicted social environment.

Again, these factors do not in and of themselves create depression; but they set women up for it. It reminds me of a stew: all the ingredients are in the pot, just waiting for someone or something to turn on the fire.

Of course, knowing we're at high risk on all fronts can itself be depressing. I choose to see it in a different light, finding a sense of strength and control first in recognizing that all these factors exist. Labeling the enemy can sometimes help render it impotent.

Women have a few even stronger weapons as well. I've mentioned that men and women experience the most severe and biologically based forms of depression at more similar rates. This would suggest that if you alter the burdensome environment, the numbers of afflicted women should diminish.

Also, women's vulnerability to minor depression may in fact be a component in an overall resiliency that is ultimately self-protective. When a woman is faced with loss of control, she becomes depressed. She bends. When a man loses control, he breaks. In the workplace, for example, when women are stressed they tend to become anxious, looking inward at their own limitations. Male workplace distress is more apt to show up in obsessive-compulsive, hostile, or aggressive actions; they explode in outward anger, often directed at others. (As someone who has spent her life in a high-stress workplace often dominated by men, my own observations concur with these findings. Moreover, I would go one step further and say, give me anxiety rather than hostility anytime.)

Men break in more profound ways as well. Worldwide, men commit far more suicides than women—by two to three times the rate.

WOMEN, INFERTILITY, AND DEPRESSION

There are now many studies that show that infertility is a major risk factor for depression in women; one study found infertile women were twice as likely to suffer depression as fertile women of the same ages. For some women, not being able to become pregnant can be as great a loss as any death.

I've said that one factor distinguishing depression from a normal grief reaction is the length of time the feeling persists. This leads me to wonder if depression triggered by infertility might not be heightened because hope relentlessly lingers in our times of high-technology pregnancy intervention. Women are not able simply to grieve and move forward; instead, they undertake long, often difficult, infertility treatments.

There is no way around the fact that not being able to have a child is a great source of sorrow for many women. Perhaps the best advice I can give here is to suggest that you have realistic expectations going in to any infertility intervention. If you must endure this loss, recognize it as such, mourn it—and try not to prolong it.

Studies of men and women (in hospitals, bomb shelters, and other conditions of extreme stress) have shown time and again that women are ultimately better able to handle severe emotional and psychological strains. In fact, the observations that more men than women are in mental institutions, have nervous breakdowns, commit suicide, turn violent, and get ulcers has led the anthropologist Ashley Montagu to expound on women's emotional strength, biological resilience, and keen intuitions in his 1954 treatise *The Natural Superiority of Women*.

TEMPERAMENT

Our temperaments are genetically determined, and certain of our tempermental traits predispose us to depression. I'm not saying our personalities are only a matter of fate or that a lifetime of depression is an inescapable result of whom we happen to pick as our parents and grandparents, but, as Peter Kramer, author of *Listening to Prozac*, says: "People don't have to be made vulnerable by trauma; they can be born vulnerable." Although there are those who would take issue, I wholeheartedly agree. Some inborn traits clearly put some people at a higher risk for depression and anxiety, traits such as being less resilient after stress, less emotionally strong, moodier—and, particularly, more dependent and more inhibited.

I differentiate temperament from character. Character is developed over time, very much acquired through interaction with the environment. Character is about instilled values, surrounding culture, expectations and aspirations, standards of good behavior, while temperament stems from biology and determines whether we are optimistic or pessimistic, energetic or lethargic, as well as our levels of introversion, passivity, empathy. Our personalities are the vector sum of character and temperament.

SOCIOECONOMIC FACTORS

Depression cuts across economic groups and travels all rungs of society. Whatever the income or educational level, however, depression is lower among those who are employed and have a sense of financial independence. Clearly, we are again seeing that any factor that contributes to your sense of dependency, insecurity, or lack of control can also put you at risk for depression.

BABY BOOMERS

All over the developed world, baby boomers are depressed. Despite higher standards of living, despite profound medical and technological advances, those born after World War II have seen a striking increase in the rate of depression.

The societal reasons for this phenomenon seem clear. Divorce, single parenthood, and simple logistics—many of us live miles from our extended families and support systems—have created clear psychic trauma. Frequency of crime (or the perception of such) and an uncertain economy filled with jobs requiring knowledge of technology that most of us don't understand add to our individual sense that we cannot control our own destinies. Our national self-esteem is battered; 76 percent of Americans polled by *Newsweek* in June 1994 thought that the United States is in a moral and spiritual decline. Baby-boom women, with more responsibilities inside and outside the home and not much real authority yet, are increasingly the beasts of burden but rarely the leaders of the pack. This is the definition of stress—and a clear risk factor for depression.

MARITAL STATUS

Those with the lowest rates of depression are happily married men and single, never married women. Those who are divorced or are living together without being married have the highest rates of depression. Why an insecure environment such as living together can be a risk factor for depression is clear; what's not so clear is why men tend to be less depressed in marriage than women.

Perhaps one reason is that unhappy marriages are still experienced as traps for women. Men can get out; women are more apt to be locked in social and economic dependence through marriage, feeling helpless.

Perhaps the reasons are more subtle and more historical. For centuries women have found their societal worth and identity in their marriages; this view is entrenched in society despite the many advances women have achieved. A married woman is often judged by the marriage, not by her accomplishments; a single woman, on the other hand, is judged on her own merit and may feel far more independent and in control of her life.

A marriage does not have to sap a woman's identity or independence, but even in a happy marriage, it is a risk we must all recognize and combat.

FAMILY HISTORY

Anyone in talk therapy for depression is likely to take a close look at family history; "Tell me about your childhood" (asked with a put-on Viennese accent) has become the stereotyped spoof of shrink talk. Early environment as a risk factor was indeed first proposed by Freud, who maintained that affective disorders in adults recapitulate infantile disappointments and loss.

While heredity does play its role, there is also clear support for Freud's notions. Obviously, parental style can be a risk factor for depression. For example, a parent may be overprotective or a good provider of material goods but indifferent and even rejecting in personal interactions. A child raised in such an environment may feel inferior, have very low self-esteem, and grow up, consequently, at high risk of depression.

LOSS

It's no wonder that the word *loss* appears in this chapter; it is the primary precipitating factor in most common depressions. Again, experiencing a loss will not in and of itself throw you into the illness of depression, but enduring a loss or a series of losses will render you particularly vulnerable (or, if sufficient other factors are already in place, can itself trigger a depressive illness). The death of a loved one, especially a child, but also a spouse or a parent, is devastating. When you are an adult, you might think that the loss of a parent is somehow easier to take; nothing could be less true. When my own father died, I read and reread the poem Edna St. Vincent Millay wrote in *Mine the Harvest* about the death of her mother:

> The courage that my mother had
> Went with her, and is with her still:
> Rock from New England quarried;
> Now granite in a granite hill.

The golden brooch my mother wore
She left behind for me to wear;
I have no thing I treasure more:
Yet, it is something I could spare.

Oh, if instead she'd left to me
The thing she took into the grave! —
That courage like a rock, which she
Has no more need of, and I have.

We experience many losses throughout our lives; some are less concrete and therefore damaging in a compounded way (we have the burden of allowing ourselves to mourn and sometimes convincing others that a loss exists, as well as having to bear the loss itself). Divorce, the breakup of a friendship or love affair; infertility; the loss of a job, a financial investment, or your home; a personal failure in school or in business; even the loss of an old identity coinciding with a very positive life transition, such as marriage or parenthood—all can threaten our sense of security and self-esteem.

Although it is natural and human to mourn any loss, the gloom should eventually pass and not take on the symptoms of a depressive illness. If you find you can't seem to sleep or get out of bed, work, or feel, don't hesitate to seek help. That does not mean, however, that one ever really gets over the death of a loved one. Grief changes you; it is one of our life experiences.

PHYSICAL ILLNESS

Depression is a common complication of other illnesses, especially major illnesses involving surgery. Such depression, once called *reactive depression* and now termed *adjustment disorder with depressed mood,* is discussed at length on page 316. For now, do note that illness is a risk factor, and take heed if you experience symptoms such as problems sleeping, loss of appetite, or low energy during your recovery.

OLD AGE

The elderly are vulnerable for several reasons. First, they are often afflicted with other illnesses—some debilitating and chronic, such as arthritis; others frightening and life-threatening, such as heart disease.

As noted above, illness alone puts everyone at an increased risk for reactive depression.

Additionally, as we age we experience other life events that engender risks, especially loss: we lose spouses and friends to death; children and grandchildren to distance; and even our ability to do some things that used to come easily to us.

Finally, there seem to be structural or hormonal changes in the aging brain that may cause depression. For example, as part of normal aging the levels of the brain hormone monoamine oxidase increases. This enzyme breaks down neurotransmitters such as norepinephrine and serotonin, thereby decreasing the levels of these important chemicals whose depletion has been linked to depression. (An NIH Consensus Development Panel on Depression in Late Life held in 1992 made a strong plea for a targeted research effort focusing on the diagnosis and treatment of biological causes of depression in the aged.)

Too often, doctors have trouble perceiving depression in the elderly. Symptoms may mirror dementia or become masked as a reaction to other illnesses. Furthermore, physicians often feel that depression is appropriate for a given condition. "If I had just been told I have Alzheimer's disease, I'd be depressed too," they're likely to think, and then do nothing to treat the problem. But even with terminal illnesses, treating the depression can help sufferers eat better and sleep better, lose their sense of hopelessness, and generally derive greater satisfaction from whatever remaining time they have. The converse is also true. After hip fracture, for example, elderly women who are depressed need longer hospitalizations and more physical therapy in order to walk again.

Depression may be understandable, but it is never good for your health. Neither is ignoring it.

PUTTING IT ALL TOGETHER

It's clear that no single factor causes depression; therefore, any single theory about it must fall short of the truth. Most research studies in related fields are by definition faulty because they are generally restricted to the specific discipline from which they arose. Study of affective disorders ultimately demands an approach that brings together the social and psychological factors on the one hand and biochemical and neuroanatomical observations on the other. In response to this need, many institutions are establishing centers of research and teaching to study the mind-brain connections.

TREATMENT CHOICES FOR AFFECTIVE DISORDERS

The causes, both environmental and biochemical, of affective disorders are complex and intertwined; so, too, are the cures. Many forms of depression benefit from a combination of drug and talk therapy; generally, though, the more severe and clearly biochemical (or physiological) are treated predominantly with drugs, using talk therapy as an adjunct, while the milder and more environmentally based types of disorders are treated primarily with talk and occasionally with drugs as well. Of course, since all lines are blurred, picking the right treatment or combination of treatments must be carefully determined and then adjusted case by case—and at times seems to be mostly an educated guess.

I'd prefer that your experience of treatment, though, be less depressing than your illness, and I know that the more you understand each of your treatment options, the better you'll feel about your ultimate treatment choice. For this reason, while I'll outline commonly recommended specific treatments for each form of affective disorder beginning on page 311, I'll first provide below a brief review of general treatment choices you're likely to encounter.

PSYCHOTHERAPY: TALK THERAPY

Psychotherapy is talk therapy. It was created, more than one hundred years ago, by Sigmund Freud; hundreds of varieties of treatment through talking have evolved since that time.

All talk therapies are based on the theory that, whatever the cause, emotional or psychological illness can be successfully treated through self-exploration and understanding: talking of past and present interactions that influence current judgment and behavior; bringing to light the fears, thoughts, and misperceptions born in cloudy and hidden memories of your past experience. As you understand why certain fears or vulnerabilities are so vivid, you also defuse the emotional charge linked to whatever has caused you to distort reality, past and present. Psychotherapy should not deny the biogical component to depression (and all of the therapies below may be conducted as one part of a treatment program involving drugs as well). Even when talk therapy is used alone, the successful treatment of depression may well result in a physical change: extraordinarily, psychotherapy may enable the biochemical processes in the brain to return to equilibrium.

While there is a wide range of talk therapy available, the following approaches have proven to be the most successful in treating depression.

(We'll take a close look at selecting your therapist beginning on page 309; for now, note that for any therapy below I strongly recommend that you begin with a psychiatrist or Ph.D. psychologist, and work with a lesser-trained therapist only under the supervision of a psychiatrist or Ph.D. psychologist.)

PSYCHOANALYSIS

Psychoanalysis, developed by Freud, is the granddaddy of all the talk therapies and provides insight into the unconscious workings of the mind. It is extremely intense, usually requiring three to five sessions a week, and lasts for years. It is based on the fundamental theory of resistance, in which the mind tries to block the emergence of painful memories into conscious thought, and may create inexplicable or irrational behavior in doing so. At the same time, the unconscious still holds the memories, and these memories or feelings, unchecked, can lend inappropriate emotional charges to present experience. In terms of affective disorders, your own emotional past—your feelings from childhood of loss, insecurity, helplessness—may be causing or increasing your vulnerability in the present, out of proportion to actual events. Classical psychoanalysis involves a deep exploration through your talk of minute and major details of your life, your personal feelings, and your experiences and relationships with others; (the therapist is generally fairly quiet, providing some guidance.)

As you relive the past, emotionally charged experiences are inevitably "transferred" to the therapist, who might become, to you, your abusive parent or sibling or your own frightened self. Through this reenactment and transference, you are able to achieve a mastery over events you have otherwise repressed.

The under-the-microscope exploration of a person's life leads to many pleasant and unpleasant psychic events being relived. It can be emotionally draining and painful. By definition the process is laborious, takes a lot of time and money, and requires the establishment of a close, long-term relationship with a trusted therapist.

Psychoanalysis is practiced almost exclusively by psychiatrists (who have attended medical school) and psychoanalytically trained

Ph.D. psychologists, who have pursued years of special training in analysis. In fact, they themselves must undergo a training analysis before being allowed to practice.

PSYCHOANALYTICALLY ORIENTED PSYCHOTHERAPY

The number of therapists currently practicing the true, Freudian psychoanalysis described above is quite small. Most analytic therapy today enlists a modified approach, taking on a decidedly less ideological and more practical bent. Psychoanalytically oriented psychotherapy shares with psychoanalysis the basic tenet that a person feeling out of control or dependent or otherwise experiencing a psychological disturbance (or an affective disorder) is struggling with repressed and destructive emotions, which can be brought to the surface and thereby rendered powerless through talking with a trusted and skilled analyst. Self-realization is still the goal. Psychoanalytically oriented therapy does not, however, involve the full exploration of personality or the re-creation of old relationships and emotional reactions through transference. It delves into the past only as far as seems necessary to understanding the present.

Psychoanalytically oriented therapy is generally practiced by Ph.D. psychologists and by psychiatrists. It can be as short-term as a few months or extend for years.

COGNITIVE THERAPY

Cognitive therapy, developed by Dr. Aaron Beck some thirty years ago specifically for treatment of depression, is also grounded in the belief that our content and style of thinking can make us more vulnerable to an affective disorder. The cognitive therapist, as well as the psychoanalyst, seeks to establish a caring, supportive therapeutic relationship that will make self-awareness possible. That, though, is where the similarities end.

In cognitive therapy, the focus is wholly on the conscious and in the present and specifically on how you *think* about what you experience. It is both interactive—your therapist will voice plenty of opinions—and very active. As a patient you would be given homework: your job would be to identify, through various exercises, current erroneous and typically negative beliefs you might not be consciously aware you hold, but which may lead you to distort interactions or situations and respond or feel inappropriately. Your therapist or perhaps other members in a group therapy session would help point out ways you view the world as an inhospitable place; for example, you might be told you are setting yourself up for depression if you hold the belief "I am completely worthless if I fail at this [this job; this relationship; this task]."

Cognitive therapy is short term, generally taking sixteen to twenty visits, although it is flexible. Along with the two following therapies, it was named by the American Psychological Association's Task Force on Women as among the three types of psychotherapy most effective in resolving women's depression. Therapists who practice cognitive therapy can come from many backgrounds, from the psychiatrist to the highly trained social worker. In addition, group therapy sessions are often led by specially trained psychiatric nurses.

INTERPERSONAL THERAPY

Like psychoanalysis, interpersonal therapy does involve a search for self-awareness; like cognitive therapy, it concentrates on the present and was developed specifically to treat depression. But interpersonal therapy has quite its own approach.

Interpersonal therapy is very concentrated and is usually limited to three months. Developed by Dr. Gerald Klerman and his colleagues about twenty years ago, this "relationship therapy" focuses on a few key but problematic relationships in your life. You and your therapist will agree on, ahead of time, which relationships the therapy will target. The idea is that you derive substantial self-esteem from your relationships; dysfunctional relationships can therefore predispose you to depression. Within this context, an interpersonal therapist will explore with you additional risk factors in your relational life: grief; dispute about roles; difficult changes and transitions; or interpersonal conflicts.

Proponents find this type of therapy far more efficient than psychoanalysis, where everything is game, or cognitive therapy, where an entire belief structure is examined and tested. Interpersonal therapy is usually practiced by a psychiatrist or psychologist, but specially trained nurse practitioners and psychiatric social workers under the supervision of a psychiatrist have also demonstrated great success.

SOCIAL AND COMMUNITY THERAPY

A new and controversial talk therapy that recently evolved specifically to treat depression is social and community therapy (or, simply, social therapy). In this approach, created explicitly for women, the focus is on revealing, facing, and coping with external risk factors, rather than on self-exploration.

With the help of a therapist, you take a scrutinizing look at the societal risk factors that, according to this theory, have both contributed to and caused your depression: perhaps your socioeconomic status or lack of independence, your family situation, disturbances in your social support structures (loss of parents, extended families, or friends), or the power relationship in your marriage.

As is cognitive therapy, social therapy is behaviorally based, short-term, and practical. Once those elements causing your feelings of powerlessness in society are identified, you would be encouraged to make practical changes, such as obtaining child care to help you get involved with more personal activities, altering your environment to allow you more ready exposure to friends and supportive interactions, or dealing directly with marital problems. By taking charge of your environment, you again render impotent the depressive feelings of hopelessness and helplessness, while increasing your self-esteem.

Social therapy for depression has not been around long enough or subject to the same kind of study as other treatments. My own belief is that it can be beneficial at the very least as an important adjunct to a more introspective or drug therapy. Social therapy can be practiced by specially trained psychiatrists, psychologists, and, under supervision, specially trained psychiatric nurses and social workers.

BEHAVIOR MODIFICATION THERAPY

Behavior modification therapy represents a collection of treatments that focus exclusively on trying to change an abnormal behavior rather than figuring out why it occurred. This pragmatic approach is grounded in animal psychology—and the work of the Russian physiologist and experimental psychologist Pavlov—which demonstrates the ability to condition certain responses by repetition through punishment-reward schemes. Behavior modification therapy is used most often in treating specific types of anxiety disorders, through gradual and methodical exposure of patients to situations that led to their anxiety disorder.

Over time, they become desensitized to the situation or the object (such as heights, bridges, airplanes, or animals). Sometimes the symptoms rather than the causes are the focus; for example, you may be given exercises to slow down breathing, take deeper breaths, and overcome the sensation of shortness of breath that accompanies anxiety attacks.

You probably won't find a behavior modification therapist in the phone book. This approach is used most effectively by psychologists or master's-level professionals with specific training in behavior modification techniques, but is often used by many types of therapists in conjunction with the other therapeutic approaches described above.

TALKING TO NONTHERAPISTS

While many affective disorders require specific treatments from trained professionals, it is possible to obtain certain types of very useful help from nontherapists: friends, religious leaders, even books and diaries. Depression can have a wide range of precipitating causes; support, affirmation, and personal insight in any form may well prevent symptoms such as low self-esteem or feelings of powerlessness from blossoming.

Talking with nontherapists can go only so far, obviously, and you don't want to place inappropriate burdens on friendships by turning a friendship into constant, one-sided mock therapy sessions. I suggest only that you do not hesitate to reach out when you feel you are on an edge; if you feel you're about to tumble over, call in the professionals (see page 308 for help in determining just when you need treatment).

BIOLOGICAL TREATMENTS

For years, psychoanalysts after Freud both resisted and ignored the biological dimensions of affective disorders. Even now, there are some talk therapists who firmly believe the only viable method of treating these illnesses is talk and introspection alone, and many non-M.D. or non-Ph.D. talk therapists may simply not have been trained to address the biological question with their patients or to recognize when medication may be appropriate (see page 309 for advice on picking a therapist).

With just a few exceptions where the patient is so severely afflicted as to be a danger to herself or others, my feeling is that talk therapy should always be the first and preferred line of attack in an affective disorder (for one thing, a certain amount of talk is requisite for the psychiatrist to come up with a diagnosis). I also strongly believe that a therapist must be familiar with the benefits and dangers of all potentially appropriate medications; if talk therapy alone has failed to provide relief, the right drugs, dispensed with a coinciding talk therapy program, can truly help. Today we have an arsenal of many dozens of drugs, each with a unique ability to change the biochemical composition and physiological function of the brain and thereby treat the full range of depressive and anxiety disorders.

Antidepressants are drugs geared toward uplifting mood; antimanic agents control inappropriate euphoria, and a spectrum of tranquilizing and calming medicines are prescribed for anxiety disorders. Virtually all of these drugs work by altering the biochemistry of the brain, specifically the level and distribution of the neurotransmitters (discussed on page 285).

A general word of caution: I recommend none of these drugs to pregnant or nursing mothers, except in unusual circumstances. If you're on any of the following medications and become pregnant or plan to become pregnant, talk with your doctor.

ANTIDEPRESSANT DRUGS

The antidepressants used today can be grouped into three general categories: *MAO inhibitors* (MAOIs), *tricyclic antidepressants* (TCAs), and a newer class called *serotonin selective reuptake inhibitors* (SSRIs). Some of these drugs are also used to treat specific anxiety disorders.

The MAO Inhibitors—such as iproniazid,
Marplan (isocarboxazid), Parnate (tranylcypromine),
and Nardil (phenelzine)

Monoamine oxidase (MAO) is an enzyme that breaks down many of the neurotransmitters, including norepinephrine, dopamine, and serotonin (see page 286). When it is inhibited, levels of the important mood shifters, norepinephrine and serotonin, rise.

For a time, MAO inhibitors were thought to be a godsend in the treatment of depression. Now, though, this class of antidepressants is reserved for special or difficult cases because of their side effects, including high blood pressure, agitation, and changes in heart rate and rhythm. Some patients were reputed to have had cerebral hemorrhage when these drugs were taken with foods containing the chemical tyramine, such as cheese, some meats, red wine, chocolate, and coffee. MAO inhibitors can increase the levels of many neurotransmitters and ultimately overstimulate the brain.

If dispensed with caution and carefully monitored, the MAO inhibitors still prove to be an inexpensive and valuable approach in treating certain resistant forms of depression and you should at least be aware of both their positive and negative potential. The MAO inhibitors are most useful when other antidepressants have failed.

The Tricyclics—such as Pamelor and Aventyl (nortriptyline),
Tofranil (imipramine), Elavil (amitriptyline),
Norpramin (desipramine), and Anafranil (clomipramine)

In the 1950s, Dr. Ronald Duhn went in search of a drug that acted like opium (which was known to relieve symptoms of depression in depressed patients but, curiously, brought on depression in healthy people). In late 1957, he found imipramine (Tofranil), a drug that achieved the central goal of relieving depression. Because of its chemical structure—it has three benzene rings—it was labeled a tricyclic, a term that unfortunately obscured its function: how it affected brain chemistry. The tricyclics block the reuptake of selective transmitters by the nerve ending, leading to a buildup of those specific mood-controlling neurotransmitters within the appropriate nerve network. Unlike with the MAOIs, tricyclic antidepressant treatment does not require dietary modification or avoidance of other medications.

Tricyclics are commonly used to treat a broad range of mood disorders but must be carefully prescribed and monitored. They can cause a number of side effects, including a sharp drop in blood pressure, weight gain, dry mouth, urinary problems, and disturbances of heart rhythm. Tricyclics must be used cautiously, if at all, in patients with known heart disease.

Selective Serotonin Reuptake Inhibitors—
such as Prozac (fluoxetine), Paxil (paroxetine)
Zoloft (sertraline), and Luvox (fluvoxamine)

Currently, we are trying to be more and more exact in the development of depression-combating drugs, searching for agents that increase available levels of one specific neurotransmitter, rather than even a limited group, as do the tricyclics. Although focused in their activity, tricyclics stimulate the acetylcholine and histamine systems, sometimes resulting in unpleasant side effects. Research zeroed in on the neurotransmitters norepinephrine and serotonin; with studies of the latter, we hit pay dirt: Prozac.

Not all great discoveries are accidental. Prozac (fluoxetine hydrochloride) was found only after a specific, exhaustive search to find just such a remedy at the Eli Lilly company in 1974. Released to the public in 1987, Prozac was popularized through the recent best-seller *Listening to Prozac*. Prozac in many ways is indeed a miracle drug in the treatment of the full range of depressive disorders and certain anxiety disorders. Prozac blocks serotonin reuptake and thus increases the local buildup of serotonin, thereby enhancing our sense of security and self-esteem. It helps us feel safe in our environment. It doesn't cause the dry mouth, lethargy, weight gain, or potentially dangerous cardiac rhythm disturbances of the tricyclics. Also, overdoses are less of a problem because its toxicity is lower. Prozac has some side effects. Some patients lose weight, develop headaches, become restless, or have gastrointestinal disturbance, and a small number have problems sleeping or have difficulty achieving sexual orgasm. There are now two other widely used serotonin reuptake inhibitors on the market: Paxil (paroxetine) and Zoloft (sertraline).

Because these compounds work so well in both severe and mild depressions and even some anxiety disorders, Prozac quickly acquired the label of panacea and was prescribed to millions of people. Some physicians, formerly leery of using drugs to treat even mild depressions, began prescribing it everywhere: to treat insomnia, premenstrual syndrome, substance abuse, appetite control, and a host of other problems for which it was not originally intended—even to improve personality. But Prozac is meant for the treatment of specific forms of affective disorders, and its long-term effect when given to nondepressed patients is simply not known.

Despite a Prozac backlash claiming serious side effects, specifically violence and suicide, the FDA concluded after September 1991 hearings that warning the public about the dangers of Prozac was not warranted. Furthermore, the FDA pointed out that problems attributed to Prozac, in some cases at least, came not from the drug but from the way some doctors were prescribing it.

Although the benefits are undeniable, we cannot forget that Prozac and all antidepressants are powerful drugs that alter the very complex chemical mix that defines who we are and how we feel and think. I don't ever advise messing around with those chemicals without a concrete therapeutic goal and unless there is a body of scientific work that shows expected benefits as well as risks. The lower the risk and apparent side effects, the greater is the temptation to try a new drug. I urge caution. Prozac and others like it should be prescribed only after careful diagnosis, and then monitored closely.

ANTIMANIC MOOD-STABILIZING DRUGS

Lithobid, Lithane, Lithonate (lithium carbonate), Lithium, Tegretol (carbamazepine), Depakene, Depakote (valproic acid)

Lithium is another serendipitous breakthrough in the treatment of mood disorders. For more than one hundred years, lithium was not taken very seriously, seen only as an alternative medicine, a "bromide" that could calm and tranquilize agitated patients. It was not until some thirty years ago, when an Australian psychiatrist stumbled upon its use for manic depression—and took the drug himself to prove its safety—that it came into mainstream medical use.

Chemically, lithium is undoubtedly the simplest of all drugs: it is a naturally occurring element, like calcium, sodium, or potassium, which is used in the form of a salt, lithium carbonate or lithium citrate. (In the past the form used was lithium bromide, hence its old-fashioned name.) And it has proven to be stupendously useful, allowing those with manic depression to function in society; previously, long-term hospitalization was almost the only option. Until very recently lithium was virtually the only drug available to treat the agitated, euphoric, hyperactive, and manic phase of manic-depressive illness; furthermore, it prevents those episodes from occurring. Lithium also is used as chronic maintenance treatment for this illness. Lithium is tolerated well because it has few side effects in the right doses. (The depressive part of the cycle is treated with standard antidepressants; see page 319.) Recently, anticonvulsant drugs such as carbamazepine (Tegretol) and valproic acid (Depakene, Depakote) have been found to be effective against manic-depressive disorder. Although lithium has traditionally been regarded as the drug of choice for maintenance treatment of this illness, a recent multicenter trial demonstrated that valproic acid was at least as good as (and in some patients may be better than) lithium.

Benzodiazepines—such as Librium (chlordiazepoxide),
Valium (diazepam), Tranxene (clorazepate),
Xanax (alprazolam), and Ativan (lorazepam), Klonopin (clonazepam)

The benzodiazepines are a powerful class of drugs used for their sedative, anticonvulsant, and antianxiety effects. They are believed to strengthen the inhibiting neurotransmitter GABA in the limbic system of the brain and thereby lessen the effect of local anxiety-promoting brain chemicals.

Both Valium and Librium are most effective in treating panic and phobic disorders; however, the drug we commonly associate with anxiety is Xanax (alprazolam), a mild and short-acting benzodiazepine. Xanax became popular when studies showed how effectively it quelled agoraphobia and panic attacks. Subsequently, however, we learned that stopping Xanax abruptly can trigger a withdrawal syndrome with hallucinations, psychosis, or seizures. If you take Xanax, taper off gradually when it's time to stop. Because stopping Xanax abruptly can cause dire consequences, many psychiatrists prefer to treat anxiety disorders with antidepressants which are also effective antianxiety agents.

Habituation can occur with any of the benzodiazepines. People can get hooked. If you carry a history (or family history) of substance abuse or alcoholism, don't add to your burden with one of these drugs.

THE MORE DRASTIC MEASURES

Antipsychotic Drugs—such as Thorazine (chlorpromazine),
Clozaril (clozapine), Mellaril (thioridazine),
Haldol (haloperidol), and Prolixin (fluphenazine)

Antipsychotic drugs are thought to exert their effect by blocking the dopamine neurotransmitter system. They are primarily used to treat psychotic behavior, including hallucinations, delusions, disorganized thought patterns, and catatonic, violent, or aggressive behavior—rare but occasional components of some severe forms of depression.

The antipsychotic drugs have many unpleasant side effects, including mouth dryness, blurred vision, problems with urination, constipation, sexual dysfunction, and a range of allergic reactions including skin rashes, and with prolonged use, they may cause a movement disorder called *tardive dyskinesia*.

Electroshock or Electroconvulsive Therapy

Here's a surprise. Although there was a time that electroshock therapy (ECT) had fallen out of favor, ECT can be impressive in its effectiveness and, employed correctly and with proper caution, safe and without side effects. I have seen severely depressed patients in the hospital, unable to eat or communicate, who suddenly come awake with ECT. In fact, the American Psychiatric Association has endorsed the regularly scheduled use of ECT, carefully tailored to the needs of the patient. In some cases, ECT is administered two to three times a week for a period of several months; in other cases, it might be given in monthly intervals.

ECT is not to be taken lightly. It is an extreme treatment for extreme cases—generally reserved for those unresponsive to other treatments and for people who are hospitalized, and suffer from delusions or are suicidal. The positive effect is virtually instantaneous and dramatic.

So how does it work? ECT is actually very similar to drug therapy in its benefits. The shocks trigger an acute release of neurotransmitters, notably norepinephrine and dopamine; increase sensitivity of receptors for dopamine, serotonin, and noradrenaline; and stimulate the hypothalamus to release many substances, including neuropeptides.

Of course, we don't know all we should or could about ECT. Studies show no change to the brain anatomy after ECT, but, as is generally true, more studies need to be done. And we don't know with certainty how ECT works or what its long-term effects might be. But it can work miracles, and to my mind, if the depression is so severe that it needs a miracle cure, ECT's benefits well outweigh the risks.

Lobotomy, or Psychosurgery

If electroshock therapy has had a bad name, lobotomy has been completely demonized and condemned. But it hasn't always been the nightmare that shocked all of us in *One Flew Over the Cuckoo's Nest*. This surgical treatment for severe depression and other mental illnesses won the Nobel prize for medicine in 1949 for the Portuguese neurologist Antonio Egas Moniz and was celebrated as one of the most important advances of the century. It was widely practiced throughout the world in the 1940s and 1950s before most drug treatments were available—and had some dramatic successes. Now a more refined, more effective and safer technique called *cingulotomy* is used as a treatment of last resort for intractable severe chronic depression that has failed all other therapy.

Needless to say, the treatment is still quite controversial, but its practice today is far more refined and limited. Rather than cutting into the frontal lobes, the seat of higher cortical function, the surgery is more selective, and in some cases focuses on the mid part of the brain, the limbic system, which is the seat of our emotions. Very tiny lesions are created by either freezing or using radiofrequency waves under X-ray control. There is still, however, an eerie quality to going in and rather blindly destroying tissue in the brain without knowing its full consequence. Not only is the result unpredictable, but in some rare circumstances unintended personality and intellectual changes can result. Hence, the surgery is performed only as a last-ditch effort with the fully informed consent of the patient and responsible family members.

My view is to stay away from this treatment unless there is some dramatic new breakthrough in our neuroanatomical understanding of depression that would suggest a novel benefit. Even then, the only way to prove the benefit scientifically would be to do some kind of carefully controlled trial, but that is highly unlikely to happen anytime soon.

GETTING SPECIFIC AND GETTING WELL

If you believe you or someone close to you may have an affective disorder, don't let the maze of available treatments leave you feeling more overwhelmed and helpless than the disease itself. Although you may find all your options confusing, you can simplify the process of getting help by thinking in terms of the following questions:

1. Do I have an affective disorder? If so, what kind do I have?
Beginning on page 311 of this section, you'll find descriptions of all common affective disorders, with recommended treatments.

2. Do I need treatment?
I think Freud had it right. Can you work? And can you love? If you can do both, then your disorder is apt to be one that will pass with time and the support of friends and loved ones. If the depression or anxiety is interfering with life functions, with study or work, concen-

tration, or effectiveness in carrying out responsibility; if it is throwing personal relationships into turmoil, making it impossible to care or respond—then I believe it's in your interest to seek professional help.

Before you embark on your search for a therapist, get a medical evaluation. It is possible that your symptoms may be a manifestation of some other illness, such as a thyroid imbalance, or may coexist with another medical problem.

3. If I need treatment, what's best?

Drugs, talk, or both? And which kind? The best type of therapy for you will depend in large part on the form your affective disorder takes and on the recommendation of your doctor. As I've said, except in those few very severe cases noted later in this chapter, always try talk first. Drugs will work more quickly, but the question that remains is, how long should the drug treatment last? If there is an underlying psychological origin of your depression, the blanket of drugs will at best be only a temporary cure. In any case, talk therapy should continue throughout the drug therapy.

My view is that therapy for an affective disorder should be a lot like therapy for any illness impairing a patient's ability to function, causing pain and putting life at risk. Make the proper diagnosis, treat acute symptoms while trying to sort out underlying cause, and embark on a course of short-term intervention and longer-term therapy aimed at preventing recurrence.

Your therapist should first evaluate you, then provide you with a diagnosis and a clear treatment plan—with a time frame. Make sure you know exactly what is being proposed; if you feel confused or ill-informed, it may be time to find another therapist who can be more clear. You must find a therapist in whom you feel confident; and trust without doubt is imperative.

Selecting a Therapist. Psychotherapy is a valuable tool; it can also be destructive and damaging. It is a treatment that is based on sound research but is anything but concrete in its application; it is intangible, reliant on the skills, experience, and even mood of the therapist. You must choose wisely not only the type of therapy, but also your therapist.

First and foremost, if you suspect you may need medication, I urge you to consult your primary care doctor for recommendations, then a psychiatrist. Ph.D. psychologists practice psychotherapy and counseling but cannot prescribe drugs. Depressed, you're already a bit lost;

you don't need the added trauma of shifting therapists midstream if you find you need medication and your current therapist isn't qualified to dispense it. After evaluation, your psychiatrist might prescribe medication and continue to supervise the process but recommend group therapy or specific therapy with another psychologist, social worker, or nurse practitioner handling your talk therapy program. Although there are many qualified but less-degreed therapists out there, I nonetheless feel your best treatment option is to see only a psychiatrist or a Ph.D. psychologist (or a therapist who is part of his or her treatment team). You'll want someone reputable with good training and appropriate experience. Don't hesitate to ask difficult and personal questions in your first session (see page 327). Personal compatibility is also important. You should feel confident that your therapist understands you and that he or she is your advocate, involved with your concerns and not aloof. If, after several sessions, you feel you've made a mistake, don't be afraid to make a change.

We've all heard stories of abuse in psychotherapy. In every field, there will be some irresponsible people; psychotherapy is no exception, and therapists can hold tremendous power over a patient who already doubts her own judgment. All I can suggest is that you trust your instincts, wobbly as they may feel at this time in your life. If you suspect at all that your therapist seems to be getting personal in a way that doesn't feel therapeutic, is coming on to you sexually, or is attempting to gather information from you for personal gain, get a new therapist. Paranoia is not a symptom of the vast majority of affective disorders, and even an unfounded suspicion can get in the way of your trusting relationship.

4. How long should my treatment last?
Most affective disorders are temporary (although they may recur); therefore, with a few exceptions noted below, no therapy need go on forever. The length of talk therapy, as discussed, will vary with the type.

We should be cautious about administering any drug indefinitely. I recommend that you stop any drug after six months, just to see how you do. There is no harm in stopping medication, provided that the treatment is appropriately tapered and you're closely monitored. And, as we've seen, most types of affective disorders are self-limiting.

The exceptions to this rule are notable. If you've had relapses of an affective disorder, longer treatment can minimize the likelihood of yet another. Eighty to 90 percent of people who have had two bouts of depression in their lives will have a third, and after a third, the likelihood of recurrence goes up to 95 percent. According to David J. Kupfer, head of psychiatry at the University of Pittsburgh School of Medicine, patients who stay on their antidepressants for five years will avoid recurrence during that period. (Also, for the lifelong types of depression described below, chemical treatment must also be lifelong.)

Do not forget, in any case, that these powerful mind-altering drugs have been in widespread use for only a few decades and that we have very little information on their lifelong use. Respect them all—including Prozac. And let me add another note of caution: Prozac and the new emerging class of mood-altering drugs that are more selective in manipulating brain chemistry are very tempting to use in milder and more minor forms of mood disturbance. These drugs can become like fast foods: too easy and not so nutritional, replacing the more time-consuming and more nourishing family meal. Talk therapy, whether it be psychotherapy or behavior modification, takes time and is hard work for the patient, surely harder than popping a pill. Remember, in his chilling book *Brave New World*, Aldous Huxley saw mood-altering drugs as a means of controlling mass behavior and stamping out individuality and creativity—even love and passion. Such pills do not develop personal insight or teach people to grow as individuals. That's what mental health is all about.

FORMS AND TREATMENTS OF AFFECTIVE DISORDERS

Thus far, I've discussed affective disorders in their broadest categories: depression and anxiety. In reality, we've discerned many subsets of this illness. The distinctions below will sound concrete—but remember that the more we learn about biology, the more likely we'll be to find even more forms or redefine old ones, based on indisputable tests such as blood tests or brain scans.

DEPRESSION

Depression is actually an illness of two distinct types. We've talked thus far in this chapter almost exclusively about the type called *unipolar depression*, meaning that the dominant symptom is, in fact, depression, without any manic symptoms offsetting the overriding lows of depression. Depression also can be *bipolar,* which is far less common. In a bipolar depression, which is generally a serious, biologically based, lifelong illness, the depressive lows alternate with manic highs.

UNIPOLAR DEPRESSION

Unipolar depression is the most frequent psychiatric illness that affects adults, with the chance of this problem coming to medical attention sometime in the course of a woman's life being close to 20 percent. The figure is surely an underestimation since the illness is typically self-limiting and often does *not* come to medical attention. It can and sometimes does recur over a lifetime, but each episode lasts only a discrete period of time. Unipolar depressions can be either minor or major; some fall into the recognized categories of dysthymia, postpartum depression, adjustment disorder with depressed mood, seasonal affective disorder, and premenstrual mood disorder, which are discussed below.

As we'll see, virtually all forms of psychotherapy discussed in this chapter have some merit in the treatment of most unipolar depressions, either with or without medication.

Major Depressive Disorder

A major depression is far more than the blues. It is a serious illness that can strike with or without a precipitating life event, rendering its victims unable to accomplish even the simplest of tasks. So how do you know if you have it? According to the American Psychiatric Association bible, the *Diagnostic and Statistical Manual of Mental Disorders* (DSM-IV), major depression exists when any five of the following nine symptoms persist without interruption for two weeks:

1. *Persistently despondent mood.* Abject sorrow and sometimes uncontrollable sobbing for no apparent reason overtakes you without warning. The more mundane events of the day, such as setting the table or putting dishes away, seem wearisome and purposeless.

2. *Loss of interest in activities usually found pleasurable.* You find little to no meaning in even the significant aspects of life; you just don't seem to care and feel no joy.

3. *Change in appetite patterns often associated with change in weight.* You have lost appetite for food, sex, or much of anything else, or may eat out of control.

4. Sleep disturbance marked by inability to stay asleep or by excessive sleeping. You wake up in the middle of the night or early morning and can't get back to sleep. Some sufferers can't gather the strength to get themselves out of bed in the morning and sleep most of the day.

5. Listlessness or excessive nervous energy. Talking feels like work. You feel you have nothing to say; your friends feel you are holding back. Or, you "run-in-place" with a frenzy of activity that is often futile.

6. Fatigue or lethargy. You feel you are moving in glue.

7. Uncharacteristic feelings of low self-esteem and inappropriate guilt. A British psychiatrist at the turn of the century called major depression a state in which "misery is unreasonable."

8. Problems with memory, thinking clearly, making decisions, or concentrating. Often, you fear taking initiative or making even simple decisions.

9. Fantasies or talk of death, possibly accompanied by thoughts of or attempts at suicide.

Major depression typically lasts a matter of months and usually less than a year. In about half the cases, it is a single event that never occurs again. In the other half, the disorder will recur, with episodes increasing in frequency with age, but each recurrence will also eventually end.

While the treatment of all major depressions will vary with the severity of the depression and the analysis of your therapist, most are treated with a combination of drugs and talk therapy. Most of the talk therapies have been shown to be effective, but strict psychoanalysis is simply too long-term for some (because the analysis would continue long after the depression has run its course). I would not recommend social and community therapy for a major depression.

Drug treatment, as always only under the close supervision of your psychiatrist or doctor, often starts with selective serotonin reuptake inhibitors (such as Prozac) as the safest. If the SSRIs fail, tricyclics and then MAO inhibitors are used. Sometimes hospitalization is required, particularly when there is a concern that the patient may commit suicide.

Dysthymic Disorder

Dysthymic disorder (or what has also been called minor depression) carries with it the same appearance as a major depression—despondent mood, sluggish motor behavior, low self-esteem—but in a more subtle way. A minor depression is not necessarily a mild depression and can be quite debilitating. It lasts more than two years, and in some individuals, can last a lifetime. It can have an impact on your over-all health as well: some primary care doctors have estimated that 10 percent of patients seeing a doctor for physical ailments such as unexplained weight loss or fatigue actually have an underlying dysthymia.

Those suffering with dysthymia are mildly depressed all the time, with no relief. They often remember feeling like this all the way back into their childhood. It is estimated that as many as nine million Americans have this inability to be happy or feel pleasure. Although historically dysthymic disorder was often written off as a neurotic depression or characterologic depression, suggesting that the depressive symptoms were due to a flawed or disordered personality and without cure, recently drug treatments have proved dramatically successful in lifting the gloom.

Milder forms of dysthymia can sometimes be treated through talk therapy alone, primarily through psychoanalytically oriented therapy, cognitive therapy, and interpersonal therapy. More severe forms of minor depression are generally treated through the same type of therapeutic approaches, but in conjunction with drug therapy.

SSRIs, such as Prozac are the drug class of choice used to treat minor depressions; the side effects of both the tricyclics and MAO inhibitors often outweigh their benefits for this illness. These newer agents are recommended only on a case-by-case basis, depending on you and your doctor. And, in some very mild cases, a minor depression will run its course and end without drugs or talk therapy.

OTHER FORMS OF DEPRESSION

Any of the forms of unipolar depression below may range from mild to severe; the treatment generally recommended will vary with both the type of illness and its severity. While all of these disorders fall under the huge category of major depression, their character and causes may be quite different, ranging from hormone imbalance to psychological issues.

Postpartum Depression

Women are especially vulnerable to depression immediately after childbirth. Hormonal shifts during and after pregnancy have been clearly linked to depression; emotional factors can often put a woman at an even higher risk.

Most women experience postpartum blues, hitting within a few days of delivery, but this feeling usually lasts a few days and promptly resolves. This is not the same as postpartum depression.

Postpartum depression is a frightening and distinct illness, usually appearing within the first two weeks of delivery. In its most severe form, the new mother can suffer confusion, delusions, and sometimes hallucinations, and it is then referred to as major depression with psychotic features. In extreme cases she may harm herself or her baby. Postpartum depression can affect women who have never been seriously depressed, but women who have a history of depression are more likely to experience it. Also, women who have had a bout of postpartum depression have a one in four chance of facing it again with each subsequent pregnancy.

Less severe forms of postpartum depression can come on about one month after delivery and last for months. It seems to be triggered by a combination of biological and societal factors: a personality that seems more hysterical, dependent, avoidant, or anxious than is typical; marital discord; ambivalence about being a mother; lack of family support; financial woes.

If a woman has experienced postpartum depression, she should be cautious about taking oral contraceptives, since they mimic pregnancy and can become a risk factor possibly leading to further depression.

Postpartum depression involving hallucinations and delusions is an acute and dangerous illness that should be treated immediately with a combination of antidepressant and antipsychotic drugs, such as haloperidol or ECT. Hospitalization is a consideration. Medication (plus talk, as always) is used to remedy postpartum depression that isn't accompanied by such delusions; in these cases the antidepressants are often prescribed and in some instances talk therapy alone, psychoanalytically oriented, cognitive, or interpersonal, is effective.

Some have tried thyroid hormone to treat postpartum depression, but this treatment has not been sufficiently studied to recommend it.

Adjustment Disorder with Depressed Mood

Symptoms of depression can be triggered by stressful outside situations: by death or divorce, marital or romantic problems, job loss, or physical illness, for example. It can run the gamut from mild to severe and lasts for three to six months. When triggered by events other than illness, such a "reactive" depression is treated as any major depression would be.

Do pay close attention to the depressed moods that can accompany a major illness. Identifying and managing it speeds recovery from acute illness or surgery and eases the disability of chronic illness. Some researchers have noted, for example, that support groups have helped breast cancer patients prolong their lives up to eighteen months.

When a depressed mood is triggered by an illness, the symptoms may come and go for a few weeks or months, then disappear as recovery proceeds or the illness becomes manageable. If the problem does not resolve itself, if bad days give way to bad weeks without letup, the adjustment disorder warrants professional attention: short-term counseling and/or antidepressant medication.

Neither long-term nor formal and scheduled talk therapy may be needed to treat reactive depression, and some have found the specific focus of social and community therapy to be quite beneficial. If the problem is truly severe, Prozac or its equivalent is the medication of choice; the tricyclics are sometimes used but are to be avoided if any type of heart disease is present. Only in very severe or refractory cases are MAO inhibitors used.

Seasonal Affective Disorder

Seasonal affective disorder (SAD) is an incompletely studied affective disorder related to time of year and rhythm of life. With SAD, you experience symptoms of depression more or less in proportion to the amount of sunlight (full-spectrum light, as opposed to light from a light bulb) in your life.

Surveys suggest that in Sarasota, Florida, only 2 percent of the residents are depressed, and in New York City, it's less than 5 percent. But in Fairbanks, Alaska, 10 percent develop severe symptoms. They feel despondent, crave sleep, become irritable, gain weight, and develop a sometimes uncharacteristically intense desire for carbohydrates. For another 15 percent, the symptoms are less severe, but they may feel sluggish, lose interest in sex, and become irritable and morose.

Some people are skeptical that SAD exists. I'm not. First, one cannot ignore the cyclic and rhythmic dimensions related to depression and depressive feelings in general. Depression is often most intense in the dark of early morning, getting better as the day goes on. We know we live in a cyclic, seasonal universe, and within our bodies are clear rhythms. Certain hormones produced by the brain play a role in biological rhythms. Theoretically, the absence of light triggers a hormone imbalance that brings on depression.

SAD treatment is by far the most unusual of all affective disorder remedies. People who experience this illness find help in a general short-term therapy, conducted by a therapist with specific training in this disorder. As supervised by the therapist, the treatment is light, specifically fluorescent light that mimics sunlight for up to three hours a day. A midwinter vacation in the Sun Belt, simple as it may seem, can also alleviate this disorder.

Premenstrual Dysphoric Disorder

Premenstrual tension has been in women's vocabulary for most of this century. The vast majority of women on occasion notice some kind of mild mood changes such as irritability, fatigue, nervousness, or just feeling blue during the few days preceding the onset of menstruation. That is entirely normal.

When premenstrual symptoms become a predictable cluster of mood and behavior changes including fatigue, sugar craving, headaches, nervousness, sleep disturbances, depression, or anxiety, we call it premenstrual syndrome, or PMS. The American Psychiatric Association reports that between 20 and 50 percent of women experience PMS at some time. Research studies, meager as they are, have failed to define any biological abnormality in hormones or brain function to explain PMS or its variability.

In a relatively small group of women (about 3 to 5 percent), PMS becomes disabling and severe, taking on the form of a major depressive illness. The DMS-IV now terms this state *premenstrual dysphoric disorder*. The point at which premenstrual syndrome become premenstrual dysphoric disorder is determined by the diagnostic formula: "Can you work and can you love?" When the mood changes impair a woman's ability to function for several days a month, whether it be going to school or work, caring for her family, or nourishing her personal relationships, she then has an illness.

Treatment varies and often calls for some trial and error. Talk therapy is a must and is also crucial to rule out other mood disorders that show premenstrual aggravation. Along with counseling, there are several options. Some women respond well to diet therapy, including reducing salt and caffeine intake, and taking supplements of vitamin B$_6$, which is thought to decrease estrogen and increase progesterone levels. Hormones such as progesterone, oral contraceptives using progestins, and agents that block the pituitary gland from stimulating the ovaries have helped some women. As a last resort, women can take the antidepressant medications, trying the serotonin uptake inhibitors first. (These drugs are not to be used, however, if a woman is planning a pregnancy or not using contraception.) Predictably, pregnancy and menopause eliminate premenstrual dysphoria.

The American Psychiatric Association has struggled for many years with the issue of classifying severe forms of PMS as a psychiatric disorder. Some have criticized their classification as either medicalizing or stigmatizing a normal state of woman's being. Nonetheless, for the handful of women who have disabling symptoms, recognizing and treating the condition has become a godsend. Their struggles have also highlighted the need for more research and understanding of this often elusive and sometimes trivialized condition.

BIPOLAR DISORDER

Unlike unipolar depression, the far less common bipolar disease (affecting about 1 percent of the population) is a lifelong recurrent illness, has a strong genetic tendency, and afflicts women and men equally. Although it may look like a major unipolar depression during its depressive phase, it is a distinctive disease that requires careful and specific treatment.

Manic Depression

Some of our most creative and productive people in the arts and sciences have been manic-depressives: the late Salvador Luria, a scientist and Nobel laureate, was quite open about his illness, acknowledging that it may have been a high price to pay for his genius. Manic-depressive illness is a lifelong presence that waxes and wanes, characterized by huge swings in mood. During the depressed phase, those afflicted behave as others with major depression do. They feel worthless, inadequate, sluggish, and are often suicidal. During the manic phase, however, they typically live in a state of euphoria, needing little sleep and talking excessively, but may also experience considerable irritability and paranoia. They see their own capabilities as boundless and often make grandiose plans. Losing all capacity for discretion, they may make embarrassing pronouncements, spend wild amounts of money, make disastrous personal or professional decisions, take inappropriate risks, drive recklessly, or participate in other activities that are fraught with danger. If they get frustrated, they can become angry and aggressive. Sometimes, the manic phase mimics schizophrenia when it is accompanied by hallucinations and delusions. The DSM-IV defines the manic episode as a distinct period lasting at least a week during which at least three of the following seven symptoms occur and are severe enough to interfere with normal functioning:

Inflated sense of self
The ability to function with substantially less sleep than usual
Talking more than usual or feeling the need to talk incessantly
Feeling as though your mind is racing out of control
Being unusually subject to distraction
A feeling of restlessness or the need to constantly be doing something
Excessive involvement in activities that hold the potential for disaster

Talk therapy is used only as an adjunct in the treatment of manic depression; a sufferer of manic depression needs a psychiatrist throughout her life to provide support and monitor the drug therapy that is a necessity. With proper care, patients with this illness are now able to lead normal lives. Psychoanalysis is not generally effective.

Lithium is the drug of choice to manage the manic episodes and sustain a state of normalcy (see page 305); antidepressants are sometimes necessary to treat the depressive phase of the illness, but should be avoided if possible. Your doctor will help you with this decision.

Cyclothymia

A mild, chronic form of manic-depressive illness is called *cyclothymia*. People who have cyclothymia experience swings of emotion that seem inappropriate but last only for days (not weeks or months) and are not as severe as seen in manic depression. Low self-esteem alternates with a grandiosity, a pattern of unevenness marks their work and productivity, and their human relationships sustain sharp ups and downs. The diagnosis is made when there is a two-year period of mild mania alternating with minor depression. What little research there is on these patients suggests that tricyclic antidepressants are risky, and that sometimes, but with great unpredictability, lithium or other mood stabilizers helps.

ANXIETY DISORDERS

Anxiety is a normal part of life and, in fact, can stimulate productivity. But if you live in a perpetual state of anxiety, if you're so uncomfortable in crowds or strange places that you avoid leaving home, or if you're subjected to panic attacks severe enough to bring on symptoms like shortness of breath, dizziness, or chest pain, you may be afflicted with an anxiety disorder (also called a *panic disorder*).

Sigmund Freud was probably one of the keenest observers of anxiety disorders; he noticed women were on the whole more predisposed to this illness and believed that the underlying cause was inner conflict related to unreleased or unsatisfied sexual impulse. Over time, this theory of anxiety's cause was broadened to include the conflict between all repressed and unsatisfied drives. In the early years of psychiatry, anxiety was seen at the core of almost any mental illness; it was viewed as a symptom, not as an illness in and of itself. With the evolution of contemporary psychiatry, anxiety disorders have taken on a more narrow definition. They are now seen and approached as distinctive conditions with their own origins and treatment.

Anxiety disorders are now subdivided into several general groupings based on the symptoms, but each has one element in common: extreme fear or panic, out of proportion to the situation. Sometimes the fear is associated with a specific thing, such as heights, germs (which can lead to an obsessive-compulsive behavior such as constant hand washing), or a shocking episode (leading to post-traumatic stress disorder). Sometimes the fear has no apparent cause: out of the blue you experience the symptoms of what is called a *panic attack*—palpitations, dizziness, chest pain, or shortness of breath.

Anxiety disorders are quite separate from depression and, if anything, tougher to diagnose and treat. What anxiety disorders do have in common with depression is that they clearly have both psychological and biological causes; therefore, treatment also involves either psychotherapy or drug therapy, or both, depending on the form and the severity.

PANIC ATTACKS

The word *panic* comes from the Greek god Pan, who was apparently a moody, anxious god. Panic attacks are indeed frightening experiences. Often, symptoms mimic those of heart disease: your heart pounds, your chest hurts, you can't breathe, you may feel as if you are dying.

There are, in fact, thirteen distinct symptoms noted in the DSM-IV, any four of which occurring at the same time constitute an attack:

Shortness of breath or feeling as though you're being smothered
Feeling as if you are being choked
Palpitations or a racing heart
Pain or discomfort in the chest
Sweating
Feeling faint, unsteady, or dizzy
Nausea or abdominal distress
Feeling detached from reality
Numbness or tingling in your hands and feet
Hot flashes or chills
Trembling or shaking
Fear that you are dying
*Fear that you are going crazy or that you might lose control of
    yourself*

Panic attacks run in families, affecting 1 to 2 percent of the population, with women suffering almost twice as often as men. These attacks may be unrelated to any obvious trigger or they may be precipitated by a distinct event (in which case it's likely you'll also develop a *phobia,* or overwhelming fear, about that event. If you experience a panic attack in a grocery store, you may well avoid grocery stores in the future—and suddenly have two anxiety disorders to deal with, not just one).

AGORAPHOBIA

Agoraphobia is related to panic attacks but is somewhat different. Literally meaning "fear of the marketplace," it is a complex disorder where fear of having a public panic attack translates into fear of going outside the home, driving, using public transportation, going to movie theaters, or attending other social functions. Obviously this is a serious condition, far more common in women than men, which restricts your ability to work, to play, and to function in your family and society. Women who have agoraphobia are more likely to come from families who are predisposed to mood disorders.

If you have four or more attacks of panic or agoraphobia in a month, or if one or more attacks leave you petrified of a subsequent attack, you would most likely benefit from professional help. Both panic attacks and agoraphobia respond well to medication in conjunction with talk therapy.

Psychoanalysis is a bit deep for panic attacks, but the other types of therapy, provided they are conducted by a therapist both well trained in behavior modification techniques and qualified to prescribe medication or under such supervision, can be very helpful. These disorders mark an exception to the rule of talk first, then drugs; drugs are often prescribed from the start and sometimes by a physician without a therapist's involvement. Xanax is the medication of choice for panic attacks; antidepressants are prescribed if depression coexists with the anxiety disorder.

OBSESSIVE-COMPULSIVE DISORDER (OCD)

Shakespeare recognized obsessive-compulsive disorders long before Freud gave them a name. His poor Lady Macbeth, tortured and unable to sleep, compulsively washing her guilty hands for her role in the murder of the king, was troubled with "fancies / That keep her from her rest." Macbeth implores his doctor to help: "Canst thou not minister to a mind diseas'd, / pluck from the memory a rooted sorrow, / raze out the written troubles of the brain . . . ?"

OCD can be very disruptive and disturbing: you know these uncontrollable behaviors are "silly," but you just can't stop doing them. An obsessive, repetitive thought (your hands are dirty, the oven is on) drives you to repeat compulsive actions (washing your hands, returning to the kitchen to check the oven) to keep from being racked with even more anxiety and torment.

Once thought to be uncommon, OCD is now thought to affect as much as 2 to 3 percent of the population, men and women equally. Freud and others thought OCD was created by defense mechanisms, as a means of overcoming an unconscious guilt, containing an uncontrollable environment, or controlling a desire to do something that is unthinkable. OCD tends to appear early in life, and about half of OCD sufferers also have a history of depression.

OCD can be treated with talk therapy, but talk alone is generally inadequate and either medication, behavioral therapy, or both are needed.

Several medications are especially useful: Prozac, Anafranil, and, the most recent addition to the pharmacologic armamentarium, fluvoxamine (Luvox).

ACUTE STRESS OR POST-TRAUMATIC STRESS DISORDERS

Post-traumatic stress disorders (PTSDs) can be experienced quite differently for each individual, but what all have in common is that they are clear responses to major traumas: rape, abuse, witnessing a murder, wartime events, a natural disaster such as an earthquake or a fire. In order to be termed a PTSD, symptoms must have persisted more than a month.

In the midst of a PTSD, you are in an anxious state continually. You may uncontrollably relive the event in your mind or in hallucinations (or even in your dreams); you may feel that whatever happened is about to happen again any minute; you may develop a phobia about going to the place the event occurred; or, you may on the other hand not be able to recall the event.

Vulnerability to PTSD tends to run in families, though an actual event is needed to trigger it; often PTSD accompanies other affective disorders such as major depressions or panic attacks.

Treating a PTSD depends in large part on the severity of the illness, but in most cases talk therapy, particularly cognitive, interpersonal, and psychoanalytical psychotherapy, has been very successful.

If the illness does not diminish with solid talk therapy, medication is sometimes used: Xanax or another benzodiazepine, depending on the degree of anxiety, and antidepressants if depression is a component of the disease. Again, Prozac is attempted, then the tricyclics, before the more dangerous MAO inhibitors.

SIMPLE PHOBIAS

Simple phobias, more common to women, are discrete fears about highly specific situations, objects, people, or things, such as a fear and consequent avoidance of dogs or snakes, closed spaces, or airplanes. They are not connected to a more generalized anxiety or even to panic attacks. (Despite its name, agoraphobia is a much more complex and serious anxiety disorder.) Phobias might make sense from an evolutionary standpoint: perhaps fear of many objects was our ancestors' instinctive internal warning system through which they protected themselves or their children.

Most of the time, phobias can be treated by behavior modification and supportive psychotherapy through which you are gradually exposed to the object of fear while at the same time reassured, learning where the fear came from. Medications should be avoided altogether in the treatment of simple phobias.

Generalized Anxiety Disorder

Women suffering this illness are constantly keyed up, jumpy, irritable, restless; they can't sleep or concentrate and are chronically worried. Their heart rate may be sped up, their mouth is dry, and they may feel smothered. Often they will simultaneously be in the midst of a major depression.

Freud felt such a chronic state was caused by a fear that what is lurking in your unconscious might break through. Whatever the cause, from a biological standpoint, the stress hormones are at constantly increased levels.

Little is known about this disorder as a discrete classification. Most treatment is highly individualized, involving talk therapy—psychoanalytical, interpersonal, or cognitive—and medication only after careful analysis. Medication generally is limited to the benzodiazepines.

COPING DAY BY DAY

Any one of the forms of depression and anxiety we've seen can be debilitating. You can go to the therapist once or twice a week, take your medication daily, and still not be able to drag yourself out of bed in the morning during the course of the illness. I'm not suggesting you'll be able to alter significantly the course of the disease by psyching yourself out of it; however, certain environmental factors are within your power to control. As you know by now, many disparate elements contribute to depression, and no one can know which single one caused that chemical shift in your brain. It's possible that you may be able to help speed up your recovery—and possibly prevent recurrences—through some very simple tools.

- *Focus on tasks and activities that reassure you of your own competence and reinforce your sense of control over your environment.* For me, caring for my daughter was therapeutic. My constant awareness of my responsibility for her kept me from dwelling on my sad thoughts. Furthermore, my work, particularly caring for patients, gave me an additional sense of mastery over my environment. Responding to these external demands gradually assured me that I was indeed capable and independent, as I saw myself acting so. You may find a similarly strengthening distraction in your work, in volunteering to help others, or even in a simple chore or hobby you can take from start to completion.
- *Take advantage of whatever gives you emotional support.* I've mentioned talking to nontherapists earlier in this chapter. This can be complicated, as you may end up reinforcing negative feelings if you choose to lean on a friend who prefers dwelling on the reasons for your depression—or hers. I did find great solace in the comfort of my dear sturdy friends Mary and Isabelle, and my newly widowed mother and I helped each other as best we could. The key is to find friends who can give you emotional support and comfort, and distract you, but who also encourage you to move forward, not focus on the past. Some people find this sort of support through religion, through community or school activities, through women's groups, and even through self-help books.
- *Eliminate environmental stressors that are risk factors for you.* You can cut back on the helpless feelings that engulf you when you take on too many tasks, set unrealistic deadlines, care for too many people, and so forth. Look at your life. Can you simplify? How can you feel less overwhelmed and more in control? Can you master even one small part of a large task? For some women, the simplest of solutions—setting priorities, hiring household help, taking stock of what must be done through list-making and then delegating or making a conscious decision to let the housework go undone or a deadline go unmet—can significantly reduce the helplessness and stress, in turn heading off a depression.

By the same token, now is not the time to pile on more stresses. If you can help it, don't initiate any other major life changes until the depression has run its course.

- *Don't self-medicate or accept any kind of antidepressant medication without the clear and careful advice of a qualified doctor or therapist.* Alcohol won't help you and will hurt you in the long run. The last thing you need to do is mask your depressive symptoms with the illusion of gaiety that alcohol can bring. Alcohol is itself a depressant, will only prolong your depression, and potentially will give you another, equally dangerous problem—addiction. It's also fairly easy to find a doctor who will give you a quick prescription for Valium, an antianxiety medication, or even a sleeping pill. Don't let these quick fixes get in the way of your getting better.
- *Exercise.* This seems a ludicrous solution to a disease whose symptoms number lethargy and exhaustion among them. Nonetheless, exercise raises the levels of your body's natural mood uplifters, the neuropeptides called *endorphins.* If you can bring yourself to take a walk, do it, and do it in the morning sunshine. The body is one unit; I believe that a healthier body contributes to overall health of both mind and spirit.
- Fill your mind with positive, pleasant thoughts when you are awake and when dozing off to sleep, day by day.

QUESTIONS FOR YOUR DOCTOR

Successful medical treatment of anxiety and depression means the therapist has helped the patient heal herself. The therapist is much like a midwife: helping, supporting, encouraging, delivering—but believe me, it is Mother who does the work. It is critical for you—however down, dependent, dejected, and despondent you might feel—to take the first step toward mastery by setting out a plan for therapy and asking the key questions below. Be sure that you do not see prescribed drugs (if any) as a substitute for understanding and insight into the psychological, social, or environmental issues that may be triggering or aggravating the depression.

For your primary care doctor:
- Could there be a physical problem behind your feelings? What could it be and how can your doctor test for it?
- Who does your doctor recommend as a therapist? Why? Does your doctor know the therapist personally? Has she seen successful results in other patients of hers who have worked with this therapist?

- Will your doctor continue to be involved in your treatment?
- What is her advice about medications? Does she prescribe them?
- Don't hesitate to bring to the attention of your primary care doctor unusual stresses in your life that may be coexisting with physical complaints.
- If you are suffering from a serious physical illness such as cancer or heart disease and see yourself as "terminally ill," wondering if it is time to call in Dr. Kevorkian, think and ask about reactive depression. Simple treatments may well lighten your burden and dramatically improve your quality of remaining time.

For your psychiatrist or other therapist:
- How long will this therapy take?
- How much will it cost?
- Exactly what medication does the psychiatrist recommend, and what are the possible side effects?
- How long should you take this medication, and what results should you expect? Are there other drugs on the horizon that you should know about?
- What are her views on drugs vs. talk therapy?
- What's her educational background and general therapeutic approach?
- Plus: Any leading question you can devise that helps you learn whether the chemistry is right—or whether you can feel comfortable and confident. For example, if you're extremely religious, you might be uncomfortable with an atheist; if you're gay, an unresponsive therapist or one unfamiliar with gay issues will be difficult for you to trust. The therapist doesn't have to believe exactly what you believe, but knowing that your therapist holds a fundamental philosophy substantially different from yours is sure to make you uneasy.

WHAT WOMEN CAN DO PERSONALLY AND POLITICALLY

Combating depression is in part about self-mastery. I am convinced that if women can take better control of their lives—both at home and at work—they will be able to deal with milder forms of depression early on. Our modern-day suffrage movement is about women's health—and women's mental health may be a barometer of our success in mastering personal well-being.

Stresses of modern life including the breakdown of family units, the erosion of bonds and values, the fast pace of modern times, and the increased demands placed on women in particular may be partial explanations for the increase in depression among those born after World War II. They must be confronted by all women. Each of us should ask how we can build a better world for ourselves and our daughters.

And we cannot forget the need for a societal commitment to medical research and its hope for millions of sufferers from depression and anxiety. The neurosciences, molecular biology, neurochemistry, and human genetics hold the key to our understanding of depression. With depression on the rise, our legacy to our children must be the transformation of a century of melancholy into a century of melancholy solved.

Edna St. Vincent Millay had depression most of her life. When she was fifty, she was hospitalized for several months with a "nervous breakdown" and was unable to work for two years after that. Back then, in the 1940s, there was little understanding and no treatment, so she suffered and her contributions to the world were diminished. A few years later, after her husband died rather suddenly of lung cancer, she fell into a state of melancholy—retreating in solitude to their farm, where she remained despondent, unable to work, and unwilling to see friends, with no one to fully understand her reactive depression and no antidepressants to lift her out of her dark hole. She wrote a poem, "Thanksgiving," which was published posthumously but may have obliquely referred to her depression: "Let us turn for comfort to this simple fact: We have been in trouble before . . . and we have come through."

A month before the poem was published, she died suddenly, alone and on the steps at her farmhouse. It was a massive heart attack. Heart disease may rob a woman of quantity of life; depression surely robs her of quality of life. Are they not, at least, equally important?

EIGHT

HEART DISEASE
A Woman's Profile

Let us then be up and doing,
With a heart for any fate.

—HENRY WADSWORTH LONGFELLOW,
"A PSALM OF LIFE," 1839

The cardiac surgeon at the other hospital had refused to operate; the patient was high risk, and as her husband was told, it would be pointless. Age was the risk factor that unnerved the referring doctor. The patient was in her late seventies and, while otherwise healthy, was clearly on the verge of a major heart attack. Her distraught husband insisted she be moved to Johns Hopkins.

Mrs. Martucci survived the transfer to Hopkins, itself a risky trip. As I walked into her room, I saw first Mr. Martucci, her husband of fifty years, hovering over his wife like a guardian angel. He spotted me and said simply, "Please, do everything for her. She's mine." I tried to calm them both as I reviewed her records, examined her, and asked a few questions. They understood the facts all too well: her age increased her chances of complications and death from heart surgery, but avoiding surgery meant almost certain death from a heart attack. To them, surgery at least provided a chance. I gave them no argument; I had come to the same conclusion.

I conducted preliminary tests and learned that Mrs. Martucci had what is called *left main disease,* an especially dangerous blockage that increased the chance she might not survive the operation. Normally a coronary bypass heart operation comes with a mortality risk of about

1 to 2 percent—at least for middle-aged men. This woman's risk was more like 10 to 20 percent, odds that many would argue are too great, putting the patient, if she survived, at great risk of a long, painful, expensive hospitalization, and the hospital at risk of losing stature in the surgical statistics game. To me, odds are only odds—they can't say what the outcome will be for an individual patient. My experience and clinical intuition told me nonetheless that this otherwise robust and healthy woman would survive.

I spoke privately to her husband. (Although I generally advocate informing a patient of all risks, I also feel that a patient going into high-risk surgery with trust, optimism, and confidence has an extra edge on surviving.) Mr. Martucci was shaken by my disclosures, but his resolve was not. The only thing I didn't tell him was how scared I was, too.

Our fears proved groundless. This highest of high-risk "old ladies" sailed through the coronary bypass operation and the surgical intensive care unit like a young champ. The day she was discharged, the two of them seemed like newlyweds or parents taking home a newborn. As they stood to leave, the gentle and reserved Mr. Martucci gave me a sudden hug and quietly said, "Thank you for letting me keep my wife." But all I had done was judge his wife's situation on the basis of what her body told me, as I would any patient, and not dismiss her on such arbitrary grounds as age.

Shortly after the Martuccis went home, one of the youngest patients I cared for during my years at Hopkins was admitted to the cardiac care unit. Jill, a college girl, had been volunteering on a farm project for the summer when, totally unexpectedly, she had a cardiac arrest while baling hay. She had been born with a very rare and difficult to diagnose congenital abnormality of one of her coronary arteries. Had her problem been picked up when she was little, it could have been repaired with a coronary bypass type of operation. But *if* is the most frustrating word in medicine. By the time Jill got to the hospital, her heart had resumed beating, but the prolonged lack of oxygen had severely damaged her brain.

Jill didn't make it. With each brain wave test, there was the hope that brain activity might reappear, but it did not. She was declared "brain dead." On a very bleak day, we turned off her respirator.

Both Jill and Mrs. Martucci remind me of a crucial lesson: the pervasive societal perception that heart disease is a man's disease is both wrong and dangerous. Most women feel their biggest threat is breast cancer, yet it is cardiovascular disease—or disease involving the blood vessels and the heart—that dwarfs virtually all other afflictions, including all forms of cancer, in sheer numbers of victims. At least one in every two women can expect to have serious heart trouble in her lifetime; 245,000 American women now die each year because of coronary artery disease alone. (The number who die of breast cancer is 46,000.) Coronary heart disease is the number one killer and disabler of women in this country. Women like Mrs. Martucci are most often its prey. We are stricken with heart attacks at a later age than men, and, because we are all living longer, more and more older women are victims of what can be a preventable disease. The implications of this fact are staggering and must be attended to, particularly at a time when as a nation we are exploring health care programs that may effectively deny treatment on the basis of age.

I devote most of this chapter to coronary disease since it overshadows virtually all other heart diseases in women (such as valve disease). Starting on page 365, I will discuss the other important cardiac problems that a woman may face in her lifetime.

ANATOMY OF A MYTH: WOMEN DON'T HAVE HEART DISEASE

Heart disease maintains the aura of being a man's disease; it's called "the widow maker." There *is* an element of truth here; younger men do have more heart attacks than younger women. The empirical evidence of this fact was undeniable during the formative years of many readers of this book. In the fifties, sixties, and seventies, the male heart attack epidemic was everywhere; middle-aged men were dropping dead at work and on the golf course, having heart attacks in the middle of the night and while raking leaves. I vividly remember the fear in my neighborhood that shoveling snow brought on a heart attack; my own father always insisted that Mom and the girls did our snow shoveling, since everyone knew men carried this special risk. In September 1955, President Dwight Eisenhower was stricken with a heart attack, and the whole country was terrified. (At that time, treatment for Ike and all others was primitive at best: morphine early on, followed by six weeks in bed. Half of those with a heart attack died within the first few hours, and another third died within the first few weeks. Ike was one of the lucky few who survived and survived well.)

The belief that men were the target of heart disease was confirmed by one of the greatest ongoing pieces of observational research ever conducted in this country: the Framingham Heart Study supported by the National Heart, Lung and Blood Institute of the NIH. This study, which began in 1948 and is still running today, has continuously followed 5,127 of the adults in the community, focusing specifically on cardiovascular disease. The first Framingham results were published in 1954, after six years of study. By that time, 98 heart attacks had occurred, 81 of them in men. Of 44 women who had complained of chest pain, none had experienced heart attacks. In 1960, the second set of findings rendered similar results: of all the men who showed any sign of heart disease, 70 percent dropped dead; in contrast, of all the women with any sign of heart disease, 69 percent had chest pain that, by all available measures, looked benign—that is, it did not lead to heart attacks or sudden death.

FRAMINGHAM "PROVES IT": WOMEN ARE HYSTERICAL

The results above seemed to confirm an already disturbing, centuries-old view of women as hysterical and hypochondriacal (while men are strong and stoic). They were moaning and groaning about nothing, turning small physical annoyances into large, unwarranted fears of heart attacks. The Framingham studies provided the hard data to support the stereotype of the complaining woman, a being to be heeded little, if at all, when she reports physical discomfort. The data appeared to prove that chest pain in women is harmless in nature and possibly psychosomatic in origin.

THE PROBLEM WITH FACTS

It all sounds awfully convincing. Only one problem: it isn't accurate. Truthful, yes; but accurate, no. The Framingham findings have to be understood in the context of the times. When Framingham began in the late 1940s, we knew amazingly little about heart disease. We barely knew the underlying causes of chest pain or heart attacks; when someone had chest pain, the only way we could figure out if it was serious or not was to wait and see what happened. If she had a heart attack or died, we knew it was "real"; if she did fine, whatever caused the pain was viewed as unimportant. The potentially dangerous—and very real—causes of pains women reported that did not lead to heart attacks were not even considered during the Framingham studies; the causes were not known.

We now know that chest pain in women can be caused by a range of problems not typically seen in men. Younger and middle-aged women, unlike men of the same age, are subject to a wide variety of other heart conditions that can cause chest pain, dizziness, and shortness of breath—symptoms to be acknowledged with respect and given credence, but which are only rarely life threatening.

What was also missed in this early study is that women do get heart attacks, but their heart attacks strike some ten to twenty years later in life than do a man's, generally after menopause. The participants in Framingham ranged in age from thirty-six to sixty-eight. So the heart disease that afflicted women, the same deadly variety men get, was virtually left out of the picture. And, because Framingham was one of a kind, other data that might call into question the Framingham findings were nonexistent for years.

The myth inadvertently perpetuated by Framingham has become more and more erroneous as time has gone on. The longer that women live, the more likely they are to develop heart disease. Back in 1948 when the Framingham Study started, life expectancy in the United States was only sixty-five years for men and seventy-one for women. Today women are living well into their eighties and experiencing this deadly disease in incredible numbers. So what was only a minor myth back in 1950—that women did not get coronary disease—has become a major myth of the 1990s.

IMPACT OF THE MYTH

When an entire culture, doctors and laypeople alike, erroneously view the world of heart disease from an exclusively male perspective, the ramifications are bound to be *significant*. If we don't believe women get heart attacks, we don't pay attention to our own symptoms, and neither do our doctors. The bias may be inadvertent, but it makes a huge impact.

This perspective has led to some misdiagnosis or late diagnosis of women's symptoms; for example, several reports have shown that women with chest pain and abnormalities in their diagnostic tests are less likely to be referred for more intensive evaluation than are men. Other studies have shown that after a heart attack, when every minute lost can diminish the effectiveness of emergency treatment, women themselves do not go to the hospital as quickly as do men. And there aren't enough of these studies! Years of medical focus and research all too often have left women out.

Once a doctor is faced with a woman having a heart attack or demonstrating unequivocal heart disease, there is no difference in the treatment she will receive. I've called this the "Yentl Syndrome," a manifestation of a broader phenomenon. Yentl, the heroine of Isaac Bashevis Singer's short story, disguises herself as a man in order to attend school and study the Talmud. Only by "acting just like a man"

DON'T THROW OUT THE BABY ...

Yes, Framingham and other early studies reinforced two destructive fallacies: women don't get heart attacks, and they complain needlessly about physical pain. But that does not mean that women have not benefited from the breathtaking advances that have occurred in our understanding of cardiovascular disease over these past four decades. Thanks to Framingham, we now recognize certain key risk factors for both men and women, such as cigarette smoking, hypertension, diabetes, obesity, and diet, and the importance of trying to lower or eliminate those risks. Also, in part because this deadly epidemic hit men so hard in the prime of their lives, at times of peak and visible productivity, robbing families of their breadwinners, a national resolve emerged to fight it. Efforts took hold in government, industry, private hospitals, clinics, and universities and research institutes to pour talent and resources into understanding, preventing, and treating heart disease. The investment has paid off. Mortality for coronary disease in the United States has decreased by more than 40 percent among men and women since the early 1960s. And, although powerful and important differences in male and female cardiovascular systems have largely been ignored and must be studied, many treatments that have been developed in men have been successful in treating women as well, even though, by and large, the outcomes of the disease and its treatments tend to differ by gender, as I'll explain, with women doing less well.

can she be admitted to the school and get the same treatment as her male peers. Until very recently a woman had to show all the signs of having a heart attack "just like a man" in order to have her symptoms of heart disease given the same credence.

HEART DISEASE *IS* A WOMAN'S PROBLEM

The heart is a muscle that pumps blood, nonstop, for a lifetime. It beats on average about 70 times a minute, 4,200 times an hour, 100,000 times a day, and some 3 billion times in a lifetime, without rest. It is a remarkable part of our bodies, among the first organs that begin to work early in fetal development and the last to quiet at the end of life. But sometimes this wondrous, life-giving organ fails us too soon.

Heart disease comes in many and various forms, some of which are more common to women than to men. Diseases that involve the valves within the heart, such as rheumatic heart disease or abnormalities of the mitral valve in the left chamber of the heart, inexplicably are more likely to appear in a woman, and women are susceptible to certain distinctive cardiovascular problems surrounding pregnancy (see chapter 3). We have as much high blood pressure as men and experience more of certain forms of heart-related birth defects.

But, just as for men, it's the heart attacks caused by coronary artery disease that are a woman's most common and deadly form of heart affliction.

CORONARY ARTERY DISEASE

Coronary artery disease is simply a narrowing or blockage of one or more of the three major arteries that supply oxygen-bearing blood to the heart. Hearts cannot function without the oxygen brought to them by a sufficient supply of blood; without enough oxygen, your heart will try to correct the problem by decreasing its own oxygen demands. Contractions become weaker, and sometimes the heartbeat becomes irregular: if the oxygen supply continues to dwindle, the oxygen-deprived parts of your heart will begin shutting down.

A heart will also try to tell us when it is in trouble. First we get pain, called *angina,* which forces us to stop whatever we're doing and therefore place less demand on the heart. If the blockages stop blood flow completely to one part of the heart, that part dies and we experience a *heart attack;* in the most drastic cases of coronary artery disease, we die.

Your arteries can be narrowed by any number of causes, such as coronary embolisms, coronary spasms, or the mysterious Syndrome X (see page 337), but by far the most likely is *atherosclerosis,* or hardening of the arteries.

ATHEROSCLEROTIC HEART DISEASE

Nine times out of ten, it's fatty plaque building up over time that narrows an artery, just like the clogging of a rusty pipe. Blood clots form in the rough inner lining of the diseased artery; eventually a large clot in a narrowed artery can cause its sudden and complete closure. Any artery is susceptible, but for millions of men and women, it is the arteries of the heart that fall prey.

Causes of coronary atherosclerosis are many and varied; while many doctors and researchers over time have attempted to pinpoint just one factor, this disease generally arises from a combination of genetic, metabolic, and environmental factors. In other words, you can't change whether or not you're genetically predisposed to atherosclerosis, but as Framingham proved and as we'll see throughout this chapter, you can make a great impact through your lifestyle choices on whether your susceptibility will grow into a full-blown disease or whether it will lie dormant as you live a long and healthy life.

We can predict which arteries are apt to have a sudden life-threatening closure by the extent or character of their narrowing. If a blood vessel is narrowed by more than 75 percent, or the narrowing is highly irregular and complex (bulging with crystals of cholesterol that can rupture the plaque), there is a greater chance that the artery will suddenly become blocked altogether.

In turn, the severity of coronary atherosclerosis depends on which of the heart's three major arteries is narrowed or blocked, how many are blocked, and how extensively within each vessel. These are the factors that will determine the amount of heart muscle at risk for damage if a total coronary blockage occurs. The more the muscle damage, obviously, the more serious the impairment of the heart, and the more difficult the recovery from a heart attack. If only one of the major arteries is diseased, your risk of a heart attack or death is substantially less than if you have double- or triple-vessel disease.

Generally, narrowings involving two particular segments of the left coronary system are the scariest. Two of the three major arteries lying atop the heart and feeding it with blood are branches of a larger main trunk artery, the *left main coronary artery*. When this trunk is narrowed, the heart is in critical danger from massive loss of oxygen. The *left anterior descending coronary artery,* which is the major branch of the left main trunk, feeds the largest territory of heart muscle of all of the arteries; that includes most of the front surface of the heart and a large part of the muscular septum that divides the right and left chambers (called *ventricles*). Three-fourths of all people who die of heart attacks have a narrowing high up in this artery; cardiologists call this the "widow maker" lesion.

OTHER TYPES OF CORONARY ARTERY DISEASE

Other types of coronary artery disease are rare, but they do exist. It's important for you to be aware of them if you have chest pain and to consider them in addition to atherosclerosis with your doctor, particularly if you are under fifty.

CORONARY SPASM

In a coronary artery spasm, seemingly normal (or near-normal) coronary arteries spontaneously contract to the point of pinching off blood flow temporarily, producing the same kind of chest pain that occurs when atherosclerotic plaque impedes blood flow. When chest pain has a coronary spasm as its origin, it is called *variant* or *Prinzmetal's angina* (the more common form of angina is discussed on page 338). Although the pain from coronary spasm is every bit as real and as frightening as the pain from an early heart attack, it rarely results in heart attacks and almost never ends in death.

SYNDROME X

With the obviously little-known Syndrome X, women experience the same kind of pain, but spasm of their major coronary arteries is not evident. Instead, this condition is due to dysfunction of some of the very small coronary microvessels that penetrate deep into the heart muscle. These little vessels, which relax and contract depending on the oxygen needs of the heart muscle, don't function properly. When this occurs, the heart itself is almost never at risk because the interruption of flow is brief and the area of heart muscle affected very small. Syndrome X is most often seen in postmenopausal women, and some physicians suspect estrogen fluctuations may be a culprit.

CORONARY OBSTRUCTIONS

There are several very rare forms of coronary blockages; virtually all of them are found more often in women than in men, possibly because of gender-related differences in the blood-clotting system. In a *coronary embolism,* a clump of material (usually a blood clot) floating in the blood gets swept into the coronary arteries, lodges, and blocks blood flow. Even less common is *primary coronary artery dissection,* where a seemingly normal vessel wall splits and causes an obstruction. This problem occurs most often in women during or just after childbirth, but only in extraordinarily rare circumstances. Sometimes the coronary arteries are *congenitally malformed,* that is, defective from birth. Over time the malformed arteries cause damage to the heart muscle by starving it of oxygen, and the result can look like a heart attack, which is what happened to Jill. Sometimes, too, rare multiple immune system diseases such as scleroderma and systemic lupus can be linked to coronary disease in young women. I mention these diseases because of their gender link, but please note that all are quite unlikely to affect you.

CONSEQUENCES OF CORONARY ARTERY DISEASE

The consequences of coronary artery disease range from chest pain to irregular or abnormal heart rhythms to heart attacks and sudden cardiac death. We all face a fifty-fifty chance of encountering one of these problems in our lifetimes.

ANGINA PECTORIS

Angina pectoris is the medical term for chest pain originating in the heart muscle, resulting from what is called *ischemia* (lack of oxygen). This spasmodic pain was first recognized as a system of cardiac disease and associated with degeneration of the coronary arteries more than a hundred years ago by the patron saint of Hopkins medicine, Sir William Osler. Of course, to Osler, angina was a man's disease; women who complained of chest pain were hysterical or neurotic, suffering from the condition of "pseudo-angina," something, he cautioned, of which doctors must be skeptical.

We now know that angina is actually more common in women than men, and that the older a woman gets, the more serious it becomes; but as recently as twenty years ago, when I was in medical school, we were still taught that angina occurred predominantly in men (by as much as six to one), and that when it occurred in women, it was generally a harmless condition. Not only is this view outdated, it is harmful; in fact, a woman's first sign of coronary disease is apt to be chest pain. Despite what you may believe and what your doctor may have been originally trained to think, angina must *always* be given attention and prompt diagnosis.

For women under fifty, angina is a very real illness, but in three out of four cases it indicates a disease other than atherosclerosis and generally less alarming. Problems that may precipitate this frightening pain include the coronary artery diseases discussed above (coronary spasms and Syndrome X), *mitral valve prolapse* (discussed on page 369), severe high blood pressure, or inflammation in the sac around the heart, called *pericarditis.* Ailments as relatively mild as a spasm of the esophagus (the muscular tube that carries food into your stomach) or indigestion can mimic angina, as can the pain of ulcers and some kinds of lung disease. These will all be considered by your doctor. But for women over fifty, the chances that the angina forewarns of serious coronary trouble are much greater than for younger women.

Angina as a symptom of atherosclerotic artery distress usually first shows up during some kind of exertion: running, walking up stairs, lifting, or carrying something. As soon as you stop the activity, the pain generally eases. The reason is that the need of the heart for blood varies depending on the workload put on it, as with any muscle. Doctors classify angina's severity by how easily it comes on and how long it lasts. The less the exertion needed to bring on the chest pain, the worse the angina. When angina comes on with no activity at all—sitting in a chair or awakening from sleep—then it is unpredictable, unstable angina and forewarns a high risk of a heart attack. Such angina, called *pre-infarction angina,* is treated as a medical emergency (*infarction* is explained in the "Heart Attack" section below). Unstable angina sometimes looks like an early heart attack even to a physician, but remember that angina can also be a symptom preceding an attack or a symptom of a number of coronary artery and other diseases—it is not a fail-safe sign of a heart attack.

Angina caused by atherosclerosis typically resolves itself within a few minutes, but it sometimes may last as long as twenty minutes. When atherosclerosis is the cause, the lengthier the episode of angina, the more severe the disease and the greater the threat of a heart attack. (Angina born of other causes such as spasms can come and go for days, but such length is not a harbinger of a heart attack.)

The pain of angina is not pleasant. My patients have described it as "sickening," usually deep in the chest toward the left side. Sometimes it radiates into the left arm or the throat and even into the back. It is the kind of dull aching pain that makes you want to stop what you are doing and catch your breath—as well you should.

HEART ATTACK

When narrowed arteries get completely blocked and a part of the blood- and oxygen-deprived heart muscle becomes injured, we have heart attacks, which the medical world calls *myocardial infarction,* or a *coronary thrombosis.* (*Infarction* refers to the damage done to the part of the heart muscle fed by the blocked artery; *thrombosis* refers to the clot, or *thrombus,* which develops on the surface of the atherosclerotic plaque already narrowing the diseased artery.)

To some people, just the term *heart attack* is interpreted as a death sentence, but this is far from true. All heart attacks are not created equal. Some engender no meaningful long-term damage to the heart; others can leave the heart weakened for life. Depending on the type of blockage, a heart attack may involve a relatively small part of the heart, perhaps 5 or 10 percent, or it may be massive, involving some 35 to 40 percent of the working muscle of the heart. The most severe attacks destroy the full depth of the heart muscle wall and increase the likelihood that heart failure will occur; almost as threatening is a large attack that involves the front of the heart (the "widow maker" discussed on page 337). Smaller attacks and those that strike the back of the heart are more apt to be mild, and some heart attacks damage just a small sliver of inner heart lining. Many people experience mild heart attacks and are left essentially with a normal heart for the rest of their lives.

If you take nothing else from this book, heed this: *if you fear you are having a heart attack, get to the hospital immediately.* One of the most important discoveries of the past decade was the realization that we can safely limit the amount of heart damage if very early in the course of a heart attack the blocked artery is opened with clot-dissolving drugs. If opened within twenty or thirty minutes, the blood-starved muscle suffers very little damage; as the clock ticks, more and more of the heart muscle that should be fed by the clotted artery is destroyed.

For a woman, quick treatment is imperative because statistically women don't do as well after a heart attack as men do. The reason may be that women get heart attacks at an older age or that elderly women are more likely to suffer from *co-morbidity*, the presence of coexisting illnesses such as hypertension, diabetes, or chronic lung disease. Whatever the reason, women who have heart attacks have more cardiac failure and almost twice the chance of having a subsequent stroke and are more than twice as likely as men to die from the attack. With the latest in medical therapy, a man faces a 5 to 6 percent chance of dying after a heart attack; for a woman, that likelihood is between 11 and 12 percent. A woman is also more likely to have a second attack than a man. This was recently confirmed through one of the largest studies ever done in the United States that included women heart patients, the Global Utilization of Streptokinase and Tissue plasminogen activator for Occluded Coronary Arteries (GUSTO) trial headed by Dr. Eric Topol of the Cleveland Clinic Foundation. GUSTO, which studied more than ten thousand women with heart attacks, also revealed that women even though sicker benefited from clot-dissolving treatment as much as men did.

Age and associated debility help explain these differences; we know, for example, that younger women who have cardiac surgery, such as valve replacement, do not show such gender differences in outcomes. It is less easy to explain why women are more apt to have so-called silent heart attacks (which are picked up on a routine *electrocardiogram,* or *ECG,* described on page 351), without any reported pain, or why they are significantly more susceptible to what is called *cardiogenic shock* once they get into the hospital (as studied extensively by Dr. Judith Hochman of Columbia University in New York). Cardiogenic shock is a dire state of cardiovascular collapse that occurs with the largest heart attacks, involving 35 to 40 percent of the heart's muscle; it carries a 70 to 80 percent mortality rate. We don't know why, but I suspect it's related to the fact that a woman's heart will change shape, bulging out in parts and weakening, after major heart muscle damage. This change leads also to an increased likelihood of suffering a ruptured heart at the site where the heart muscle has been damaged. Rupture is a dramatic event that usually strikes in the first few days after a heart attack and is almost universally fatal. There is, to me, a sad poetry in the fact that women are more susceptible than men to broken hearts.

SUDDEN CARDIAC DEATH

In a sudden cardiac death, the heart goes into an abnormal rhythm called *ventricular fibrillation* (see page 365). It is unable to pump blood to the brain and the rest of the body, causing a person to lose consciousness within seconds and experience what is called a *cardiac arrest,* dying within minutes. Only the lucky few will be in the vicinity of someone who can administer life support with CPR (*cardiopulmonary resuscitation*) long enough to activate electric shock *defibrillation,* which jump-starts the heart before irreversible brain damage occurs; only those lucky few can survive this cardiac catastrophe.

All too often sudden cardiac death occurs in people who seem perfectly healthy. Remember the exercise guru Jim Fixx who died suddenly while jogging? Nonetheless, its cause almost always is clogged arteries—atherosclerotic coronary disease. While sudden cardiac death is good news for no one, women do experience it far less frequently than do men, especially men in middle age and beyond.

WHO'S AT RISK FOR CORONARY DISEASE?

Many of the risk factors for coronary artery disease are now common knowledge: high-cholesterol diets, lack of exercise, high blood pressure, diabetes, and obesity. But wait—what was common knowledge about coronary artery disease twenty years ago has now been turned on its ear, and what we now take for granted about the "obvious" risk factors and their relative importance may not turn out to be so true, after all . . . if you're a woman, that is.

ESTROGEN DEFICIENCY

Women get heart attacks after menopause (including surgically induced menopause in the form of a hysterectomy with ovary removal) because they lose the benefits of female hormones that protect the arteries from the scourges of atherosclerosis. When you go through menopause, the level of the hormone estrogen that your body produces drops drastically. Without estrogen, your risk of heart attack increases to that of a man of the same age (see page 185). In brief, loss of estrogen may be the single most important risk factor for women.

CHOLESTEROL

Everybody knows that you are at great risk for a heart attack if your cholesterol levels are too high. But sometimes what everyone knows can be wrong. You *are* at great risk—if you're male. If you're female, the issue is far trickier.

Many studies document the benefits of lowering cholesterol. The only problem is that they have been done almost exclusively on men! Studies of men from all over the world document the dramatic results of lowering cholesterol: for those in middle age with what is called "borderline elevated" total cholesterol levels in their blood, a reduction of 10 percent in cholesterol through changes of diet leads to at least a 20 percent decrease in heart disease, provided the lowered level is sustained for five years or more.

High cholesterol in a woman is *not* in itself dangerous but is a risk factor only in very specific scenarios.

In both men and women, cholesterol can be broken down into two types, LDL and HDL (see page 36). HDL is a "good" cholesterol, cleaning up the "bad" cholesterol, LDL, from the bloodstream by taking it to the liver where it is destroyed. The similarities end here. For men, it is the high LDL levels that pose the most danger, and a man can combat the LDL enemy through simply bringing down his total cholesterol. Ideally, LDL should be under 130 milligrams per deciliter (mg/dl); an LDL over 160 is deemed very high risk. HDL levels for a man don't have that much practical impact because it is hard for a man to bring up his HDL cholesterol. Although intense exercise, olive oil, and alcohol may have some small effect, estrogen seems to have the greatest power to raise HDL. (An acceptable HDL cholesterol is one that is over 35 mg/dl.)

Thus the story is different for a woman. It is the level of HDL, the good cholesterol, that determines her risk in large part. Most women have an HDL cholesterol over 50, and many approach 100, amounts that can inflate the total cholesterol levels substantially. For example, total cholesterol in the 200 to 240 range is deemed borderline high and therefore worrisome by the National Cholesterol Education Program. But if a woman has a relatively high HDL of 85, a total cholesterol of 220 to 230 is very good. Women's total cholesterol—even if borderline high—may be a reflection of high HDLs and low LDLs, a healthy profile by any measure. (To be precise, total cholesterol is the sum of the HDL, LDL, and one-fifth of the serum triglyceride level, which is discussed in its own section below.)

Lowering total cholesterol significantly—below 150—may in fact pose a danger to women. A pooled analysis of twenty-four studies observing the relationship of total cholesterol levels to all varieties of cardiovascular disease in some 125,000 men and women, with follow-up periods of as long as thirty years, showed that lowering cholesterol in women did decrease the chance of dying from a heart attack—but it did not save lives. There were more strokes in women, which offset the death rate decline from heart attacks. Possibly there is a correlation between low cholesterol and the risk of an uncommon type of stroke caused by bleeding in the brain. In addition, very low cholesterol seems to correlate with death from other causes, such as cancer, digestive diseases, and violence, including suicide (although this observation has recently come into question in a cholesterol-lowering drug study from Scandinavia.) I therefore question some of my colleagues who promote for themselves and their patients drastic total cholesterol reduction to the range of 110 to 140. It's hard to achieve and may do more harm than good.

You can get a good and simple picture of your cholesterol risk readily and inexpensively, by calculating a ratio of total cholesterol to HDL. Your doctor will obtain these measures from a routine blood test taken after you've fasted for about twelve hours. A ratio of total cholesterol to HDL of under 3.5 to 1 (or simply stated, 3.5) is most desirable. A ratio of 3.5 to 6.9 is borderline, and anything above 6.9 is high. This range takes into account the good effect of a high HDL: the higher the HDL, the lower the ratio, and the lower your risk. And before you get panicked about those home cholesterol tests that have just been approved by the FDA to be sold over the counter in your local drugstore, remember they tell you only your total cholesterol. If you feel compelled to test yourself, consult your doctor about the results and factor in your own HDL.

SERUM TRIGLYCERIDES

Like cholesterol, triglycerides are forms of circulating fat in the bloodstream (see page 36). There isn't much we can do about our baseline

SEXIST SCIENCE

I see no justification for the consistent and purposeful exclusion of women from cholesterol studies. Some may try to rationalize the choice by saying the inclusion of women would have skewed test results, since women's cholesterol naturally rises from age thirty-five on, whereas men's cholesterol stays fairly level; also, because of the protection offered by their female hormones, women tend to be older when they get heart disease, so including women would have skewed the results. These differences mark the very reason to keep women in the studies in adequate numbers to determine a woman's different risks and different treatment.

In a move compounding the problem, the National Cholesterol Education Program, in the late 1980s, reduced its recommended cholesterol levels, advising all American adults to strive for total levels under 200 and warning that cholesterol levels between 200 and 239 are borderline high, with levels over 240 spelling big danger. A conscious decision was made to keep its recommendations simple and easy to remember and therefore not to have different advice for women and for women of different ages—despite the fact that the NCEP advisory groups were well aware that such advice was inadequate for women. More recently, the NCEP has modified the advice by stressing the need to obtain separate measures of LDL and HDL and to monitor the total-cholesterol-to-HDL-cholesterol ratio. As yet, however, they still haven't stressed publicly the different needs of men and women, particularly as women get older. In fact, there is recent evidence, sure to be controversial, that cholesterol bears little relationship to the risk of heart attack or death for women over seventy.

Two medical embarrassments—near-total neglect of controlled medical studies on this key risk factor for cardiac disease, one of a woman's biggest health problems, paired with hefty, expensive research done on the disease's effects in men only—have combined to leave us with a legacy of ignorance that fails to help the legions of aging women with rising cholesterol levels and increasing risk of heart disease.

triglyceride levels, i.e., those levels obtained while we are fasting, but I note them here because some studies suggest that triglycerides may be a more important female risk factor: chronically elevated triglycerides (over 150 mg/dl) correlate with heart disease in women more than in men of the same age group. Triglycerides go up temporarily in all of us after we eat any fat, and their levels show rapid swings depending on the content of each meal. Most studies show that a high triglyceride level is not an independent risk for heart disease; it usually comes tied to other risk factors such as obesity, diabetes, and a lowered HDL level. While it is difficult to reduce chronically elevated triglycerides either by diet or medication, cutting out alcohol and losing weight may help.

DIABETES

Diabetes, specifically juvenile-onset, insulin-dependent diabetes (Type 1), is a male-female risk equalizer for coronary disease. When a woman is diabetic, her chance of heart disease leaps to become identical to that of a diabetic man—a risk several times higher than even that of an average nondiabetic man. The disease leads to across-the-board elevations in LDL cholesterol and triglycerides and the lowering of the protective HDL cholesterol. Long-term diabetes causes degeneration of the small arteries of the kidneys and eyes and accelerated atherosclerosis throughout the body. Curiously, more women have diabetes than men, and it does them more harm than it does men. If a diabetic woman has a heart attack, her chances of complications and dying are substantially worse than that of a male diabetic. Diabetes *must* be a top women's health research priority!

On the brighter side, diabetes that shows up later in life, called adult-onset diabetes (Type 2), has fewer complications and is far easier to manage. Careful diet and regular exercise can control its risks, and weight loss can often completely resolve it.

FAMILY HISTORY

We know coronary heart disease runs in families. If you have a parent or sibling with this disease, particularly when afflicted earlier in life (at less than fifty years old), you're at risk. Sometimes we know the risk relates to an inherited abnormality in cholesterol processing that causes very high blood lipids. But often there is no evident reason why heart disease seems to run in some families.

One of the most exciting areas of cardiovascular research today involves human genetics. It is likely that the risk for coronary artery disease relates to many different genes and that in time we will be able to predict the gene or genes that predispose you to heart disease long before symptoms develop. This means that you can tailor your lifestyle and medicines to your own personal health needs or in some circumstances even take a preventive medication.

HIGH BLOOD PRESSURE

High blood pressure, or hypertension, is not sexist; it is a clear risk factor for coronary artery disease in both women and men. High blood pressure is a silent condition that sabotages the heart and blood vessels for years without symptoms—but it doesn't have to. Once diagnosed, it can be kept under control through changes in lifestyle and/or medication; its risk can be minimized to almost nothing (see page 385).

Of course, nothing is totally straightforward or simple. While severe hypertension is a clear risk factor requiring medication, mild hypertension does not necessarily lead to either severe hypertension or heart disease; therefore, your decision on treating your mild hypertension has to be discussed thoroughly with your physician. I rely heavily on my patients' first keeping a careful home blood pressure diary, using a home blood pressure monitoring device that can be purchased in any drugstore (see page 403). While a woman's blood pressure may be up in the stress-filled environment of the doctor's office, perhaps her home diary will show me that she has no need for medication, with home readings mostly in the normal range, with occasional mild elevations.

STRESS

Worry, anxiety, emotional turmoil, pressure, and frustration are normal human reactions to the traumatic events that life lays at our feet. But for some of us, these emotions are not occasional experiences; they are a way of being. If this is true for you, if you create your own major stress out of what for many people would be a minor inconvenience, you are, male or female, at an increased risk for coronary artery disease.

As pointed out by Dr. Meyer Friedman and Dr. Ray H. Rosenman more than twenty-five years ago when they coined the phrase *type A personality,* your innate personality very much determines how you react to life's challenges. The type A personality is always under stress—and, according to Friedman and Rosenman, prone to coronary disease. They describe the type A person as one who is consistently involved in some kind of struggle to extract from the environment the greatest amount in the shortest time period and against all odds. The type A personality is demanding, time conscious, aggressive, dissatisfied, and perfectionistic. Type A's often speak louder, talk faster, and listen impatiently. There has, however, been some challenge to the premise that these characteristics (which some might say describe New Yorkers) are a cardiac risk, unless they are also combined with a hostile, ever-in-conflict dimension.

Indeed, most psychologists agree that the most malignant form of type A by far is a hostile and angry personality. Although any one of us who is striving to build a home, raise good kids, do well at work, keep physically fit, and responsibly follow the rules of society may have certain dimensions of type A, the angry, frustrated, hostile, dismissive temperament that allows for little joy and makes for higher risk need not be part of that striving. (See page 364 for more information on how to modify type A reactions to the world.)

Is Working a Risk Factor for Women?

I am often asked whether the movement of women into the male workplace over the past few decades has increased our chances of getting heart attacks. Actually, there is no evidence at all to suggest that working outside the home leads to more coronary artery disease. It produces stress, especially since the home responsibilities for women don't diminish, but it can also relieve stress by bringing a needed social outlet or a sense of fulfillment and control over our own destinies.

I also remind questioners that the stress linked directly to coronary problems is the kind engendered by inappropriate reactions to stressful situations, which are experienced differently by each of us depending upon personality. Simply being in the workplace won't change anyone's personality into a type A; a woman prone to react with hostility to a stressful situation will be at greater risk in whatever environment she inhabits.

MULTIPLE BIRTHS (MULTIPARITY)

We do have some growing but only observational information about some moms' unique cardiovascular stresses. A rather provocative group of commentaries recently surfaced in the *New England Journal of Medicine* and elsewhere that demonstrated that women who have five or more pregnancies and births have a substantially increased risk of coronary heart disease—in the range of 50 percent or more—over women with fewer children or none. These observations were described in multiple populations and corrected for educational and for socioeconomic levels, as well as for most heart disease risk factors. Possible explanations include sustained lower levels of HDL cholesterol in such women, changes in glucose metabolism, and increased levels of emotional stress. Although some studies showed that men with four or more children had a somewhat higher risk for heart disease, it was not nearly as great as that which women faced. Is grand multiparity a special kind of risk factor for women that has been largely overlooked in an androcentric research world?

OBESITY

Obesity is a risk factor for heart disease in both men and women. People who are obese (as determined by you and your doctor, not just a few extra pounds) tend to develop high blood pressure and diabetes, which are precursors for cardiovascular disease and add to the risk of certain treatments such as surgery. There is also plenty of evidence that leaner women live longer and have fewer heart attacks.

EDUCATION

One of the most important pieces of information regarding women's health that came out of the Framingham studies is that education level is among the best predictors of cardiovascular health. Women who did not have a high school education had almost four times the risk of getting coronary disease as did high school graduates. This reinforces a general and little-known medical fact of life: healthy women are educated women. And educated healthy women pass their habits and knowledge onto their families. Education brings with it health awareness and lifesaving information that will have an impact on generations, not only on individuals.

Smoking

Last but by no means least on the list of risk factors is smoking. There is no question that smoking equals puffing your life away; if you have any fatty buildup in your arteries, smoking will speed up the life-shortening effects, damaging your blood vessels and accelerating atherosclerosis. When I ran the coronary care unit at Johns Hopkins, I would often say that a young or middle-aged woman presenting with a heart attack was most likely a smoker. And she usually was.

If you have no atherosclerosis, smoking will still cause you coronary problems. Smoking has an acute toxic effect on normal blood vessels, causing them to contract or even spasm. That can cause angina and increase the chance of your forming blood clots. Perhaps the most disturbing fact about smoking in this country is that more teenage girls and young women are starting, although the habit is declining overall. There is only one prescription for smokers: STOP. And only one for non-smokers: DON'T START.

DETECTING CORONARY HEART DISEASE: INVASIVE AND NONINVASIVE TESTS

When a woman concerned about possible heart diseases gets to the doctor and the hospital quickly, she will in all likelihood be given concrete information to reward her efforts—not the vague "we're not sure; we don't know why" nonanswer usually offered before diagnosis of so many other illnesses. There is almost no heart dysfunction that we can't figure out with astounding precision through quick tests.

Exercise Stress Test

The exercise stress test is a simple yet powerful means of detecting narrowing of the coronary artery; it's called a noninvasive test because it is entirely external. In the most common and least expensive form of an exercise stress test, you simply exercise on a treadmill or sometimes on a stationary bicycle while a doctor carefully monitors your heart. Throughout the exercise you are attached, through wires taped to your chest, to an electrocardiograph, a machine that measures the electrical currents that normally and consistently run through the walls of your heart during its contraction and relaxation. The ECG (or EKG) will reveal abnormal currents and can sometimes even pinpoint which part of the heart is in trouble. If you get chest pain and the electrocardiogram starts to show abnormalities with the pain, the test is stopped immediately, termed positive, and you may well have coronary narrowing.

A "normal" test, for both men and women, is a reliable indication that the coronary arteries are either normal or at most mildly diseased. However, this test is better at accurately reporting abnormalities in men than in women: for men, a positive test means coronary blockages about 90 percent of the time. The more severe the narrowings of the coronary arteries, the more likely it is that the exercise test will show an abnormality. Women are much more likely—one in four—to get a false positive reading (the test says she has the disease when in fact she doesn't). We do not know why; perhaps it's related to specific nerves and reflexes during exercise that behave differently in women.

If you take the exercise stress test and receive a positive result, you and your physician have several options to consider in choosing which test you wish to take to confirm the findings or how you may want to otherwise proceed. If there's a minor abnormality in the ECG, your doctor may elect simply to keep an eye on you for a period of time, as you investigate together the many preventive measures you can take through lifestyle changes. The doctor will use her clinical judgment; she may put you on medication as well. Together, you may also opt for a more elaborate version of the exercise stress test, a *thallium* heart scan: a radioactive compound called a *radionuclide* is injected into your vein, and a special camera obtains an image of either the heart muscle or the heart wall as you exercise. But this test, too, is more accurate for men than women (perhaps it is difficult to read because a woman's breasts may cast a shadow), and, more to the point, I'm concerned about the radioactive exposure to the internal organs, particularly the ovaries. I think the value of this test for a woman is limited, too often a waste of money. Recent studies done at the Cleveland Clinic and elsewhere suggest that using echocardiography (see page 369) combined with the stress test increases the accuracy of the test in women, poses no radiation exposure, and is also about half as expensive as a thallium stress study.

CORONARY ARTERIOGRAPHY (CARDIAC CATHETERIZATION)

As you read about this test, certainly a more invasive procedure, you may feel a bit squeamish. But most of my patients claim coronary arteriography is not uncomfortable. Invented by Dr. F. Mason Sones at the Cleveland Clinic Foundation some thirty years ago, coronary arteriography represents the single most crucial turning point in the history of cardiovascular medicine. The test to this day is the "gold standard" of detecting coronary heart disease, since it allows us actually to see the functioning coronary arteries and predict what is likely to happen to a woman and her heart. We have arrived at our modern-day understanding of both chest pain and coronary artery disease in women only through the early arteriographic studies of women with heart symptoms that were conducted in large numbers in places like the Cleveland Clinic.

Cardiologists perform coronary arteriography by carefully threading a *catheter*—a little hollow tube about the width of a strand of angel-hair pasta—through an artery in either the arm or the groin, until it reaches and is inserted directly into the heart. The doctor then injects an inert dye into the catheter, and the dye travels into the coronary arteries so they can be seen on X ray. During the injections, moving pictures are taken that show in precise detail the anatomy of the heart and its blood vessels.

When a woman is experiencing angina and the results of an exercise stress test are questionable (particularly if she is past menopause) and all other possible causes have been tested for and eliminated, the only way to be sure about the symptoms is with coronary arteriography. The procedure is not to be taken lightly. It is costly, invasive, involves some X-ray exposure (as with all X rays, the pelvic area of women of childbearing age should be shielded), and carries a small risk of stroke or death, especially in older patients who have heart muscle dysfunction or severe arterial disease.

Good judgment on the part of your physician is essential in deciding to recommend the arteriography or any diagnostic test for coronary disease, for that matter. (See page 372 for questions to ask your doctor.) For example, chest pain in premenopausal women usually does not mean atherosclerosis and rarely requires cardiac catheterization. For postmenopausal women, however, coronary disease should be suspected in the face of a positive stress test more often than it is. Until more reliable noninvasive tests are developed, we have no choice but to rely on angiography. The potential benefits of identifying disease and stopping it in its tracks more than offset the test's slight risk and expense.

CORONARY DISEASE TREATMENT: CHOICE AND GOOD JUDGMENT

Not long ago the approach to treating coronary artery disease was what I called Darwinian: survival of the fittest. Now, thanks in large part to the intense funding of research prompted by the great American male heart attack scare of the fifties and sixties, we have three good treatment choices: medication, angioplasty, and surgery. Each approach works somewhat differently, but each accomplishes the same goal: increasing blood flow through the coronary arteries and thus protecting the heart muscle. Once your disease has been diagnosed, your treatment should not vary with your sex. (I'll discuss preventive measures more fully on page 360.)

Treatment Through Medication

In general, when disease is mild, medication is the appropriate first choice. "Mild" refers to the number of coronary arteries affected and the degree to which they are narrowed. Remember, mild disease does not always correspond to mild symptoms; furthermore, some people with very advanced coronary disease have few or no symptoms. So long as the medication relieves symptoms and permits a normal life, and the blockages are not severe, it is a reasonable choice. Some trial and error will be required to find the appropriate kind and amount of medication. (Medications are also frequently used along with more invasive treatment as needed.) However, take note: none of these medications eliminate the underlying disease. You must also make the lifestyle changes suggested beginning on page 360 in order to stop its progression to the extent possible.

Heart medications work on a variety of levels; some dilate, or enlarge, the narrowed coronary arteries so that sufficient blood can once again reach the heart; others slow or decrease the actual intensity of each contraction, thereby lowering the energy the heart expends, and thus the blood and oxygen it requires to handle its work of pumping the blood out into the vessels throughout the body. Some medications overlap in their functions.

The heart medications used most often are nitroglycerin, calcium channel blockers, beta-blockers, and anticoagulants—all discussed below. (Many of these are also useful in treating hypertension; see page 405.) Your doctor will decide which of these agents and in what combination are the best for you, but you should remain in close dialogue about them.

Nitroglycerin

Nitroglycerin has been around a long time. When some character in a B movie is about to collapse into the death throes of a heart attack and gasps "My pill, my pill!" nitroglycerin is the miracle medication popped into his mouth for an instant recovery (or perhaps not administered, allowing the villain to stand by and smirk). These scenes are both surprisingly accurate and fundamentally wrong. Nitroglycerin does work like magic in instantly relieving the excruciating pain of angina; it dilates the coronary arteries and at the same time decreases the workload on the heart. But although it may stop the pain and lessen the severity of a heart attack, it will not stop a heart attack from happening.

In reality, we don't have to wait for an attack of angina for nitroglycerin to work its wonders; you can now use nitroglycerin around the clock to prevent many, sometimes all, episodes of angina from occurring. Nitroglycerin, in the form of nitrates, can continuously reach your arteries and heart through sustained-release daily tablets, a transdermal patch, or even skin ointment. Otherwise, the effect of nitroglycerin is very short-lived; a pill under the tongue will have the strongest impact but lasts only a few minutes. Because of its effects on the arteries, it can also cause a pounding headache and sometimes dizziness. Isordil is a nitrate form of nitroglycerin that is far longer acting—each pill lasts about six hours—and can be taken by mouth.

Beta-Blockers

Beta-blockers act like a brake on the heart, slowing down the heart rate and the intensity of heart muscle contraction. They are used to combat angina and also may decrease the size of a heart attack as it occurs; for heart attack survivors, they can decrease the chance of dying from complications of heart disease or of having another heart attack. The beta-blockers are a class of drugs that work by interfering with the action of adrenaline, a chemical element that is a part of the sympathetic nervous system (see page 386)—thereby slowing the heart rate, decreasing the intensity of heart contractions, and lowering the blood pressure. The best known of the beta-blockers is propranolol (Inderal); others include Tenormin, Lopressor, and Blocadren. Beta-blockers can sometimes cause tiredness and fatigue or interference with sleep, wheezing in asthmatics, and vivid dreaming.

Calcium Channel Blockers

Calcium is the key element that stimulates contractions of muscles and is particularly important in maintaining blood vessel tone. When calcium is selectively blocked from reaching cells in a narrowed blood vessel through a medication called a calcium channel blocker, the vessel relaxes and dilates, growing wider. Calcium channel blockers were developed for use in heart disease in the early 1980s. Given their ability to relax all muscles, including the heart muscle, it was hoped that they would be useful in acute heart attacks, but this has not proven to be the case. They are powerful arterial dilators, though, and quite successful in combating angina and coronary artery spasms. These blockers include nifedipine (Procardia), verapamil (Isoptin), and diltiazem (Cardizem). They have few side effects, mostly minor, such as swelling of the ankles.

Anticoagulants, or Blood Thinners

The anticoagulants work at multiple levels to interfere with the process of blood clotting. This effect is often called blood thinning, although that is not a precise word because blood doesn't thin—it just becomes less apt to clot. Nonetheless, the term has taken hold. Anticoagulants have been shown to decrease the risk of heart attacks, protect against the development of coronary disease, protect vein grafts to the heart from plaque formation, and decrease the chances of having a second heart attack.

Aspirin is one of the oldest medicines known to woman. It is a powerful anti-inflammatory agent and analgesic and is still the best treatment for headaches. It is also, perhaps surprisingly, one of our most powerful cardiovascular drugs. Its mild but effective anticlotting properties are extraordinary and may be an effective preventive agent, protecting against the development of coronary disease. For a further discussion, see the section on heart disease prevention (page 360).

There are more powerful blood thinners, but they come with

greater risks of causing you to bruise easily or to bleed excessively from an injury. Coumadin (sodium warfarin) interferes with the liver's synthesis of certain blood-clotting proteins and thereby "thins" the blood. Because of its power, it is now used instead of aspirin to thin the clot-prone blood of patients who have mechanical heart valves. There is growing interest in the use of low-dose Coumadin for preventing coronary disease progression, but even in low doses, Coumadin must be carefully regulated by frequent blood tests.

Heparin is a third blood thinner, which works immediately when given through the veins. (It cannot be given orally.) Used primarily in coronary care units of hospitals as a follow-up to clot-dissolving drugs to prevent the dissolved clot from re-forming, this powerful agent is not a medication likely to be prescribed by your doctor for home use.

TREATMENT THROUGH INVASIVE PROCEDURES

The medications above can prevent or at the least reduce your episodes of angina, but they are only the front line of defense. When your pain persists or increases despite these medicines and a cardiac catheterization shows clearly dangerous narrowings, it is time for you and your doctor to consider a more invasive procedure, one that mechanically restores blood flow.

Most physicians will recommend angioplasty as your next alternative, unless the severity of the illness precludes it, and most people would prefer this nonsurgical procedure to facing an operating room. But both angioplasty and surgery hold special risks and benefits for a woman—in some cases similar risks with fewer rewards—so I urge you to consider your choices carefully.

Angioplasty: Dilating and Disrupting the Blockages

Angioplasty, also called "the balloon," is an oddly nonmedical-appearing procedure—and yes, it really employs a balloon. It's not surgery; instead it uses an approach similar to arteriography except that the catheters not only introduce dye into the arteries but also are specially designed to treat the arteries, too. Under local anesthesia, a catheter with a collapsed balloon at its tip is inserted into your leg and fed up into the coronary artery that is blocked. At the point of the blockage, the balloon is inflated to compress the plaque and widen the channel for blood flow.

Angioplasty is still an emerging technology and, as such, is not without its problems. Some of these problems are serious enough for you to consider forgoing the procedure entirely and instead opting for what may appear to be a scarier choice, open-heart surgery. It should be recognized that angioplasty carries a risk of stroke, heart attack, and death—a risk quite similar to surgery itself. The biggest problem with angioplasty, though, is that the narrowing returns within a few months fully 30 to 40 percent of the time. This return of the original disease, called *restenosis,* happens when blood clots and local tissue growth build up at the site of the balloon dilation; whether it occurs is somewhat related to the severity and type of blockage. Some of the most dangerous narrowings—of the left anterior descending coronary artery (the "widow maker" artery) or of all three arteries—engender the greatest risk of restenosis after angioplasty.

Research efforts are exploring means of preventing restenosis, including whether or not the application of high concentrations of medicines that block the deposits of blood products or the growth of cells at the same site of the angioplasty will keep the treated arteries open longer. We are awaiting the major breakthrough, but it is a procedure you must discuss in detail with your cardiologist.

Angioplasty can be repeated if a vessel develops restenosis. I feel strongly, however, that when restenosis occurs for a third time, it's time for the next step: surgery. Not everyone agrees with me. Some cardiologists will almost endlessly repeat angioplasty each time the blockage returns—sometimes seven or eight times. Remember, each repeat angioplasty carries the same risk of stroke, infarction, and death as the original procedure. Each also carries a large economic cost. (Once you start considering a third angioplasty, the total dollar cost begins to exceed the cost of a bypass operation.) Unfortunately, the ease and speed of the procedure can sometimes be deceptive to the woman who sees it as a way of avoiding the operating room and a longer convalescence.

In a small number of cases, the blood vessel at the site of the dilation closes up immediately after the angioplasty, because of either a blood clot or a tear in the artery. This complication can lead to a heart attack and usually requires emergency surgery. Therefore, if you are to undergo angioplasty, be sure to ask your cardiologist who will be on standby for surgery. Some hospitals doing angioplasty don't have backup surgical teams on-site, which I believe is totally unacceptable; in other cases, backup help is on call, but available only after a delay. You must ascertain not only the availability of a ready surgical team, but also who specifically would perform your surgery if necessary. Remember, women run a higher risk of complication from these procedures than do men, so for you these questions are doubly important.

I am optimistic that we will see major improvements in angioplasty in the future. There are a host of technologies in development, including miniature drills and atherectomy devices to cut out plaque, which enable angioplasty to reach more and more elusive narrowings. Another new technology now sometimes used along with angioplasty is a *stent*. Stents are like the spiral in a notebook; they are permanently inserted into an artery if it looks like it is about to close. Stents and new platelet-inhibiting drugs also offer promise for decreasing restenosis. (Even these newer approaches are consistently less favorable for women, perhaps because women have smaller coronary arteries or more coexisting disease.)

Coronary Artery Bypass Surgery

Sometimes the best choice to treat coronary artery disease is the most invasive treatment option, coronary artery bypass graft surgery. (It is often known by its initials, CABG, pronounced "cabbage.") Depending upon how advanced the disease is, where the blockages are located, how many exist, and how severe they are, surgery can offer the most protection from heart attack and the best outlook for vigorous, pain-free living. When I have a patient trying to choose between angioplasty and CABG surgery, I always consider surgery if disease is extensive or the narrowing is a risky one: a blockage high in the left anterior descending coronary artery, especially if tests find that one other artery is narrowed as well; a three-vessel narrowing; or a main trunk narrowing.

Coronary artery bypass surgery is time-tested, having been around for more than twenty-five years, another innovation for heart treatment developed at the Cleveland Clinic Foundation. CABG surgery involves the sewing of a new vein into the central artery, the aorta, and then "downstream," into the damaged artery below the point of narrowing, forming a new conduit that allows blood flow to "bypass" the obstruction. The new vein is generally taken from a patient's leg; if an artery is used, it is usually a mammary artery (technically known as the internal thoracic artery), taken from the inside wall of the chest. Mammary arteries are already connected at one end to the arterial circulation and only have to be sewn into the heart at one end; veins have to be sewn at both ends. Over the years, dramatic improvements in protecting the heart during surgery have made this a safe procedure with a mortality rate of less than 1 to 2 percent for all patients in most good centers. But women still face twice the chance of dying as do men. We don't know why women face higher risk for these cardiac procedures; some in the field suggest that there is some kind of mysterious "female factor." I doubt it. More likely the reasons are that women have smaller hearts and arteries (and are therefore simply more difficult to operate on) and that they are older and sicker than men by the time they have surgery.

Notwithstanding the sex differences, long-term surgical results are superb and getting better. For several years following such operations, more than 90 percent of patients get angina relief and improved quality of life. The chance of heart attack is decreased, and for many, life is lengthened. There is a marked difference, though, in the *long-term* outcome depending on whether a vein graft or an arterial graft is used.

The benefits of vein grafts are long-lasting—but not permanent. Atherosclerosis can attack vein grafts; after ten years close to half of vein grafts show narrowing, and about 10 percent of patients need a repeat operation, which carries a risk that is about double that of the first operation (and higher still, of course, for women). After fifteen years almost a third of the patients need a repeat procedure.

Arterial grafts last longer and for some reason are resistant to atherosclerosis. More than 95 percent of the time, arterial grafts are wide open and working well when studied after ten to fifteen years. The operation itself is more difficult than a vein graft, however; therefore the skill of the surgeon will be a key consideration for you.

Choose Your Doctor Well. In these invasive procedures there is no turning back; they simply have to be done right the first time. The success of your surgery is dependent on your surgeon's judgment, acquired experience, and technical ability, as well as the skill of the surgical team and surrounding hospital support systems. The more difficult and complex the procedure or the sicker you are, the more critical these factors become. A first-time CABG operation is vastly easier than a repeat procedure; angioplasty to dilate a single narrowing is simpler than one for disease involving many arteries. As a woman, with your inherently higher risk and smaller margin for error, the choice of the doctor who will be doing an invasive procedure is every bit as important to your health as the decision to have it. (See page 372 for questions to ask your doctor and surgeon.)

This point was vividly brought home to me by a seldom-mentioned study done more than a decade ago, involving more than ten major and rather famous academic medical centers from around the country. The study was intended to compare coronary artery bypass surgery with drugs alone in the treatment of fairly mild atherosclerosis, but what it revealed instead was the importance of plain old talent. When all the patients were analyzed together, there turned out to be little difference in outcome between patients who had treatment with drugs alone and patients who underwent surgery. But when surgical patients were compared center by center, the results were dramatically different: the best surgical teams had a mortality rate of less than 1 percent, the worst over 7 percent. Some complained the findings were due to the fact that some hospitals had tougher cases, so the groups were compared again, carefully adjusted for the difficulty of each operation. The result? The spread was even wider: the better centers did better and the poorer centers did worse. (Similar findings have been made with angioplasty and other catheter techniques.)

These studies only put into numbers, however, what every doctor knows and every patient suspects. The only answer to this problem is to have access to information, and to find for yourself a trusted medical mentor who can get this kind of information for you. But you first have to ask, to investigate, and to listen carefully.

PREVENTION: HOW TO TAKE CARE OF YOUR HEART FOR A LIFETIME

Because of the myth that women don't get heart disease, a whole generation of women didn't focus on heart disease prevention as part of their prescription for better health. For years the American Heart Association entreated women to look after their husbands and fathers and brothers and sons, with nary a word of warning for the women themselves.

This lack of focus is tragic because cardiovascular disease can be prevented and even existing coronary disease can be diminished when both men and women adopt a low-fat diet, exercise regularly, and stay away from cigarettes. Indeed, it was through cardiovascular research that we developed our strongest evidence that healthy living makes a difference.

Yes, the risk of heart disease for a woman in her childbearing years is minimal, but it is present. And the rewards of preventive planning are clear: when women and men assume the same healthy habits, the women's risk profile improves more. In addition, the natural course of heart disease in women is more gradual. These truths suggest that with healthy living, good medical care, and some actions based on the unique biology of being female, women can take powerful steps toward preventing death and disability from cardiovascular disease.

HORMONES

As we've seen, it is the lack of estrogen after menopause in particular that most exposes you to the perils of coronary artery disease. You do have an option: you can replace the missing estrogen through hormone replacement therapy and thereby significantly decrease your risks. (Recent studies have shown that adding the hormone progesterone to the estrogen sustains the positive effect of estrogen on both blood cholesterol levels and on the blood-clotting factor called *fibrinogen*, which, in high levels, is associated with vascular disease.)

Hormone replacement therapy is not as simple a choice as it may appear; many women past menopause have strong reasons for avoiding it. I take a close look at this confusing issue beginning on page 189. Nonetheless, based on what we know now, I suggest you give serious thought to taking hormone replacement therapy. Through this simple preventive option, you can mitigate one of your single largest risk factors for heart disease.

DIET AND CHOLESTEROL

A high-fat diet goes right to your coronary arteries. This we now know from comparing cultures around the world. Although our genes and our hormones can protect us to a degree, the importance of diet is reinforced time and time again by studying immigrants from parts of the world like China and Japan. When they adopt Western habits, they develop Western heart diseases. My recommendation, for every adult, is to keep the number of calories you consume as fat—especially fat you can see, like butter or fats in meats—down to 20 to 25 percent of your total calories. A balanced diet, rich in fruits, vegetables, and whole grains, can prolong your life (see page 57).

Cholesterol is clearly a more complicated issue for women. If you are generally healthy, I cannot say with certainty you will lower your risk of coronary disease if you lower your cholesterol intake. The stakes are different, however, for women at high risk of getting heart disease and who have LDL cholesterol levels substantially above 130 mg/dl (see page 343). Your doctor may advise reducing your total cholesterol if your LDL (bad) cholesterol is in the danger zone, through diet or even through medication. There are many choices of drugs, both new and old, that will reduce cholesterol by as much as 20 to 30 percent. A number of agents including gemfibrozil (Lopid), lovastatin (Mevacor), colestipol (Colestid), cholestyramine (Questran), and newer drugs such as simvistatin (Zocor), are effective. Simvistatin improves survival *in men* with coronary disease.

The decision to treat will depend on the specific level of your cholesterol, the form it is in (HDL:LDL), your age, and your overall medical history. But remember, for all women, it is the HDL that counts. If your ratio of total cholesterol to HDL is in the appropriate range (see page 344), just watch your fat intake, and you'll be protecting your heart.

A lean body weight is good preventive medicine for your heart. As we eat healthfully and exercise regularly (see page 363), these problems tend to disappear. Risk profiles—which are aggregate measures of low HDL cholesterol, high blood pressure, diabetes, smoking, and obesity—improve, and the likelihood of developing heart disease diminishes.

Almost daily we are learning about other nutritional factors that may lessen the high occurrence of heart disease in our population. For example, deficiencies in vitamin B_{12} and folate have been linked to an increase in the amino acid *homocysteine,* which at high levels injures the lining of blood vessels and stimulates growth of plaque. High levels of homocysteine in the blood (which can result from a genetic problem or a poor diet) have also been correlated with heart attacks and stroke. Increasing the levels of folate, vitamin B_{12}, and also vitamin B_6 lowers homocysteine rather easily by converting it into another nontoxic amino acid, methionine.

I am also convinced that certain vitamins known as the *antioxidants*—C, E, and beta-carotene (see page 45)—may decrease our chances of getting atherosclerosis. I can recommend all these supplements only in the context of a healthful diet; you can't gorge on fats and hope to compensate by popping a vitamin pill.

EXERCISE

When it comes to preventing coronary artery disease, diet cannot really be separated out from exercise. Being lean and active are both linked to a heart-disease-free life. They are both equally important means, easily available to you, of drastically lowering your risks. Make exercise a priority for you and your family. Regular aerobic exercise trains the heart, reduces blood pressure, reduces body fat, moderates the craving for nicotine, improves the cholesterol profile—particularly by elevating the good cholesterol (HDL) so essential to a woman's health—and improves the metabolism of carbohydrates, helping to control non-insulin-dependent diabetes. Regular exercise also alleviates stress, helps to prevent depression, and often brings a general sense of well-being. If that is not enough, it is good for bone health and has been shown in some studies to be associated with a decreased cancer risk. Finally, once you start exercising, you'll find you have more energy, not less. You'll be more likely to walk that extra block or take the stairs instead of the elevator, thereby getting even more exercise and more of the protections a well-exerted body affords.

If you are without symptoms of heart disease and, after checking with your doctor, learn you hold no major risk factors such as high blood pressure, you can safely embark on a moderate exercise regimen without any concern. It's never easy to fit exercise into a busy life or to stick to it; for you to succeed, it must be fun, become a pleasant habit, and be tailored to your own lifestyle. Whether you like to walk or jog, ride a stationary bicycle, jump rope, Rollerblade, do aerobic dancing, or some combination thereof, just sustain it for at least twenty minutes three times a week, and you've done enough. (Take five extra minutes on each end to stretch, warm up, and cool down.) Encourage your children to do likewise. The example we set as moms and the habits our children develop early will serve them well through the years.

ASPIRIN

As Americans, we have benefited from the many studies reported recently about the wondrous preventive properties of aspirin in regard to heart disease. The results have indeed been remarkable; sadly, these studies were conducted only on men. The major study of more than twenty-two thousand healthy male physicians, called the Physicians'

Health Study, determined that a low dose of one aspirin tablet per day, taken over a period of five years, decreased cardiovascular mortality—in men—by more than 40 percent. I can't tell you to extrapolate these results to yourself. While it's likely that your heart will benefit from an aspirin a day, it's possible that your head may not. As women get older, their risk for strokes caused by bleeding in the brain increases; chronic use of aspirin, with its "blood-thinning" properties, may exacerbate that risk. As a group, postmenopausal women stand to benefit most from aspirin's preventive magic but are also most at risk for this hemorrhagic type of stroke. Consult your doctor and stay tuned. (This issue is now being explored in a study of a large group of nurses, conducted by Dr. Charles Hennekens and others at Harvard. It is unlikely that we will see the results before the end of the decade.)

SMOKING

Smoking is a crucial risk factor; stopping smoking is a key prevention. STOP SMOKING! It is the *single biggest modifiable risk factor* for heart disease in both men and women—to say nothing of its other health benefits. You will save your own life and be a better role model for your children.

STRESS

While stress itself does not make a woman more likely to suffer coronary disease, certain reactions to stress, born in personality type, absolutely do. You can't change your innate temperament; if you're a type A, you're a type A—and you may be at greater risk.

But you can modify your behavior in anticipating and responding to stressful situations. You don't have to react according to your natural predisposition; although it isn't easy, you can attempt to respond to life in a way that makes your own life last longer.

Being sensitive to where you are emotionally vulnerable is a good first step. In particular, try to avoid those situations that will inevitably deteriorate into conflict and turmoil. Don't stop striving, but start striving with joy. Be exacting, but do it with a sense of humor, mostly laughing at yourself. Modulate impatience with kindness toward those around you, and be kind to yourself. When you feel angry or hostile, try to alleviate it through physical exercise, rather than exploding at an unchangeable situation. (For further discussion, see page 348.)

OTHER FORMS OF
CARDIOVASCULAR DISEASE

Coronary artery disease is the big worry, but there are other heart problems that can affect women—and, in some cases, more than men. They are important, even if less frequent types of heart ailments.

ARRHYTHMIAS

Arrhythmias, abnormal heart rhythms, can be a symptom of almost any kind of underlying heart disease, and they can also sometimes occur for no apparent reason or a very benign reason such as stress, caffeine, or alcohol. The consequences of rhythm abnormalities range from nil—an occasional extra heartbeat or a run of extra beats (called *palpitations*)—to serious and life-threatening.

When hearts beat too fast and in an irregularly irregular pattern (a condition called *atrial fibrillation*), the result, while not necessarily lethal, can be heart failure and blood clots. More serious yet is the pattern of the ventricle taking off on its own, unregulated by the normal heart pacemaker (see the following paragraph) or the beating of the atrial chambers, disturbances called *ventricular arrhythmias*. With *ventricular tachycardia* the ventricle is beating so fast that it doesn't have time to fill with blood and therefore has no blood to pump out. With *ventricular fibrillation* the heart not only beats too fast but also in a completely rhythmless pattern. (The heart muscle looks like a "bag of worms," the pattern is so chaotic.) If not corrected quickly, these rhythms are lethal.

The rhythm of the heart is normally moderated by the heart's own electrical system. Our hearts actually contain a natural pacemaker, which electronically stimulates the heart to beat, and a branching system of specially adapted nervelike fibers much like the electrical wiring in a house. Occasionally the system misfires; sometimes the cause is a heart attack or one of the heart diseases discussed beginning on page 367. Sometimes, as we get older, the conduction system just wears out, even though the rest of the heart is perfectly fine.

We now have sophisticated means available to us for both diagnosing and treating arrhythmias. ECGs can spot momentary abnormal rhythms, and another form of ECG test, called a *Holter Monitor,* can continuously measure the rhythm of your heart for a complete twenty-four-hour period as you go about your normal daily activities. A special form of cardiac catheterization, called an *electrophysiological study,* can accurately evaluate the electrical workings of the heart and identify certain abnormal sites within the heart that may be misfiring and triggering abnormal rhythms.

The treatment of arrhythmia depends on its type. To treat patients who have very slow heart rates and whose own internal pacemakers have ceased to function reliably, we can actually implant electrical circuitry that works almost as well as the original. These artificial pacemakers, developed in the 1950s by Earl Bakken and Dr. Walter Lillehei in Minnesota, have become a mainstay of treatment for arrhythmia. (I serve on the board of a company Mr. Bakken founded, Medtronic, which is now the world's largest maker of artificial pacemakers.)

When an artificial pacemaker is implanted into a patient, electrodes are fed into the heart (much like a cardiac catheterization) and attached to a small electrical box that is placed under the skin in the upper part of the chest; believe it or not, this is now an outpatient procedure. The mechanical pacemaker is run by a battery. It can both sense (detect the heart rate) and pace (electrically stimulate) the heart. Recent developments in sophisticated computer circuitry enable artificial pacemakers to sense body activity and speed up or slow down the heart rate in response—the same way our inborn pacemakers work.

When the problem involves very fast and/or irregular heart rhythms, the first line of defense is often medication. Numerous drugs can be employed on a trial-and-error basis to bring the heart back to its normal rhythm, including procainamide (Pronestyl), disopyramide phosphate (Norpace), amiodarone (Cordarone), and lidocaine (which is given only intravenously). These drugs unfortunately have many side effects, and sometimes can even make heart function and heart rhythms worse. None are prescribed to pregnant women. Other drugs—including digitalis, the beta-blockers, and the calcium channel blockers—also have milder antiarrhythmia effects.

When medicine fails to slow down a too-fast heart, we now have available to us a range of alternative therapies. Sometimes if there is just one small locus in the heart that seems to be triggering the very rapid heart rates, that locus can be eliminated by surgery or with a special heart catheter that identifies and then removes the irritable site. There is also a new type of pacemaker, developed only recently using technology based upon pacemakers, designed to correct very rapid heart rates including ventricular tachycardia and fibrillation. The very latest pacemakers not only sense heart rhythm but can also detect the potentially lethal beginnings of ventricular fibrillation or ventricular tachycardia—and in the next second can automatically deliver a life-saving electrical shock that sets the heart rhythm back to normal. This device is an *automatic inplantable cardioverter defibrillator* (AICD), used in patients who have a history of near-lethal arrhythmias that have not responded to medicines. Defibrillators have proven most effective in preventing sudden cardiac death.

The type of defibrillator with which you may be familiar is the external defibrillator, used by emergency medical personnel. This machine gives an electric shock to the heart through two electrode paddles placed on either side of the chest. It can literally bring a patient back to life when ventricular fibrillation has caused the heart to stop. These defibrillators are used in emergency rooms, operating rooms, most ambulances, and on hospital floors—wherever patients are at risk for cardiac arrest.

VALVULAR HEART DISEASE

As we learned in grammar school, the heart is a pump with four chambers—the left and right *ventricles,* and the left and right *atriums*—and four valves. The blood the heart pumps through the body has to move in one direction, and it's the valve system in the heart that keeps the blood from moving backwards.

The two valves on the left side of the heart, which is the side that receives oxygen-filled blood from the lungs, then pumps the blood into all parts of the body, are the *mitral valve* and the *aortic valve;* on the right side, which receives oxygen-depleted blood from the body and pumps it back into the lungs, are the *tricuspid valve* and the *pulmonary valve.* One of Mother Nature's most intriguing mysteries is that valve disease shows gender preferences. When a woman gets valve disease, it is most likely to involve the mitral valve; a man will more likely get aortic valve disease.

The mitral valve is located between the left atrium and the left ventricle (it is this left ventricular muscle that we worry most about being damaged in a heart attack). The two diseases of the heart valves especially troublesome to women involve the mitral valve. One, rheumatic heart disease, is old and vanishing; the other is newly discovered and the most common valve problem of women today—prolapsing mitral valve.

RHEUMATIC HEART DISEASE

In rheumatic heart disease, which affects women more than men, the valves of the heart become inflamed and swollen; over time they become either leaky or so thickened, scarred, severely disfigured, and narrowed (*stenotic*) that they cannot function properly. When women get rheumatic heart disease, it's the valves on the left side of the heart, particularly the mitral valve, which are most often and most severely affected. *Rheumatic mitral stenosis* can be a deadly disease, leading to severe heart failure, abnormal heart rhythms, and, sometimes, stroke.

The problem is caused by repeated episodes, mostly in childhood, of rheumatic fever evolving from certain types of strep throat, and, I'm glad to say, has virtually disappeared in this country and in most developed countries. The success has come through a magnificent partnership of science, good medical practice, public health studies, and the efforts of mothers. The breakthrough was penicillin, the magic bullet developed during World War II, which cures strep throat and prevents the lingering infection from setting up an assault on the heart as an aftermath. The banishment of rheumatic heart disease in our country is due primarily to the mothers who learned to fear strep throat and bring their children in quickly for treatment.

Rheumatic heart disease is still present in many parts of the world, including parts of South America, the Middle East, and Africa, and from time to time it shows up in developed countries as well. In the late 1980s we saw a resurgence of rheumatic fever among higher socioeconomic groups and involving some young college-age adults; we are not sure why. We must stay vigilant. When I was growing up, my next door neighbor died in the last month of her first pregnancy due to severe heart failure from rheumatic mitral stenosis. Our whole block mourned her and her unborn baby; we were told nothing could have been done. When I was in medical school and even in my early cardiology training, young women in their twenties and thirties who otherwise seemed fine were suddenly stricken with severe heart failure. How far we have come since then. Today we would have repaired or replaced the defective valve (see page 369); even better, today these women would likely not have gotten sick with childhood rheumatic fever in the first place.

MITRAL VALVE PROLAPSE

Just as we thought we were getting rid of mitral valve disease, we began to see more and more patients with a condition called *mitral valve prolapse*—a condition that can be quite painful but fortunately is almost never dangerous. Prolapse, which sometimes runs in families, occurs when the mitral valve billows backwards as it closes (almost like a parachute), often causing a snapping or clicking sound and a short heart murmur; these can be detected by listening with a stethoscope. Rather than being too tight, as in rheumatic heart disease, a prolapsing valve may become leaky, so that blood flows backwards into the left atrium, and, if the prolapse is severe enough, back into the lungs. In less than 1 percent of all cases, this condition can be life-threatening because the valve develops a major leak that strains the heart or becomes infected or torn, or because dangerous disturbances in the heart rhythm occur.

Mitral valve prolapse is about twice as common in women, especially young, slender women, as it is in men; its symptoms often mimic the angina caused by a coronary artery disease. Prolapse can be a miserable condition, or it can be "silent" and pain free. Curiously, the signs of prolapse come and go, often spontaneously resolving with time. During pregnancy, for example, prolapse may entirely disappear.

DIAGNOSIS AND TREATMENT OF VALVE DISEASE

It was not until the last half of the twentieth century that we developed the capability to understand, detect, and treat valvular heart disease. Valve disease is a mechanical problem within the body's blood pumping system, and figuring out the problem is a bit like analyzing any other mechanical malfunction. Now, though, we have both invasive and reliable noninvasive technologies available to look under the hood, so to speak, and figure out what is misfiring.

One of the biggest breakthroughs in the diagnosis of valvular heart disease was the development of *echocardiography*—the use of ultrasound to detect blood flows and show images of the motion of the heart and its valves on a monitor (not to be confused with *electrocardiography*—ECG—described on page 351). Thanks to echocardiography, by placing a pencil-sized probe on the surface of the chest, we can watch the chambers of the heart pumping, its valves opening and closing, and blood moving through them. With "echo," we can diagnose valve disease, congenital defects, and heart failure. With a specially adapted ultrasound technique called echo Doppler, we can get precise measures of leaks and pressures, virtually as good as those that can be obtained by placing catheters in the heart.

If, for some reason, the echo is not conclusive enough, we can use the technique of cardiac catheterization (discussed on page 352) to measure how badly a heart valve is working; with that technique we can also figure out whether the pressure buildup or the leaks are great enough to cause permanent damage to the heart muscle itself or to places where the blood can back up, as in the lungs, and cause pulmonary congestion (also called *congestive heart failure*).

Heart Valve Replacement or Repair

It is one thing to diagnose a problem; it is quite another to be able to fix it. Traditionally, correcting heart valve problems has meant replacement, not repair. Over the past forty years, surgeons have replaced faulty valves with artificial ones made out of every material from metals, carbon, silicone, and fabric to natural tissues like pig valves or even transplanted human valves. Nontissue valves last a long time, but require chronic and fairly strong blood-thinning medication due to the risk of clot formation on their synthetic surfaces. Tissue valves are not as sturdy and need to be replaced after about ten years, but they do not require the heavy-duty and at times dangerous blood-thinning medications.

More recently, a surgical technique has emerged in which a torn or overstretched and leaky valve can be repaired, not replaced, using the patient's own valve tissue. Successful repair means no anticoagulation drugs and a likely long-term fix.

The decision whether to repair or to replace your problematic valve, as well as which type of valve to use if you opt for replacement, is one you must discuss at length with your doctor. Your age and future plans may be important considerations. For example, if you plan to have children, you and your doctor might well prefer a tissue valve to eliminate the complications that blood-thinning and anticoagulant drugs pose to a pregnancy, despite the fact that the tissue valve will probably have to be replaced in the future. Make sure in any case to ask your cardiologist about the newer option of repair before undergoing any type of heart valve replacement. Note carefully, though: only some heart surgeons and certain heart centers are experienced and skilled in performing heart valve repairs. As with any coronary surgery, choose your surgeon well (see page 359); these operations must be performed correctly the first time, for there isn't often an opportunity to try again. Any good cardiologist should provide you with the information to choose a center that is competent to do this surgery.

CARDIOMYOPATHY: HEART MUSCLE DISEASE

Sometimes the heart muscle itself becomes damaged or diseased and starts to fail; when this very rare problem, called a *cardiomyopathy,* occurs, the outlook is usually dreary. Cardiomyopathies, generally considered to be caused by a virus, attack men and women equally. However, there is a distinctive form of heart muscle disease, unique to women, called *peripartum cardiomyopathy.* Shortly after delivery of a baby, mostly after multiple or high-risk pregnancies, heart muscle failure ensues. Often the heart returns to normal size and function within a few months, but if the condition persists much beyond six months after delivery, the outlook is poor.

People with heart muscle disease of any type are short of breath on exertion; they have low energy and sometimes swollen ankles and irregular heartbeat. The disease tends to be progressive, often developing in the childbearing years, and women who have a preexisting cardiomyopathy are generally advised not to become pregnant.

Medical treatment for heart muscle disease mainly helps alleviate the symptoms of shortness of breath and swelling of the ankles. The mainstay of cardiomyopathy medications are still the old-timers— digitalis and diuretics. Digitalis (in the past called *foxglove,* after the plant that manufactures it naturally) has been a heart muscle disease treatment for hundreds of years and is used to this day as a means of perking up a sluggish heart. Diuretics help to clear the lungs and other tissues of the body of the fluid that builds up because the heart muscle cannot pump properly. Sometimes, especially when there is a risk of a blood clot dislodging and moving to the brain, blood thinners are used as well.

The horizon looks brighter than the past for the treatment of cardiomyopathy. There are newer medications available; one of these, called captopril, has been shown not only to relieve symptoms and improve heart function but also to add years to life expectancy. (Captopril works by dilating arteries, helping to make the heart a more efficient pump.) Finally, for people who are deathly ill with no other choice, transplantation is a consideration. But this remains a drastic therapy that is severely restricted by the relatively few healthy hearts available from deceased donors.

QUESTIONS FOR YOUR DOCTOR

Whatever your health issue, your choice of physician is crucial, but as you've surely noted throughout this chapter, I can imagine few instances of medical intervention where *your* thorough research can have a greater impact on the outcome and your health. When it comes to coronary surgery or angioplasty, it is your life that rests in the hands of one trained professional: do your best to get the best. Here are questions for both doctor and surgeon that should help you become the informed patient you must be.

- What is your risk for coronary heart disease? Is your HDL:LDL ratio acceptable? What is it? How is your blood pressure? Can your doctor give you some advice about your diet? Any cookbooks to recommend? What about your weight and level of exercise?
- If you have chest pains, what is your doctor's overall plan for your evaluation? If the pain reoccurs, should you go to an emergency room? Which one?
- Ask your doctor to go over the details of your stress test with you. Were there changes in the ECG? Can you be confident that you do not have coronary artery narrowings? Ask her to explain why she might believe a more intensive stress test will be more conclusive. Should you have a cardiac catheterization instead?
- What can you expect from the medication she has prescribed? What are the contraindications? Why has she chosen these particular medications? (Make a list of your medications, and keep it with you at all times.)
- Where should you go for emergency care if you develop symptoms of a heart attack? Which is the best hospital in the area? Does it have backup support, including a catheterization laboratory and cardiac surgery? What is the quality of its surgery?

- If your doctor advises angioplasty or surgery, ask him to tell you what hospital he would recommend if you were his spouse, mother, or sister. Also, what doctor would he recommend?
- What is the experience of the hospital and the surgeon who will be doing the procedure? Specifically? How many cases has he or she done? How complex were the cases? What have the outcomes been? What is the hospital's overall record on similar cases? (If your doctor advises angioplasty, surgery, or pacemaker implantation, be sure to seek out a second opinion.)
- Ask whether there will be a backup cardiac surgery team on call and ready in the hospital during your angioplasty.
- Discuss what kinds of grafts your doctor recommends for coronary artery bypass surgery: veins or arteries? Why?
- What are your options in your valve replacement? Has he considered repairing the valve? What are his reasons for his recommendations? What centers perform valve repair?
- Ask your doctor to discuss this major procedure (catheterization, angioplasty, heart surgery) with responsible members of your family. (They must understand what is about to happen and why, what to expect, how long the recuperation, and what kind of support you will need.)
- Don't forget to ask your doctor about the *latest research:* Can we learn to do cardiac surgery through a fiberoptic scope without opening the chest? To repair valves, bypass coronary arteries, remove clots from the heart? How can we prevent atherosclerosis from returning after angioplasty? How can we prevent vein grafts from becoming obstructed? Can we learn to regrow damaged heart muscle tissue or selectively transplant heart tissue only where there is damage? Can we develop mechanical hearts that work?
- What does your doctor know about the Women's Health Initiative and its research on hormones and heart disease, or about PEPI (see page 192)? Other studies are slated to examine the risks and benefits of hormone replacement therapy in women who have had heart attacks or have known heart disease; how does she think these studies impact HRT use? Will she start hormone replacement therapy or stop it in a woman who has had a heart attack?

WHAT WOMEN CAN DO
PERSONALLY AND POLITICALLY

It is critically important that we keep political and personal pressure on the system to sustain the research efforts that have made the cardiovascular field one of hope and optimism. Work with your local American Heart Association, contact your congressman and write to your local newspapers (op-ed pages and letters to the editor), and maybe even call a talk radio show to discuss the importance of what has happened in research and technology development regarding this disease that is the biggest killer of women, and men. The dramatic payoff of research for patients with heart disease should be a model for other fields. And, each time you speak out, be sure you emphasize the need for *women's* heart research; there is a large knowledge gap yet to close.

Since cardiovascular disease has been so prominent and the advances so breathtaking, it has been a major focus in the health care debate that has deeply touched this country. You should keep in mind two things: progress that's costly and patient access.

Our great progress in this field has been dogged by increasing costs. Every patient should become personally involved in the benefits and costs of his or her care. Ask your doctor and hospital about costs and ask for comparisons from other institutions and other medical centers. Sometimes the best doctors are far from the most expensive; the best hospitals may not charge the highest fees.

Many countries in the world have targeted cardiovascular care for rationing, either through long lines or by age. I have seen one country, Finland, in which both occur. After your sixty-fifth birthday, you are generally ineligible. Good-bye, Mrs. Martucci; good-bye, most women victims of heart disease. How can we possibly make blanket decisions to treat or not to treat—or not to treat aggressively—based upon such inexact measures as chronological age? And since women get their heart disease some ten to twenty years later than men, they do very badly on age rationing; it becomes de facto sex rationing.

Of course we must address costs in our current medical system, but not in a sterile vacuum. Tests are overused, technology is overprescribed, and prevention needs more focus. We need scrutiny of practice patterns and guidelines—not regulations—to help both doctor and patient make decisions. Guidelines cannot be inscribed in government or insurance company rule books; rather, they must be flexible and evolving. We must hold doctors and hospitals accountable, but not in a capricious and unjust way. Inefficiencies and redundancies must be weeded out, and cost-effectiveness must become part of our vocabulary. Incentives must be there for all of us to consume wisely these precious resources. All the while, however, we cannot lose sight of the individual patient at the center of medicine.

By all means, keep informed of any changes that the government will be making to our health care system, whether at the state or federal level.

The cardiovascular field represents what is great about American medicine—its innovation. I went into cardiology in the 1970s because in this field a doctor could really *do* something to help a patient. Whereas in the fifties, cardiology meant watching, caretaking, and explaining (typical of most medical treatment at that time), by the time I made my choice of specialty the field had become dynamic and powerful. Through constantly expanding frontiers, including the development of technologies we now take for granted—such as coronary care units, defibrillation, echocardiography, cardiac catheterization, bioengineered drugs, valve surgery, heart transplants, and more—we can effect real change in people's lives.

NINE

STROKE
The Endless Day

It requires more courage to suffer than to die.

—*NAPOLÉON BONAPARTE*
AT ST. HELENA, 1816

My Aunt Sarah grew up in Hoboken, New Jersey, then a working-class town whose residents repaired ships, transported goods, and made machinery, clothing, and pencils. After ninth grade, Sarah started doing clerical work in a trucking company office, where she met her husband to be, Bob, who was a helper on a truck. Aunt Sarah and Uncle Bob went on to live a life that was common in that place at that time. Bob liked to hang out with the guys, while Sarah stayed home and took care of the four kids. They were very religious, ate poorly (except on Friday, when fish was the staple), had the usual family arguments, rarely concerned themselves with their health, and constantly worried about making a better life for their family. Each morning, they looked across the Hudson River to see the sun rise over the towers of Manhattan.

If someone called Sarah a tough Irish matriarch, I suspect she would have considered it a compliment. She took pride in her role; toughness and a certain starch meant survival in a harsh world. But a staunch character couldn't protect her from the devastating stroke that paralyzed her entire left side when she was sixty-two. She would never walk again; for a long time she could barely speak. She was a survivor, though, physically helpless but mentally strong as steel. Her indomitable spirit and incredibly sharp mind never deserted her. She finally died in her eighties of the same illness that had so disabled her, yet another stroke.

Far from Hoboken, in the middle of the Pacific Ocean, is an island called Kitava. Its twenty-two hundred inhabitants work hard as well, fishing and tending their fields; like my Aunt Sarah and her brood did, they live in close-knit family units. They, too, celebrate religious holidays, laugh with their children, endure family arguments, but—as described by Dr. S. Lindeberg and colleagues in a 1994 issue of the *Journal of Internal Medicine*—they never suffer strokes.

The people of Kitava live in tranquility: no electricity, telephones, fax machines, or cars. Their diet consists mostly of boiled yams supplemented by tropical fruits, nuts, beans, and fish. Each morning they see the sun rise over the Solomon Sea.

My Aunt Sarah and the women of Kitava were much the same physiologically. The drastic differences in their health were engendered by the mid-twentieth-century culture in which Sarah was stuck, dead center: poor diet, difficult lifestyle, stress, and a general ignorance of health basics. Much of this can be easily altered. With the help of medical advances not available to Sarah and with our new knowledge of the things we can do to lessen our susceptibility to strokes, we can adopt for ourselves the serenity and health of Kitavan women.

HOPE FOR THE DISEASE WITHOUT HOPE

Stroke is without a doubt one of our most frightening and disturbing illnesses. Unlike Alzheimer's, where the victim cannot remember another way of being, a stroke sufferer bears keen witness to the alteration in her brain that has left her so diminished. Stroke lags behind heart disease as the third leading killer of both men and women in the United States, but ask any group of elderly women which they fear most—heart attack or stroke—and the majority will invariably respond stroke. A heart attack is a decisive event with a decisive outcome; you either die or recover. A stroke is a decisive event with an ambiguous outcome. You either die or you can linger for years with a disability that steals your autonomy and may well be your ticket to long-term nursing home care and extensive rehabilitation therapy.

Perhaps it is this unpredictability that made stroke a frustrating area for researchers and scientists over the years. Whatever the reason, stroke is one disease where you won't find me pontificating on the male-female inequities in diagnosis, credence given women, or treatment; instead, the big problem historically with the illness lay in its nontreatment. Men and women suffer strokes in close to equal numbers (young women and old women have slightly more strokes than men; middle-aged men have more strokes than middle-aged women); medical research has ignored both equally. For centuries, stroke (called *apoplexy* in the past) was viewed as the disease that is easily diagnosed but impossible to prevent, intercede in, or cure.

We are now in a far different place from twenty years ago. No one suddenly decided this illness was worth examining, but thanks to advances in other related fields, inadvertent discoveries about stroke forced the medical community to recognize hope in what had so long been dismissed as hopeless. Through our massive efforts in preventing heart attacks, we learned about the dangers of high blood pressure, high-fat diets, and stress; for reasons having nothing to do with stroke, radiologists invented diagnostic devices through which to look inside the body, devices that, wholly accidentally, have ended up being critical in the detection and early treatment of stroke. Our treatment breakthroughs in cardiovascular disease led to new medications and complex catheterization and surgical techniques that are now invaluable in the treatment of stroke. The result: a few short decades after Sarah's stroke, the incidence of this illness has been cut by almost 60 percent.

These advances have come just in time. Baby boomers are moving in large waves into the decades when they are susceptible to stroke and heart attacks; thanks to medical science, a large percentage of this cohort is expected to survive into their ninth and tenth decades. The risk of stroke has been brought down to 6 percent for men and 3 percent for women in their fifties; but for those in their eighties the chance of stroke rises to more than one in five for both women and men.

It's therefore time for another, crucial shift in our study of stroke. Stroke hits the elderly much harder than the young, and it's there that we must concentrate our research efforts. While researchers predict a continuing decrease in the overall number of strokes, they also predict an increase in *major* strokes, that is, those strokes that leave their elderly victims permanently handicapped or dead. Stroke takes a vast economic toll as well: calculating medical and nursing care, rehabilitation, and lost income, a Duke University study estimated that the annual cost of stroke to our country was thirty billion dollars a year, with more than 95 percent of the medical cost being hospital and nursing home care. The National Heart, Lung and Blood Institute has estimated that the lifetime cost for a first stroke is between forty-five thousand dollars and ninety thousand dollars, and far more than that for those over age sixty-five.

As you read through this chapter, I hope you'll think, as I do, of Kitava. We now have very exciting surgical and medical treatments available to us with which to fight stroke; but the bulk of the battle remains in your hands. You can, through your attentiveness to your own health—including your diet, stress, blood pressure, and exercise—do much to prevent this once hopeless disease from robbing you of your sunrises while you're young; and, in cooperation with your physician, you can stop it from destroying the quality of your life as you age.

WHAT IS A STROKE?

A stroke happens when a part of your brain is temporarily or permanently deprived of the constant supply of blood it needs to function and sustain itself. Blood flow to part of the brain is blocked: for this reason the technical term for stroke is *cerebro* (brain) *vascular* (blood vessels) *accident,* or CVA. A more recently used term is *brain attack.* The extent of the damage a stroke can do is dependent on many factors, including the type of stroke you experience, but a key factor is which specific part of your brain doesn't get its blood flow. This in turn often depends on which blood vessel is damaged; different blood vessels feed different parts of your brain.

STROKE AND THE BLOOD VESSELS

Blood gets to our brains from our hearts through two major systems of arteries: the carotid and the vertebral. You can feel your carotid arteries pulsing in your neck. Most often involved in the common forms of stroke, they branch out at the level of your jaw and carry blood to most of your head and to the higher parts of your brain. The vertebral arteries, as you may have guessed, come up the back of the neck alongside the spine, supplying the back part of our brain and the cranial nerves off the base of the brain with blood.

The carotid and the vertebral systems communicate with each

other through an elaborate connective network of smaller blood vessels encircling the brain, called the *circle of Willis*. Through this connection, your brain can still receive blood flow top and bottom even if one of the arteries becomes obstructed; if, for instance, a vessel in the carotid artery system is blocked extra blood may come in through the vertebral arterial system. It's sort of nature's back-door connection—an elaborate food and oxygen supply protection for this lofty organ, the brain.

STROKE AND THE BRAIN

The brain is a three-pound wonder, the control center of our minds and bodies. It's also a high-maintenance organ—ounce for ounce, the biggest continuous consumer of our body's blood supply. It averages less than 3 percent of our total body weight but demands about 20 percent of the blood pumping out of our hearts with each and every beat.

Our brains are made up of millions of nerve cells (neurons), the vital but fragile units through which the brain functions. When a nerve cell dies, it cannot grow back. It takes only about fifteen minutes or so at normal body temperature for a nerve cell, starved for blood by a stroke in the brain, to die (longer if a trickle of blood manages to get through). As nerve cells die, they release a flood of neurotransmitters and other chemicals that can overwhelm perfectly healthy nerve cells nearby and lead to their death—even if they themselves have a good blood supply. It is a sort of neurological avalanche.

The impact of this neuron destruction varies with the region of the brain that becomes oxygen starved or damaged. The carotid arteries supply blood specifically to the cerebrum, two oval-shaped lobes at the top of the brain. The cerebrum is the seat of your intelligence, your consciousness and thought, voluntary movements of your arms and legs, your facial expressions, and the fine movements of your hands as you write, play the violin, or perform delicate neurosurgery. These cerebral lobes of about one pound each are the part of our body that most differentiates us from each other and from lower animals. Different geographic locales within the cerebrum control very specific functions. For example, the frontal lobe, or front part of the cerebrum—just beneath the forehead—is the seat of your personality, your ability to be creative, to think complex and abstract thoughts, to worry. Our higher brain functions are there, fighting it out with the impulses and emotions popping up from time to time from deep within a part of the midbrain called the *limbic system*, which is also fed blood mostly by the carotid artery system. Farther back in the cerebrum is the area that controls movement, and beyond that—the occipital part of the cerebrum lobes—is the complex part of our brains that processes vision.

Sitting beneath and behind the cerebral lobes is the cerebellum, a part of the brain that controls our ability to stand erect, to be coordinated, and keep our motor balance. This part of the brain is supplied with blood by the vertebral arteries.

Both the cerebrum and the cerebellum are attached to a bulbous stalk, which contains the midbrain and the lower brain, both leading off into the spinal cord. The lower brain and the brain stem, also fed primarily by the vertebral arteries, control the automatic bodily functions like breathing, heart rate, and blood pressure as well as touch, temperature sensation, and pain perception.

A doctor typically diagnoses a stroke backwards, deducing which blood vessel is in trouble and which part of the brain is at risk by assessing the physical or mental problems the stroke has caused. For example, paralysis of an arm and/or leg (*hemiplegia*) or difficulty speaking, writing, reading, or understanding (*aphasia*) means a cerebral injury involving a block of the carotid artery and damage to the cerebrum. If the vertebral artery is blocked or bleeding, damaging the cerebellum, you might experience dizziness, problems with balance and coordination (*ataxia*), slurred speech (*dysarthria*), disordered fine hand movements, and tremor, without any specific paralysis.

The fact that our brains mirror the symmetry of our bodies adds to the ease of pinpointing the exact locale of a stroke. When one side of the brain is damaged, the opposite side of your body is affected. That means, for example, if a stroke hits the part of the left side of the brain that controls arm and leg motion, it causes paralysis on the opposite (contralateral), or right, side of the body. This is called a right hemiplegia.

In addition, for each of us, one side of the brain dominates, controlling key functions such as the understanding and formulation of language. The left side of the brain is dominant in most right-handers; therefore, a stroke that damages the left side of the brain will commonly be more damaging, with respect to communication, for instance, than a stroke on the right side.

TYPES OF STROKE

All strokes are not the same. They come in different intensities, strike different places in the brain, and have different underlying causes. Knowing a bit more about what a stroke is and how it is caused can help to make sense of the new and better therapies that are coming along—both to prevent and to treat.

Sometimes a stroke is not a stroke at all. We speak of strokes as being "completed"; that is, strokes that leave some sort of permanent damage. There is one type of episode whose symptoms mimic those of a stroke but is actually more of a "threatened stroke," a warning sign that a full-blown stroke is on the way. We call this a transient ischemic attack.

TRANSIENT ISCHEMIC ATTACK: A THREATENING STROKE

Transient ischemic attacks (TIAs) are very ominous and frightening experiences, but thank goodness for them. When you suffer a TIA, your body is sounding an alarm that worse may be ahead. Just as angina warns of an impending heart attack, TIAs are telling you that you have a significant chance of experiencing a full-blown stroke within a month and an even greater chance of enduring more TIAs over the years and then eventually suffering a stroke.

Ischemia means blood flow deprivation bad enough to limit oxygen to a part of the body; with a TIA the flow of blood to the brain is blocked or reduced to the point where brain cells undergo the first paroxysms of starvation—but only momentarily. The symptoms of a TIA are distinctive and dramatic, such as a sudden and nearly complete paralysis of the muscles in one side of the face or one side of the body. You may go numb or experience tingling or odd sensations on one side; one eye may go blind (*amaurosis fugax*), or the world may grow darker as if the sun were eclipsed. Your speech slurs and you may become dizzy. TIAs have dozens of ways of announcing themselves, depending on which region of the brain is being deprived of blood. Worst of all, you never know if you're experiencing a TIA, which by definition lasts less than twenty-four hours (and generally disappears in one or two), or the real thing—which lasts a lifetime—until it is over and you have recovered the lost functions that defined the attack.

THROMBOTIC STROKE

Thrombotic strokes, the most common form of stroke, develop over years but happen in minutes, often seconds. The cause of this true, completed stroke is much the same as that of a heart attack born from severe atherosclerosis. This time the atherosclerosis, or fatty plaque, builds up in an artery traveling to the brain rather than to the heart. Much as it occurs in a heart attack, the plaque-lined, diseased blood vessel becomes abruptly blocked by a blood clot. More than half of these thrombotic strokes come with a prior TIA warning, but a good 40 percent of them give no advance notice whatsoever.

A far less common type of thrombotic stroke caused by atherosclerosis that we are just now beginning to recognize, is the elusive *mini-stroke*—or stroke without symptoms—which happens when tiny blood vessels in the brain become blocked off. These strokes are evident only after they have occurred, and their damage isn't clear until enough of them have occurred to create many scattergun scars throughout the brain. They cause otherwise mysterious symptoms such as language difficulty, mood disturbances including depression, abnormalities of posture and gait, and loss of reflexes; after Alzheimer's disease, they are the second most frequent cause of dementia in the elderly. When ministrokes are detected early, treatment is low doses of aspirin to thin the blood and cut down on the risk of clots.

EMBOLIC STROKES

The second most common type of completed stroke, causing about 15 to 20 percent of strokes, is known as *embolic*. An embolus is a particle—it might be an air bubble, a piece of fat, or a fragment of clot—floating in the blood that should not be there. It follows the flow of blood through increasingly smaller arteries until it gets stuck. The outcome varies with the vessel blocked; if the vessel is in the brain, the impact can be sudden and deadly, like a bullet. Instantaneous and complete weakness may strike one side of your body, speech may be disrupted; in severe cases you may be completely paralyzed or lapse into a deep coma.

In nearly a third of embolic strokes, pressure behind the blockage builds up, causing artery walls to burst and flood the affected region of the brain with blood, damaging it even further. The most common origin of these biological bombs is a diseased heart. Otherwise healthy people can also be afflicted, but only on extremely rare occasions.

HEMORRHAGIC STROKES

The least common of the completed strokes can also be the worst: a spontaneous hemorrhage into the head, caused by either the rupture of small arteries deep within the brain or by the rupture of an *aneurysm*, a saclike dilation caused by weakness of a portion of an artery wall. These strokes occur without warning, usually causing the most damage, and carry the greatest risk of death.

When the hemorrhage is caused by the rupture of small blood vessels, it is most often related to long-standing high blood pressure and usually occurs in people over fifty. A person suffering a stroke caused by this hypertensive hemorrhage will complain of a sudden and severe headache or perhaps a feeling of something odd going on inside her head. Many will lose consciousness, even if only briefly. Typically within minutes, one side of her face may sag, her speech will become slurred, an arm or leg or both may weaken, or she may have a convulsion. The buildup of blood in the brain increases pressure inside the skull; that generalized increased pressure can by itself cause damage or loss of function and lead to mental confusion or loss of consciousness.

Rarer and more dramatic than hypertensive hemorrhage is the rupture of aneurysms in the brain. Aneurysms are unpredictable, bringing death to more than half of their victims; they can occur at any age, although they are most likely to show up during and after midlife, and are more common in women than men. Aneurysms are of two types—those you are born with and those, like hypertensive hemorrhages, that develop over the years from wear and tear.

A related blood vessel abnormality associated with hemorrhagic strokes in young people are *arterial-venous malformations,* in which the vascular tree is not properly developed.

RISK FACTORS

You'll find many of the risk factors for stroke are the same as for heart disease, but a factor that may be small in the one disease can turn out to be quite significant in the other. By far, the largest risk factor for stroke is a disease in itself: high blood pressure (or hypertension). Hypertension, in turn, carries with it its own cast of risks; too little exercise, for example, can increase your susceptibility to high blood pressure, which in turn heightens your risk for stroke.

HIGH BLOOD PRESSURE

Although we are all born with normal blood pressure, we Americans are expert at putting our lives in danger by building up the force of hypertension. It is extraordinarily common in this country: some fifty million of us, or about one-third of our adult population, are affected. Men have more hypertension than women through middle age, then women take the lead. We don't know why, but hormones or the lack thereof may play a role.

High blood pressure dwarfs all other risk factors for stroke. This killer is devious, generally keeping itself unknown while it goes about its work of silently but relentlessly wearing out the large and small arteries of your body. You may experience some unclear symptoms such as headaches or nosebleed, but more often there is no external evidence of the havoc being wrought just under your skin. Your blood vessels are degenerating, your heart muscle is thickening, your kidneys are scarring and shrinking, the retina of your eyes may become damaged, and, most critically, your brain's blood vessels may leak, burst, or clot.

Hypertension can range from mild to severe, but even a sustained mild elevation in pressure can bring with it an increase in your chance of a stroke. A sustained blood pressure rise of about 20 percent over normal increases your risk of a stroke by three times. If you have longstanding, untreated high blood pressure, your chance of a stroke is about seven times greater than that of a woman without hypertension.

As we will see, high blood pressure can be treated quite successfully. Familiarity with the body's blood pressure regulating system will help you to understand your treatment options. Every organ in your body needs a regular supply of oxygen brought to it by the blood in order to function. To reach all the organs, the heart has to pump out blood with a certain optimal amount of force. Although the force needed varies with your level of activity, over the centuries we've determined a fairly consistent desirable range for that force; with a force too great, your blood vessels can be damaged by the impact; with a force too light, all the organs won't be reached.

Blood pressure is generally overseen by the part of your brain that runs the automatic body functions (like digestion and heart rate), called the *autonomic nervous system*. This system in turn includes a sort of yin-yang response network: the *sympathetic* nervous system, when stimulated (as in times of danger or stress or pain), increases your blood pressure and heart rate; this system is opposed by the *parasympathetic* nervous system, which lowers blood pressure, slows the heart rate, and can even cause a faint. (The swoon that comes with sudden shocking news is evidence of the parasympathetic system becoming overstimulated.) Both systems rely on neurotransmitters to operate: norepinephrine in the sympathetic and acetylcholine in the parasympathetic (see page 285).

Over the years we have discovered that the specific regulation of blood pressure is an elaborate interplay between the nervous system, the heart, the kidneys, the blood vessels, and a small molecule called *angiotensin,* which circulates in the blood and carries messages to each organ. Angiotensin is a hormone produced in inactive form by the liver and regulated by the kidney. Blood pressure is actually measured by the kidneys, which, like a thermostat, activate the angiotensin in our bodies when the blood pressure gets too low by pumping out a compound called renin that activates angiotensin. When activated, angiotensin causes the arteries throughout our bodies to constrict and the kidneys to retain salt and water, both of which raise our blood pressure. Angiotensin is the critical link communicating proper blood pressure needs between our brain, heart, blood vessels, and kidneys.

How High Is High?

We're all aware that blood pressure is measured through two variables; it's always some number over some other number. These numbers refer to the pumping and resting phases of your heartbeat. The top number you hear from your doctor, called the *systolic* pressure, is a measure of the pressure with which your heart ejects blood from its chamber and out through the rest of your body. This number varies quite a bit with activity, and for years physicians didn't pay too much attention to it. Systolic pressure has a tendency to rise as we age, and we are just now learning that a too high systolic number is an important risk factor to note and combat (see page 405 in this chapter). The second number, called the *diastolic* pressure, refers to the pressure within your blood vessels when your heart relaxes. This number reflects "resistance" in your blood vessels. It tends to be quite consistent, elevating only if there is a problem. A healthy blood pressure means a systolic pressure of about 120 and a diastolic pressure close to about 80, or 120/80.

Normally, in the course of a day our blood pressure may fluctuate some 20 to 30 points or more, depending on our activities. If we strain ourselves by heavy lifting, exercise vigorously, or become frightened, the heart pumps harder, and blood pressure rises temporarily. When we sleep or are completely relaxed, our blood pressure tends to fall. But for those with hypertension, blood pressure creeps up and stays up, not fluctuating with several readings. If your blood pressure gets to the range of 140/90 or higher and stays there, you have high blood pressure. The higher the pressure, the greater its potential complications. Most people with high blood pressure today fall into the mild to moderate range: mild being in the 140/90 range; moderate when blood pressure exceeds 160/100; and severe when it exceeds 180/110. A blood pressure is very severe if it gets over 210/120. When the pressure moves toward the 300/140 range, you are facing a state of medical emergency called malignant hypertension and are likely to experience symptoms such as violent headaches, blurred vision, and vomiting, and sometimes sleepiness, outright mental confusion, or coma.

ESSENTIAL HYPERTENSION

Most of the time, high blood pressure falls into a category called *essential hypertension,* or *primary hypertension,* meaning that it is a disease unto itself; it doesn't have its origin in another problem.

While we still have not found the absolute cause of essential hypertension, we do know some important things about it. First, it seems to run in families; as many as 40 percent of people with high blood pressure have immediate family members who also have high blood pressure. Recently, studies have shown that some families with hypertension also have a variation in the coding of the gene for the angiotensin hormone, discussed on page 386. I find this discovery very encouraging; if there is one specific gene in our bodies that causes hypertension, there may also be a way to screen people at risk and provide them with early preventive measures, stopping the disease well before it does harm. Second, for both those people with a clear genetic risk and those whose elevated blood pressure may have several causes, lifestyle choices can make a big difference in whether the tendency will erupt into full-blown hypertension or will stay dormant.

SECONDARY HYPERTENSION

Other, far less common types of high blood pressure result from some other condition and hence are called *secondary hypertension*. Most of the time, this kind of heightened blood pressure goes away if you can correct the underlying problem.

There are several types of secondary hypertension found in both men and women; possible causes are abnormalities in the endocrine system (such as tumors or other interferences that can create hormonal disorders, raising blood pressure) or kidney problems. The following types of secondary hypertension are predominant in or unique to women.

Fibromuscular Hyperplasia

Younger women are the major targets for a rare form of kidney problem called fibromuscular hyperplasia, which causes the small muscle fibers periodically to thicken along the length of the arteries, which then take on the appearance of a string of beads. If you are under fifty and suddenly develop high blood pressure, your doctor will consider this disease of the arteries of the kidneys as a possible cause.

Estrogen-Related Hypertension

Estrogen therapy first became linked to high blood pressure back in the late 1960s when oral contraceptives came into widespread use. We now know that estrogen treatment in oral contraceptives raises blood pressure a little in most women: about 5 points in systolic pressure and 2 points in diastolic pressure. This elevation is not generally significant, although in rare instances some women do develop persistent elevations that require stopping use of the Pill. Invariably, blood pressure returns to normal. (However, if you smoke and take oral contraceptives, the scene changes; your risk of a stroke increases markedly. I suggest changing forms of birth control if you smoke. Better yet, quit smoking.)

Elevation of blood pressure due to estrogen is less evident in women on hormone replacement therapy, probably because the dosages are lower. The recent PEPI study (see page 192) showed no blood pressure elevation in several hundred women on a variety of hormone preparations.

If an increase in your blood pressure coincides with your taking estrogen, however, either stopping the hormone for a while or modifying its dose or schedule of administration should help sort out the underlying cause. Preexisting high blood pressure, though, is not a reason for denying a postmenopausal woman hormone replacement therapy, the benefits of which far outweigh the risks (see page 195).

Pregnancy-Induced Hypertension (Preeclampsia and Eclampsia)

If you ever wondered why obstetricians are so careful about monitoring the blood pressure, weight gain, and urine protein of pregnant women, it is because of the threat of pregnancy-induced hypertension, which includes *preeclampsia* and *eclampsia* (also called *toxemia*). Normally, blood pressure falls during pregnancy because the arteries dilate. A blood pressure of 130/80 is the highest level acceptable during pregnancy.

With preeclampsia, blood pressure rises, blood vessels constrict, water retention occurs, and the kidneys start to leak protein. In advanced eclampsia, a pregnant woman will experience violent headache, seizures, mental confusion, and symptoms that sometimes look like a transient ischemic attack. The mother is at risk of a stroke or heart failure, and the baby is at risk of death.

Pregnancy-induced hypertension usually develops late in pregnancy and can be prevented by prompt attention to even mild blood pressure elevation and sudden and excessive weight gain. Often the cure is the delivery of the baby, either through a C-section or an induced labor. Women who have a history of high blood pressure or kidney disease face increased risk for toxemia.

NONHYPERTENSIVE RISK FACTORS FOR STROKE

While no other single factor carries the great risk of stroke that high blood pressure does, some of the following catalysts are a double whammy; they increase your chances both of developing the hypertension that leads to stroke and of suffering a stroke itself.

Smoking

After high blood pressure, smoking is your best way to buy yourself a stroke. The more you smoke, the greater the risk. While smoking has not been tied directly to high blood pressure, it does have a long-term degenerative effect on the blood vessels themselves. In the Framingham Study of heart disease (see page 332), cigarette smoking more than doubled the risk of both thrombotic and hemorrhagic stroke in women; the Nurses' Health Study (see page 46) of 120,000 women found that two-pack-a-day smokers were at four times the risk of those who didn't smoke.

As noted above, smoking is especially risky for women who are on birth control pills. Women who use oral contraceptives and also smoke are at forty times the risk of stroke compared to those who use neither cigarettes nor oral contraceptives.

LIFESTYLE AND DIET

Your lifestyle is to a large extent under your power to control. Your food and exercise choices can have a direct impact on the likelihood you'll encounter this destructive disease. *Obesity* is a risk factor for high blood pressure and stroke and, as we've seen throughout this book, travels along with many other illnesses.

A diet rich in saturated fat and the wrong types of cholesterol also increases your chance of having a stroke (see page 343 and the section on dietary fat beginning on page 34 in chapter 2). Atherosclerosis, the fatty plaque disease that clogs arteries, doesn't just threaten your heart. Thrombotic stroke is caused specifically by fat-narrowed arteries leading to the brain. Of course this plaque is not all due to diet, but why increase your risk?

Other dietary risk factors include not enough *calcium*, too much alcohol, and, while perhaps few of you readers would consider ingesting this substance as a part of your three daily meals, cocaine. Insufficient calcium in the diet has been linked to both high blood pressure and stroke, and excess consumption of *alcohol*—in the range of three drinks per day or more—can also both increase your blood pressure and raise your chance of a stroke three to four times. *Cocaine* use carries with it an all-too-little-known risk of stroke, particularly in young people. Cocaine not only raises blood pressure abruptly but also causes arteries to go into spasm and pinch off. It can and does cause blood vessel damage and sometimes a lethal cerebral hemorrhage.

Perhaps surprising to many is the fact that *salt* in our current diets is not a great risk factor, at least when used in moderation. As discussed on page 47, for many years there was considerable emphasis on salt as the culprit in high blood pressure, but some of this misconception stemmed from an earlier era in which salt was abundant in the diet because of a lack of refrigeration and to the use of salt-cured foods. In reality, today stringent reduction of salt has little effect on blood pressure most of the time; unless your doctor informs you that you have a very specific salt-sensitive form of hypertension, moderate salt intake should place you at no higher risk.

A recent study from California observing lifestyle patterns in women over fifty showed a direct correlation between lower *physical activity* level and higher levels of blood pressure and therefore stroke. Also, a study from Denmark examining lifestyle factors and risk of cerebrovascular disease in women linked lack of activity during leisure time to a greater risk of stroke.

STRESS

Stress as a risk factor for stroke is difficult to prove. It's clear that people with essential hypertension show an exaggerated increase in blood pressure in response to stress (and, fortunately, a greater response to blood-pressure-lowering relaxation exercises as well). These so-called hot reactors have to be particularly cautious in stressful situations, which can raise already elevated blood pressure.

It's true that stress by definition causes the "fight-or-flight" response in all of us, temporarily raising our blood pressure and increasing our heart rates in response to any experience we interpret as threatening. Theoretically, people under sustained stress would also experience a chronic elevation in blood pressure and therefore a greater risk of stroke. Proving this, though, has been tough, probably because of the complex nature of determining what stress really is, both physiologically and experientially.

The few studies done seem to show a correlation between temperament and the type of stress that raises blood pressure and increases stroke risk. Unlike the personality that is at risk for heart disease, though, it seems that type A (see page 348) is not as big a risk for high blood pressure and therefore stroke as is a personality that tends to suppress anger and emotion. As intuitively obvious as all this seems, we have yet to prove it in any reliable scientific study.

RACE

People of different races experience stroke in different numbers. African-American men and women have about twice as many strokes as Caucasians, and certain Asian populations, particularly when they live in Japan, also fall prey to stroke in larger numbers. For blacks, this relates in part to the fact that blood pressure and diabetes occur more frequently. We don't know the underlying reason for these differences, and the obvious genetic component is one that must be fully explored—and soon.

HEART DISEASE

Here's a big cloud to a silver lining: as our population ages, and medical advances enable more and more women to survive heart disease, stroke will become an even more dire threat. An aging woman faces a large risk of heart disease; then, when she survives the heart disease, her chance of having a stroke increases by as much as fivefold. That's because heart disease sometimes can prompt a blood clot to form within the heart, break off, and travel to the brain, causing an embolic stroke.

DIABETES

A woman who is diabetic from childhood or young adulthood is at as much as five times the risk for stroke as a nondiabetic woman. Diabetes is a disease characterized by diffuse abnormalities in the way sugar is handled throughout the body. It damages the arteries over time and causes premature atherosclerosis, even in premenopausal women who would otherwise be protected through estrogen. Women with the milder adult-onset diabetes are at far less risk, provided they take action to manage the illness with strict regulation of their blood-sugar level and weight control.

FAMILY HISTORY

As we've noted, essential hypertension has a strong genetic predisposition; therefore, stroke precipitated by hypertension also tends to run in families. More than one irregularity in the gene for angiotensin has been found in families who also report a high incidence of high blood pressure and stroke, but there are certain to be other genetic explanations as well.

FIBRINOGEN: A NEW RISK FACTOR?

A chemical that our bodies produce naturally has increasingly gained attention as a possible risk factor for clot-related diseases, particularly for women. While no one has proved that this blood-clotting factor produced by our livers, called fibrinogen, actually causes strokes, heart attacks, or TIAs, we've seen in several population studies, including the Framingham study, a clear relationship between higher levels of fibrinogen and the illnesses: as fibrinogen levels rise, so does the incidence of these health problems. Fibrinogen circulates in our blood without doing any damage; it's when the levels go up that the factor gets worrisome, for it increases the thickness of blood, promotes clot formation and growth, and causes plaque to grow. Smoking, age, diabetes, stress, menopause, and oral contraceptives have all been shown to increase its levels.

There is much we don't know about this blood-clotting factor; it may well be an effect, not a cause, of plaque-filled arteries—a "marker" chemical that increases only after arteries are injured. We also don't know the risks of lowering it in healthy people even if it could be done safely. I suspect we will be hearing considerably more about this molecule in the near future.

DIAGNOSING AND TREATING STROKE

The best stroke is a stroke prevented; the best treatment is action taken early to ensure that a full-blown stroke never happens. Later in this chapter (page 403) we'll examine the many means of stroke prevention available to all of us. Unfortunately, completed strokes do happen and must be diagnosed and treated, quickly and efficiently; those issues will be discussed now.

DIAGNOSING STROKE

As I said earlier, a transient ischemic attack can be a very good thing in that it serves as a crystal clear warning of an imminent, full-blown stroke—and is therefore a call to diagnostic arms. Any treatment for a TIA is more a measure taken to prevent a completed stroke from occurring than it is a means of fixing a TIA, which is by definition temporary. I'll explore TIA treatments at more length beginning on page 409; for now, let's take a look at the diagnostic techniques a TIA can inspire.

The most important issue a doctor must resolve in treating any stroke is determining its cause, for treatment of the different types of strokes are diametrically opposed (pages 382–84). If your physician suspects your TIA to have been caused by an embolus, the diagnostic devices will involve a look at your heart itself. He will probably undertake a complete cardiac evaluation, looking for rhythm disturbances (atrial fibrillation especially), valve disease, or clots in your heart. (See pages 365–70.)

There are a host of noninvasive technologies through which your physician can get an accurate picture of exactly what is going on in your brain: if there is bleeding, where it is, and how much; if there is brain swelling; whether there are dangerous narrowings of the arteries; or even where there is an aneurysm. Even when a stroke hits without warning, an increasing number of hospitals have on hand highly sophisticated machinery to help diagnose the cause of your illness—provided you get there without delay.

CAROTID ULTRASOUND, DOPPLER, AND ARTERIOGRAM

These techniques, described in detail in chapter 8, are used to determine if your TIA was caused by narrowings of your arteries. Carotid ultrasound and Doppler (which use sound waves to examine the artery and measure blood flow using a probe placed on the neck) together provide information about the carotid arteries and the degree of arterial narrowing. To get the clearest images of the blood vessels that feed the brain, though, you'll need an arteriogram. The arteriogram, an invasive procedure involving dye injected into your body vessels through a catheter, provides the clearest image, just as it does in diagnosing atherosclerosis in the heart.

TRANSCRANIAL DOPPLER ULTRASOUND

Transcranial Doppler (TCD) is an evolving technology that uses externally applied sound waves to measure blood flow inside the head (similar to echo Doppler used elsewhere in the body, but here the sound waves have to go through the skull). Its application, so far, has been in research studies of the physiology and patterns of cerebral blood flow under different conditions, but, in time, TCD is likely to be used more widely in the evaluation of stroke patients.

CAT SCANS

After a TIA, or while a stroke is in progress, we now can noninvasively determine its type—TIA, embolic, thrombolic, or hemorrhagic—and, therefore, prevent serious treatment errors. One way of doing so is by doing a CAT scan.

The CAT scan, short for *computerized axial tomography* or just *computed tomography* (CT), was developed in 1972. It uses X rays and computer technology to produce an actual three-dimensional, cross-sectional reconstruction of parts of the human body. Multiple narrow-beam X rays are swept through the body at different angles; the pictures they take are combined by computer into an extraordinary image. It can reveal exactly where there may be bleeding into the brain, without ever invading your body. CAT scans, however, may be normal early in an ischemic stroke, with changes evolving over twenty-four to seventy-two hours. The only risk of a CAT scan is the small dose of radiation that accompanies any X rays, and appropriate shields should be worn. A CAT scan should never be done on a pregnant woman.

MRI

Even more recently, scientists have developed another nonsurgical technique called *magnetic resonance imaging,* which can provide information similar to that obtained from a CAT scan without even the risk of radiation. (MRI also may be more sensitive in detecting certain kinds of strokes, such as those in the lower part of the brain.) An MRI machine reconstructs into a picture the signals coming from the atoms that make up the molecules of our body tissues, reflecting the different densities of the molecules themselves. There is no known risk to an MRI, but it is expensive and the process can make some people feel claustrophobic; you're placed into a large coil that is actually a magnet.

TREATING FULL-BLOWN STROKES

We now know that early treatment within the first few hours of a completed stroke can limit the damage to the brain, and that after those first few hours there is little anyone can do to reverse the destruction the stroke has caused. But the treatment, beyond careful monitoring of breathing and blood pressure, varies dramatically with the type of stroke you experience.

THROMBOTIC OR EMBOLIC STROKES

Quick treatment of a thrombotic or embolic stroke (a stroke caused by a blockage or blood clot) can clearly limit or even prevent irreversible damage from occurring. The key is to get the clot or blockage dissolved, and fast.

Most treatment of such strokes begins with a strong blood thinner, or anticoagulant, such as the drugs heparin or Coumadin (described on page 356). These drugs cannot dissolve the clot, but they do prevent other clots from forming. Actual clot dissolving requires more powerful agents, drugs such as urokinase, streptokinase, and tissue plasminogen activator. These drugs have not been fully studied; researchers are in the process of learning their optimal doses, combinations with other medications, and best use. But the work that has been done shows marked improvement in stroke victims who were given these drugs within the first ninety minutes of the onset of their strokes. The risk is hemorrhage into the brain.

The use of anticoagulants is primarily risky if the stroke diagnosis is wrong or incomplete—if the stroke has been caused by a hemorrhage in the brain, not by a blood clot. Clot-dissolving drugs will make a hemorrhagic stroke worse or can even cause a damaged vessel in an existing thrombotic stroke to begin bleeding.

HEMORRHAGIC STROKE

Once a CT scan or MRI shows the existence and cause of bleeding in the brain—a hemorrhagic stroke—treatment is basically either watch and wait or brain surgery. Anticoagulants are never used. Generally, if the bleeding is caused by hypertension and is not too extensive, the doctor will regulate your blood pressure, sedate you, and cross her fingers. (Some researchers are now investigating the use of steroids or *hyperosmolar* agents, which could cut down brain swelling, but the benefit has not yet been proven.)

If the hypertensive bleeding is so large that considerable pressure is exerted on the brain or if the bleeding is caused by a ruptured aneurysm, a doctor will most likely opt for surgery to repair the vessel and remove blood that has built up. Although the chance of dying from a hemorrhagic stroke is high, people who survive frequently recover remarkably well. In this type of stroke, it is often the pressure in the brain that has prompted the devastating symptoms; when the swelling is cleared, many symptoms disappear.

TREATING A STROKE THAT HAS ALREADY OCCURRED

No surgery, no anticoagulants, and not even a lazaroid can reverse the actual damage of a stroke once it is completed and the nerve cells are

STUDIES TO WATCH FOR: NEW APPROACHES TO MINIMIZING A STROKE'S DAMAGE

There are several experimental drugs on the horizon, designed to halt the neurological avalanche that a stroke sets off in the brain, thereby saving brainpower. Research laboratories across the country are investigating drugs that inhibit the release of destructive brain chemicals and prevent them from binding to receptors on healthy nerve cells (thereby causing the nerve cells to self-destruct by hyperexcitement), and other agents that interrupt the destruction of cell membranes by compounds like oxidants or too-high levels of calcium. One particularly promising experimental drug is called tirilizad. It is one of a new class of drugs, called the 21-aminosteroids, which may ultimately reverse certain death by protecting the cell membranes by scavenging for damaging oxidant compounds. They are also called, rather poetically, lazaroids.

Damage from a clot-induced stroke doesn't end when the clot is dissolved. These drugs and others such as calcium channel blockers (see page 406) would also help heal, protect, and preserve the cells that have been injured through oxygen deprivation.

destroyed. The region of the brain fed by the blocked artery has died. Will there ever be a time when we can retrain surviving cells or repair or replace those destroyed cells or grow back new neurons? Probably yes, but that is yet a long way from today. Without a doubt, one of the most extraordinary breakthroughs in all of medicine will be the ability to repair and retrain and maybe even regrow destroyed nervous system tissue. These are vital pursuits: they will offer more than hope to stroke victims, to paraplegics, and to patients with Alzheimer's disease. Our children may live to see this kind of discovery or may live longer because of it.

For now, once the stroke is done, we must continue the monitoring and support of the stroke victim and almost immediately embark on plans for her long-term rehabilitation. The brain is, after all, a large and utterly incredible contraption; the death of a part of it doesn't mean other neural pathways cannot be taught, to some degree, to perform the functions that have been lost.

AFTER A STROKE: MAXIMIZING RECOVERY IS THE GOAL

The ultimate goal of rehabilitation is to return the stroke patient to society as an independent person. In a majority of instances, fully half or more of those who suffer a stroke can expect to return to work within six months; most will return within three months. The number of stroke victims who will require long-term institutionalized care is in the range of 5 percent or less.

PHYSICAL REHABILITATION

Although the nature and severity of the stroke will determine the rehabilitative approach and specific rehabilitative procedures, neither the nature of the stroke nor its severity per se necessarily determines success with rehabilitation. Other factors that are not always easily measured come into play. Among these are the patient's self-image, her resolution or determination, the perception by her and her family of her disability and chances for recovery, and the understanding by all concerned of the disease and the demands of the rehabilitative process.

The severity of the stroke and the region of the brain damaged create the *character* of the disability. There is usually some degree of hemiplegia, altered muscle tone, on one side of the body in an arm or leg or both. For instance, in the leg, some muscles may be weak while others are under tension. The patient can stand on the leg, but when she begins to walk, the interplay of tension and weakness causes the leg to rotate in a semicircle away from the body. If the arm is affected, *subluxation* of the shoulder (a dislocation of the arm from the shoulder) may occur, and the arm is usually carried close to the chest in a flexed position because certain muscles are under tension while others are slack. A lack of tension or tone in the musculature on one side of the face will produce the drooping eye and slack cheek seen in many who have suffered stroke.

Aphasia, or speech impairment, affects many stroke patients. Impaired communication is one of the more serious disabilities and impediments to rehabilitation. It is not unusual to find depression in patients with aphasia. But the exact character of the disability is as individual as the patient, and the recovery in large part depends on the patient's attitude and determination. Since rehabilitation cannot restore neurons in the region affected by the stroke, instead, new neural pathways are exercised and taught to instruct legs to walk and the tongue to articulate language.

The rehabilitative process can be long, arduous, and uncertain, and retraining the brain is an area in which we have much to learn. In physical therapy, arms and legs are moved and stressed and reschooled in very specific ways; occupational therapy concentrates on activities of daily living (i.e., hygiene, dressing, feeding, etc.); and speech therapy teaches patients to read, speak, and think again. These therapies can continue for many months, sometimes years.

PSYCHOLOGICAL REHABILITATION

These physical remedies are far from sufficient to help a woman recover from a stroke. Never forget that a stroke is devastating in many ways, psychologically and emotionally as well as physically. The woman who is one day happy, attractive, and a source of energy and strength to her family looks in the mirror a few days after the trauma of a stroke and sees a disfigured stranger with slurred speech who will be a burden to her friends and family for an endless time. Depression can affect a third or more of stroke patients.

Not all depression after a stroke is situational. Some mood swings involving, for example, uncontrolled crying or unhappy outbursts of rage or sadness result from the damage to the brain itself. Strokes damaging the left hemisphere of the brain have been linked to depression, while those involving the right hemisphere seem to correlate with indifference and a lack of concern about recovery.

INTEGRATING CARE

A careful multidisciplinary evaluation is necessary to determine the nature of a patient's impairment, but such evaluations are not wholly reliable in determining the success of rehabilitation. Even age is not necessarily a factor; although the elderly suffer worse strokes, they are also quite resilient and often quicker to recover than younger victims. Dr. Vinod Sahgal, a renowned physiatrist at the Cleveland Clinic, stresses the importance of skilled and experienced efforts in rehabilitation that take into account a holistic approach rarely practiced in day-to-day medicine. Rehabilitation of the stroke patient must include general attention to all the medical needs of the patient, including non-stroke-related problems that may affect progress. Heart disease commonly coexists with stroke, so a cardiac evaluation is important since it may alter the plan for a taxing rehabilitation effort. (The risk of a heart attack is greater than the risk of a recurrent stroke.) Rehabilitation programs must be structured to meet the needs of the elderly as well as the young. A 1990 Report of the NIH Task Force on Medical Rehabilitation Research noted that all too often rehabilitation services are geared to younger people.

It's the environmental and psychological factors, not always easily measured, which seem to make the biggest difference. A multidisciplinary rehabilitation program, structured to meet the needs of the elderly and the young, based on an interdisciplinary team approach, must all at once provide psychological evaluation and support, vocational training, education, nutrition, family involvement, and encouragement and attention to the patient's self-esteem and social support systems. The therapeutic team typically consists of the physiatrist, the nurse, the physical, occupational, speech, and recreation therapists, the social worker, the psychologist, the case manager, the orthotist, and the chaplain. Of all these elements, few have more impact on the sufferer's good recovery than the participation and love of the family.

REHABILITATION: A FAMILY AFFAIR

A stroke can handicap its victims; when such an event happens, the ripples extend far beyond any individual's recovery. An educated and supportive family can mean a quick recovery; an uninformed or unhelpful family can mean disabilities linger for a lifetime.

Education of the family and of the stroke victim herself may play a greater role in recovery than do drugs. Everyone should learn

- What caused the stroke, and how another stroke can be prevented.
- What needs to be done to the patient's home so that it is now safe for her new physicality. Is it wheelchair-ready? Can all necessary appliances, tissues, towels, clothes, medicine, food, drink—everything necessary for a comfortable life—be reached? Do hire a rehabilitative specialist to assess the home in advance. An expert can tell at a glance that the sugar bowl is too far back on the countertop for a person in a wheelchair to reach. This may seem simplistic, but consider that every time a woman has to ask for help, even if it is something as simple as a request for sugar for coffee, she is reminded of her disability. She feels helpless and she loses a tiny bit of the dignity that she is trying so desperately to regain.
- What emotional and physical consequences everyone in the family should expect, and a plan for coping with those changes.
- Complete information about medications, their purpose and effects, dosages and side effects (for details in this chapter, see 405).
- The details of all rehabilitative techniques, why they are important, and the goals to be reached. Do not underestimate the capacity of a child to understand what has happened to a parent or grandparent. In a society in which all the adults in the family probably work, it is not unlikely that children might spend more time in the home with a handicapped parent or grandparent than does any adult. This is not necessarily a drawback; children can be a tremendous source of inspiration and encouragement.

Family support is a two-way street. If you're caring for a stroke victim, you and your family will find you need plenty of advice, hope, and encouragement yourselves. Don't ignore your own needs. You can find, through your hospital or rehab specialist, one of the many support groups now dedicated to helping stroke patients and their families. Such groups can be sources of emotional support and practical services as well. Through them, you should be able to find adult day care, housecleaning services, grocery delivery services, home health care operations, and the best sources for specialized products such as wheelchairs and seating devices.

You and your family will make a real difference in the quality of your loved one's life after stroke—but it won't necessarily be easy. Victim and family together will experience shock, denial, depression, frustration, and, finally, acceptance and adjustment. How you handle your feelings will determine, to a large extent, how the patient handles hers. Eventually, a certain degree of disability may have to be accepted. Knowing when this plateau has been reached can be the most difficult challenge a patient and her family can face. Families who see the impairment created by stroke as a challenge to be overcome a day at a time will boost the patient's determination, hope, and self-image. Families who accept impairments as a tragic fate, an inevitable step along the road to death, can spawn the same negative attitude in the patient. Right along with everyone's plummeting self-esteem fall any chances of improvement.

Stroke and the ensuing disability must not be seen as a continuing tragedy. Even though my Aunt Sarah was confined to a wheelchair and needed enormous help for the most simple tasks of daily living, with her family's support she kept her spunk for more than twenty years. When her laughter, emotions, and spicy commentary filled the room of their small apartment, believe me, no disabled person was present.

REHABILITATION MUST BECOME A RESEARCH AFFAIR

And we must learn more about ways to rehabilitate the brain damaged by a stroke. Studies are being done now on brain plasticity, that is, how we can recruit living nerve cells in the vicinity of the damage to take over the job of those destroyed by stroke. We need to learn what rehabilitative techniques will enable us to tap into brain reserves. Can we regenerate damaged or dead neurons and reestablish proper functional connections? These kinds of advances will completely revolutionize our notion of "rehabilitation" of a stroke victim.

The clinical application of biotechnology to ease the burden of disability should be further developed. The goal of this comprehensive approach is to ensure that functional disability does not become a personal or societal handicap.

THE BEST TREATMENT: PREVENTION

Stroke is clearly a depressing chapter in any woman's life; it's been a depressing chapter to write! The exciting treatments now available and on the horizon make it much less so; even more inspiring to me are the huge strides we've taken in our ability to prevent stroke from happening in the first place. We can lower our risks considerably, as I've repeated, and they are words worth repeating, through attentiveness to our genetic predispositions and straightforward lifestyle changes. Even when time, age, and heredity play their high card and we experience the frightening alarm of a TIA, medical science has developed surgical means of preventing full-blown strokes from following. There is much we can do to stop this dread disease in its tracks.

HIGH BLOOD PRESSURE: TREAT IT AND PREVENT THE STROKE

By keeping track of your blood pressure, you control the risk of stroke. This is not very hard to do. Monitor your pressure at your doctor's office or at one of those free blood pressure booths in drugstores, shopping malls, county fairs, and health festivals. Remember the recommended levels on page 387. If you have an elevated reading or two, you can buy blood pressure kits at your local drugstore and take your blood pressure at home. Try to take readings a couple of times in one day, as your pressure will fluctuate with your daily activities. If the numbers concern you (and they should if they are above 140/90), begin taking your pressure every day, and keep a log for a week or two.

Notify your doctor if your log shows consistent levels above 140/90. Together, you'll work out the proper systematic and personal steps to take to get your pressure down to a healthy level. Make sure to bring your log and your home kit so that your doctor can ascertain that your readings were correct. (Obviously, if your blood pressure is in the danger zones, your doctor will recommend stronger and more immediate measures.)

The first step I would suggest you take would be to focus on lifestyle changes, such as controlling your weight, beginning programs of relaxation, stress reduction, and exercise, mildly restricting your salt intake if you overindulge, making sure you get adequate dietary calcium, and reducing your alcohol consumption if you drink more than you should.

You have available to you some alternative means of effecting these lifestyle changes. For example, I find *biofeedback* an intriguing method for relieving stress. It teaches you to control your own blood pressure. You are hooked up to a machine that monitors blood pressure and sometimes brain waves, making a noise or blinking a light when your blood pressure rises. This is a signal for you to begin breathing or relaxation techniques or meditation—whatever works for you—to get unstressed and thereby reduce your blood pressure. Biofeedback is designed to show you your own patterns of stress and tension so you can alter them; you can certainly try it without special equipment simply by monitoring your own heart rate, paying attention to your feelings and sensations, and finding personal ways to unwind.

Some practitioners believe that vegetarian diets lower blood pressure; others believe that specific foods, even less well studied, will help healthy people to decrease their chance of stroke. For example, Japanese studies show that people who drink more than five cups a day of green tea have a markedly lower incidence of stroke and cerebral hemorrhage than those who drink less. While you should take recommendations such as these with a grain of salt (forgive the pun), we shouldn't turn our backs on these lessons from other cultures and alternative approaches. I wouldn't tell you to run out and buy green tea, but I believe that none of us, in the medical community or not, should scoff at what someday may prove to be lifesaving recommendations.

The lifestyle changes you make with the intention of lowering your blood pressure will help minimize your risk of stroke in other ways. If you're diabetic, a disciplined control of blood sugar through diet and close attention to new and sophisticated glucose monitoring devices can lower your risk. Lifestyle changes that minimize your risk of heart disease (described beginning on page 360), which include a prudent low-fat diet and exercise, will also minimize your risk of stroke.

If you alter your lifestyle and your blood pressure stays high or does not come down enough to keep you safe, it's time to move on to medication. Lifestyle changes are a lifetime commitment, though; don't go back to your old habits just because the medication seems to be working. Even if you couldn't sufficiently reduce your blood pressure through the changes you worked so hard to make, these changes will make a powerful impact over time and can help you get off medication in the long term.

MEDICATION TO REDUCE BLOOD PRESSURE

When I began practicing internal medicine, most of the drugs available to treat high blood pressure had terrible side effects, including impotence and depression. It is in large part due to the tremendous and very recent advances in obtaining safe high blood pressure medications that stroke itself has become so much less common.

Nonetheless, I believe that the fewer external chemicals you introduce into your body, even medication, the better. We now prescribe medication to blood pressure patients only gradually, starting with the lowest doses of the least powerful, then incrementally moving toward heavier dosages and more potent drugs, adding drugs in combination if absolutely necessary.

Diuretics

The most commonly prescribed medications for controlling high blood pressure are called diuretics, which increase the excretion of salts and water through our kidneys and relax blood vessels, thereby effectively decreasing the amount of total liquid in our circulatory systems. Gentle, well-tested, and good for long-term use, diuretics come in different strengths. The most commonly used chemical class of diuretic are the thiazides, such as hydrochlorothiazide (Esidrix) and chlorothiazide (Diuril).

The thiazide diuretics are very inexpensive and have few side effects (your doctor will need to watch your potassium, cholesterol, and uric acid levels, and you'll probably have to eat a banana a day to make up for lost potassium). A real plus of the thiazides for women is that they don't increase calcium excretion, as do most other diuretics. Don't think this ease of use correlates with ineffectiveness; a recent study showed daily administration of a simple thiazide diuretic at a relatively low dose brought down systolic blood pressure in elderly patients and decreased their chance of having a stroke by 36 percent. (This treatment also decreased the risk of a heart attack by almost that much.) It has been estimated by the NIH that we would decrease the number of strokes in this country by about twenty-four thousand if only about half of the eligible elderly with systolic hypertension were treated with this mild medication.

Over the past several years we have seen the development of a host of more powerful diuretics (known as loop diuretics because they paralyze a specific part of the kidney's blood-filtering mechanism called *Henle's loop*, strongly inducing sodium and chloride excretion). These more powerful agents, including furosemide (Lasix) and bumetanide (Bumex), are also commonly prescribed; I find them particularly useful in emergency situations or in the treatment of heart failure, or with co-existing kidney disease where milder diuretics are not working.

If the diuretic isn't working well enough, your doctor will probably keep you on it, adding one or more of the following medications, depending upon your particular circumstance.

The Beta-Blockers

Beta-blockers are powerful and important drugs that came into use in the early seventies primarily to treat angina (see page 354). They block receptors in the sympathetic nervous system, discussed early in this chapter (see page 386), where the brain chemicals norepinephrine and epinephrine would otherwise bind and thereby stimulate the heart to contract and the blood vessels to constrict. Your doctor now has a wide range of beta-blockers to choose from, including propranolol (Inderal), atenolol (Tenormin), and metoprolol (Lopressor). While beta-blockers do have unpleasant side effects such as insomnia, fatigue, and impotence in some patients and can bring on wheezing if you already have asthma, your doctor can generally find a beta-blocker that's just right for you by changing dose and preparation.

Calcium Channel Blockers

Also developed to treat heart disease, the more recently developed calcium channel blockers do just what you'd imagine: they prevent calcium from binding to receptors in certain tissues, relaxing the heart and the blood vessels. They do have side effects, but these are fewer than for the beta-blockers; calcium channel blockers can make the ankles swell and cause skin rashes. Common names of the calcium channel blockers include nifedipine (Procardia), verapamil (Calan and Isoptin), and diltiazem (Cardizem).

ACE Inhibitors

I've talked about the importance of that one little molecule, angiotensin, in the regulation of your blood pressure. *Angiotensin converting enzyme*

(ACE) inhibitors work directly to prevent angiotensin from becoming active by blocking the enzyme that triggers their conversion. This discovery has been an incredibly important addition to our blood pressure medication arsenal. By decreasing the amount of angiotensin in the bloodstream, blood vessels stay more relaxed and blood pressure comes down. (These drugs have also been shown to be valuable in treating those with weak hearts, even improving survival of those with heart failure and after heart attacks.) Side effects are minimal, such as a change in taste sensation, but there are some infrequent risks of which your doctor will be aware. For example, ACE inhibitors should be avoided by people with advanced forms of kidney diseases associated with potassium retention. Commonly prescribed forms of these inhibitors include captopril (Capoten), enalapril (Vasotec), and lisinopril (Prinivil).

Other Medications

The four classes of drugs listed above are not the only medications available to treat high blood pressure, but they are the best, with the fewest side effects. If your physician prescribes for you any of the following medications without first trying the drugs I recommend above, ask why before taking them: the *alpha receptor blockers,* such as Prazosin (Minipress), or other antihypertensive drugs including reserpine, methyldopa (Aldomet), and clonidine (Catapres). Many of these agents are harsher acting and have more troubling side effects.

QUIT SMOKING

If you stop smoking, you can celebrate reducing your risk of stroke and cardiopulmonary diseases the day after you toss your last pack away. On your fifth anniversary, bake a great big (nonfat) cake: your risk is now the same as someone who has never smoked in her life. You've eliminated what might be the most significant health risk in your life—and saved close to ten thousand dollars by not buying increasingly expensive cigarettes. There aren't very many medications around that can produce these kinds of results.

ESTROGEN REPLACEMENT THERAPY

Although a perfectly controlled study has yet to be done, the studies I have seen comparing women on hormone replacement therapy (see page 189) with those who are not have convinced me that replacing estrogen after surgical or natural menopause lowers a woman's chances both of having a thrombotic stroke and of dying from one. For example, the recent Copenhagen City Heart Study, which studied women at high risk for stroke, revealed that hormone replacement therapy reduced strokes *even* in women who were smokers. The explanation is simple: estrogen protects women from getting atherosclerosis. The Women's Health Initiative should give us more concrete data in the next several years (see pages 10 and 193).

ASPIRIN AND OTHER BLOOD THINNERS

The most common blood thinner in use in the world today is aspirin, also known as *acetylsalicylic acid*. It binds to platelets and decreases their efficiency in clumping together in the formation of an early clot. Low-dose aspirin in healthy men reduces the risk of stroke by 20 to 30 percent when taken in modest daily doses—one baby aspirin a day or one-half of an adult aspirin (150 mg). Unfortunately, the study has yet to be done in women, and there are some hints that aspirin may not be as beneficial to women as it is in men. One report demonstrated a favorable interaction between aspirin and testosterone as the major reason for the effect in men, suggesting that aspirin selectively benefits men.

Even if aspirin is not as helpful for women, low-dose aspirin comes with little risk and few side effects for most of us. Until we know more, and if you have no contraindications, such as a history of ulcers or an allergy, my advice is it won't hurt and might help, especially if you are over the age of fifty. But keep an eye out for the results of the Harvard study (see page 364), which will give us the final word on aspirin and stroke and heart attack prevention in women.

Ticlopidine is a new aspirin-like drug that is just coming into use. Ticlopidine (Ticlid), the first oral agent to act on platelets since aspirin, is a broader-spectrum inhibitor of platelet function, which prevents them from clumping, an early step in thrombus formation. Several clinical trials—but not all—have suggested that ticlopidine actually may be more effective than aspirin in preventing strokes and in preventing death among those who have already had a stroke. It also appears to be effective in patients who cannot tolerate aspirin. The drug is clearly promising.

Anticoagulation markedly reduces the risk for embolic stroke in patients who are at risk because of heart disease. In the case of patients with abnormal heart rhythm called atrial fibrillation, which puts women at a greater stroke risk than men, recent studies have shown that strokes can be prevented by chronic anticoagulation with lower and therefore safer doses of the blood thinner Coumadin (see below).

TREATING A TIA

A successful treatment of a TIA means a probable stroke prevented. Treating the TIA means getting rid of whatever caused it; since the majority of TIAs are thrombotic events, getting rid of the thrombus or clot or in some cases the severe narrowing in the vessel is central to its treatment. This can be achieved through drugs or, if the drugs aren't effective, through the surgical methods discussed below.

BLOOD THINNERS

Aspirin has been especially effective in both the prevention and the treatment of transient ischemic attacks. In those with known atherosclerotic disease, aspirin can cut the risk of TIAs in half. It appears to work better in the elderly than in the middle-aged, and better in men than in women (page 408).

The new aspirin-like drug ticlopidine may actually be more effective than aspirin in treating TIAs, in preventing a stroke after a TIA or prior stroke, and in preventing death among those who have already had a stroke. (Some clinical trials do contradict these findings.) Although ticlopidine is new to the United States, it has been approved for such use in Japan and Europe for about fifteen years (a common story for pharmaceutical availability in this country). Interestingly, women seem to benefit from ticlopidine more than men.

Other more powerful anticoagulants are available, such as heparin and Coumadin (warfarin), but with increased power comes increased risk. While we may be preventing a stroke caused by a thrombus, there is greater chance of causing a hemorrhage. There is, however, increasing interest in using low-dose heparin or Coumadin to treat TIAs. If your doctor finds such medication to be your best choice, make sure she carefully monitors your blood-clotting levels to minimize any bleeding risk.

PREVENTING STROKE THROUGH SURGERY

If you experience a TIA caused by atherosclerosis or your doctor otherwise determines that you are at high risk of suffering a completed stroke, it's far from the time for you to give up the ghost. Surgery can actually prevent the stroke from occurring, by removing the plaque narrowing the arteries that lead to your brain.

The procedure most commonly used to get the plaque out, called *carotid endarterectomy,* was developed in the 1950s. Endarterectomy entails cutting open the artery and removing the obstruction and, if needed, patching the artery with a piece of vein tissue. This operation requires a good bit of skill to perform, and for many years was practiced without consistent forethought and with erratic outcomes. The death and stroke rates from this preventive operation were so high that it came close to being discredited, but the medical community itself came to the procedure's rescue. Recognizing that the problem lay not in the procedure itself, but in its inappropriate or unskilled use, prominent figures in the neurology and vascular surgery fields convened a group of physicians and researchers across the country to develop stringent guidelines for the procedure, including specifying acceptable experience and complication rates. This self-monitoring prevented a lifesaving operation from disappearing and all but eliminated its inappropriate or poorly competent use. The numbers of endarterectomies performed have since fallen, but the success rate has skyrocketed. And now we know that in good hands the procedure is not only lifesaving but stroke preventing.

A series of controlled clinical studies supported by the NIH confirmed these benefits over the past few years. In one 1991 study, patients who had symptoms such as a TIA or mild stroke and a narrowing of the carotid artery of 70 percent or more showed a marked decrease in subsequent strokes with surgery compared to blood-thinning medicine alone. In late 1994, a study of people with severely narrowed arteries (detected through a doctor's routine examination with the stethoscope, detecting a *bruit,* or whishing sound, in the neck at the narrowing) but *no* symptoms at all, was suddenly and publicly cut short because the results of surgery were so dramatically positive that researchers felt it would be unethical to keep the control group (who were treated with standard medical therapy) from receiving the endarterectomy, since the operation cut the risk of stroke just about in half.

One curious fact has not yet been explained: while men's risk was reduced by 55 percent, women's risk was cut by only 16 percent (still quite significant—I calculate as many as thirty-six thousand women would be spared a stroke each year with this surgery). It will take many years to sort out this gender difference.

Whether or not you should undertake this operation is a matter for you, your physician, and your loved ones to decide. Weigh the odds carefully—and don't forget to add the track record of the surgeon to the equation. As the vascular surgeon Dr. Norman Hertzer calculates, people with a blockage of 80 percent or more face a 5 to 8 percent risk of stroke, so a surgical procedure with a risk of only 2 to 3 percent is a chance worth taking. (At my own institution, the stroke rate has been 1.3 percent in the last seventeen hundred patients, with a mortality of 0.3 percent.) If, however, your surgeon's track record shows a stroke rate higher than these or a mortality of more than 2 percent, I'd say opt out—or, better yet, find another surgeon and medical center.

Which brings me to a point that I repeat over and over again to my patients, and now to you. When considering a risky surgical procedure such as endarterectomy, you must examine the credentials and track record of the prospective surgeon or surgeons and the institution in which the procedure will be performed. Moreover, a surgeon should share with you his own personal track record for his last one hundred cases—not just the team or hospital results reported upon in the literature. What were his mortality rates and his stroke complication figures? How did those other patients' illnesses compare to your own? Many women feel uncomfortable asking these questions and pressing for answers, but my view is that in assessing a major operation that could spell joy or disaster for your future quality of life, you have every right to be both choosy and demanding about your medical care. And that is why we should never take away a woman's freedom to choose her doctor.

NEW APPROACHES TO UNCLOGGING CAROTID ARTERIES

Several surgical techniques currently used in coronary surgery are now being explored as less invasive, less risky means of removing plaque from arteries leading to the brain. These technologies, discussed at length in the chapter on heart disease (page 356), suggest great opportunities to reach blood vessels within the head through catheters, without actually opening the skull. Through balloon angioplasty, a balloon threaded through a catheter is inflated in the narrowed artery, thereby disrupting and condensing the plaque. Other instruments, also fed through catheters, include tiny drills that cut through plaque and lasers that vaporize it.

These procedures, while exciting, are still unproven. When these catheters are used in the carotid arteries, the risk of stroke may be as high as 5 percent. It will be a while before we know their full benefits and risk or how to prevent the material that is dislodged by the catheter from floating up to the brain. As I hope we in the medical community learned through the lesson of endarterectomies, inappropriate use of any new technology might not only harm patients but also ultimately prevent an otherwise valuable technology from saving lives.

QUESTIONS FOR YOUR DOCTOR

At every medical visit you should be mindful of the kinds of questions to ask, such as those below, that will in the long run keep you from a stroke.

- What are your risk factors for a stroke, based on your own health profile?
- What is your blood pressure? If it is elevated, how much so? Should you monitor blood pressure at home? Is the blood pressure evaluation due to primary or secondary causes?
- If your blood pressure needs treatment and a diuretic is prescribed, ask about the less expensive and effective thiazide diuretics. Do you need to take them every day?
- Discuss with your doctor what in your lifestyle needs to be changed: stress, diet, exercise? (You know them, but we all need reinforcement.)
- What is the latest on low-dose aspirin for stroke prevention and treatment of TIAs? Are the newer antiplatelet medicines available yet? Do they still look favorable for women?
- If you have disease in your carotid arteries and surgery is being recommended, what is the profile of the surgeon? Morbidity, mortality, stroke rate in his or her last one hundred cases? And what about those same results in the last one hundred *women* patients?

- If you are at high risk for stroke, which hospital in your community is the best to go to—with the latest in stroke treatment and good backup surgery?
- Are there any centers specializing in stroke rehabilitation in your community? If not, why not? (If yes, you need to know how many patients they treat, what the functional outcomes are, the length of stay in the center, the discharge destination, and the cost.)
- Do community programs exist to back up rehabilitation goals (such as a swimming pool at a nearby school or YMCA)?

WHAT WOMEN CAN DO PERSONALLY AND POLITICALLY

There is much you can do to encourage further research nationally, to improve your own community services, and to ensure the best health care for yourself. On a national level, be aware of the work coming out of the National Institute of Neurological Disorders and Stroke, the institute at NIH that deals with stroke research, and the American Heart Association's efforts to reduce stroke by educating the public. Support these research efforts and activities through volunteer participation in your local AHA chapters and by asking your local congressional representative about the work being done and the resources being allocated at the NIH for the prevention, treatment, and rehabilitation of stroke patients. If you are a member of advocacy groups such as the AARP, write to them to spur their interest and commitment to stroke prevention.

In your community, learn about local rehabilitation services. Meet with your local hospital board and medical society. If you're not satisfied with what you hear or see, you can get behind a volunteer effort to see that rehabilitation centers are developed or expanded. Every community needs to have good rehabilitation and home health care services.

For yourself, keep aware of the breathtaking advances that are occurring in stroke prevention and treatment. And mind the many risk factors we already know about, especially blood pressure. There is no excuse for not knowing your blood pressure or for not taking medication if your doctor has recommended you should. Don't ignore the key warning sign of a stroke—the TIA—and if you or a family member does have a stroke, become informed and become involved in the rehabilitation. Your involvement is critical to the best possible outcome.

Stroke is a devastating disease that grows in frequency as women age. As we look forward to our later years we must imagine what kind of life we want to lead and endeavor now to make it happen. And if a stroke or the threat of one appears, we can draw strength from the fact that our brains will benefit from new drugs and technology to restore normal blood flow, and our entire bodies will benefit from better means of rehabilitation. The holy grail we must continue to search for is the ability one day to retrain brain cells near damaged ones and even regenerate dead brain cells complete with their memory banks, complex interconnections, and developed pathways that have taken a lifetime to build. This will be an even greater gift than bringing Kitava to Hoboken.

TEN

OSTEOPOROSIS
Fragile Bones

To live is to function. That is all there is to living.

—OLIVER WENDELL HOLMES,
ON THE OCCASION OF HIS
NINETIETH BIRTHDAY, 1931

*I know I have the body of a weak and feeble woman;
but I have the heart . . . of a King.*

—QUEEN ELIZABETH I, 1588

My mother-in-law has taught me more about osteoporosis than my many years in medicine. Marie Dorullis Loop—Nonie, as we call her —was born in 1900 in Sac City, Iowa. The daughter of a minister, she became a schoolteacher, and eventually taught romance languages at Purdue University. Nonie is a tall, handsome, dignified, and independent woman with a core Victorian elegance about her. She still writes letters, long flowery letters in perfect feminine filigree script, quoting Keats and Butler to make the perfect point. Nonie has been a widow for a quarter of a century, living alone in a little apartment in Lafayette, Indiana, in the very neighborhood in which she was married and raised her only son. Her mind is sharp; her memory, eyesight, and hearing are seemingly perfect, her heart and soul robust.

But Nonie lives in chronic pain and growing fear about which bone will break next. Her tall straight back is now a compressed "C," making it hard for her to move about, to sit comfortably, and even to take a good breath. Walking now makes her pant. In the course of a decade, she has broken her foot stumbling on a short step; broken her wrist; and endured several stress fractures of her spine—one caused only by turning over too quickly in bed. She has just recently given up driving, and it took her ninety years to hire someone else to help clean her house.

Nonie steadfastly refuses to give up her final claim to independence, her tidy apartment. My husband and I stand by, controlling our instincts to jump in and take over; we know that, despite the latest that medicine has to offer, we cannot make her better or even ease her pain.

Nonie's bones have turned into eggshells through osteoporosis, a largely preventable (we now know) disease that afflicts elderly women. Her story is similar to those of millions of American women, made all the more tragic because it is a story of pain born of medical ignorance and bred through research neglect.

More than twenty-four million women in the United States are affected by osteoporosis; as a woman, you have a fifty-fifty chance of breaking some bone due to osteoporosis in your lifetime. More than 300,000 people fracture their hips each year because of osteoporosis. For older women, hip fractures carry a horrendous toll: some 25 percent die within a year of the fracture. If a woman is lucky enough to live to ninety, she faces a one-in-three chance of breaking her hip—an event that is likely to end or drastically alter her remaining years of life. Yet, as recently as the 1960s, this debilitating disease was considered merely a normal part of the aging process, not worth preventive attention.

The economic toll of osteoporosis is staggering—osteoporotic fractures in the United States are estimated to cost about ten billion dollars, the entire annual budget of the NIH. The human toll among elderly women is even greater: pain and suffering, loss of independence, and an increased risk of other illnesses, such as pneumonia. One psychological consequence for elderly women is that they become frail and fragile, fearful of going out or doing things, of bad weather or strange places, making them truly the weaker sex physically, and soon emotionally. All too often the disease sets in at a time when a woman is widowed and living alone, and the first fracture is the first step in a lonely trek into a nursing home.

As our population ages, and more and more women live into their ninth and tenth decades and beyond, the consequences of osteoporosis will become more visible, and more frustrating. Women have achieved equality because of brain power, not muscle power or brawn. It is thus sadly ironic that in the end we face a large risk of being overtaken by a failing, weak, and vulnerable frame, defeated by a loss of brawn and bone after all.

UNDERSTANDING OSTEOPOROSIS

The bones of all women become weaker over the years. This is inevitable, and not necessarily debilitating. But when the bones become so weak they can shatter through an act as simple as lifting a bag of groceries; when the bones of the spine compress so that the back becomes deformed and curved in upon itself; when walking, sitting, lying in bed, even breathing, becomes difficult—this is the disease of osteoporosis at its worst.

Some of us are genetically predisposed to this curse, and all of us are vulnerable to it. But weaker bones don't have to mean osteoporosis, and osteoporosis itself can be, if not completely prevented, delayed and diminished. A clear understanding of the role our bones play in our bodies, the way our bones are structured, and the manner in which they normally function provides the tools with which to halt osteoporosis before it reaches its most destructive form. I am confident that in time, if we resolve to do so, we will also develop the tools to restore strength to even the weakest of bones.

THE BARE BONES

Most people think of bones as inert and everlasting, since they are the sole survivors of ancestral life found at archeological digs. Actually, our skeleton is a dynamic living tissue in a constant state of flux, carefully regulated by a complex orchestration of our internal hormones, our eating habits, and gravitational forces.

Bones have two major functions. One is the obvious, the holding of our bodies against gravity, allowing for locomotion, and providing a scaffold to encase and protect our soft and sometimes fragile internal organs. The second function is just as important—bones serve as a giant reservoir, holding and releasing calcium and other minerals critical to the function of virtually every cell and tissue in our bodies. Osteoporosis interferes mainly with the first of these functions.

Bones not only hold minerals; they themselves consist of about 70 percent minerals, and 30 percent water and connective tissue (called *collagen*). The minerals in our bones are primarily calcium, phosphorus, and magnesium (and sometimes, if there was earlier exposure, certain toxic minerals, like lead and mercury). All three major bone minerals are important to the functioning of our bodies and our bones, but calcium is absolutely crucial. Without calcium, our muscles don't contract, our cells can't reproduce or repair themselves, most of our enzymes don't work, most body functions cease. Without calcium, our bones crumble.

Bone is built with a magnificent architectural design suited to the work the bone has to do. The long, weight-bearing bones of our bodies, such as the ones in our legs and arms, have a callous, dense outer layer called *cortical* bone and a spongy inner layer called *trabecular* bone. The vertebrae of the spine, which function as shock absorbers, not surprisingly are made up mostly of spongy trabecular bone and have relatively less of the sturdy cortical bone; the ribs are also composed mostly of spongy trabecular bone.

The two functions of bone work beautifully together during much of our lives, keeping us sturdy and upright, and supplying our bodies with vital calcium through an intricate process called *bone remodeling.* In this process, calcium (with other minerals) constantly flows in and out of our bone's reservoirs, the bone itself breaking down and building up to supply calcium on demand. The spongy trabecular bone is the part of the skeleton where the flow of calcium into and out of bone is most brisk.

This bone breakdown or *resorption* is executed by *osteoclasts,* giant bone cells which produce powerful enzymes that make pockmarks in bone, dissolving away minerals and underlying connective tissues. The dissolved calcium then gets released into the bloodstream. Conversely, *osteoblasts* lay down collagen, creating the complex structural matrix in the holes in the bone, and help to attract calcium and other minerals back into the bone—to "mineralize" or strengthen the bones by increasing their actual density. These processes result in bone *deposition.* Osteoblasts also produce certain factors called *cytokines,* which in turn influence osteoclast formation and function, so that these two different cell types actually "talk" to each other.

Osteoblasts and osteoclasts do their work in response to a complex stew of external hormones and other chemicals that bathe them continuously and give them their marching orders, either to tear bones down or build them up. The four central hormones that regulate the minerals in a woman's bones are *parathormone* (from the parathyroid gland, which sits on the thyroid); *calcitonin* (from the thyroid gland itself); *calcitriol* (1,25 dihydroxycholecalciferol), which is the chemically active form of vitamin D in our bodies; and *estrogen,* which comes mainly from the ovaries.

These are the key players in the regulation of a woman's body minerals, but other players modulate the net effect of these four, and may come into play at various times during the course of a woman's life. For example, cortisol, a steroid stress hormone made by the adrenal gland, leads to bone demineralization. Other hormones, including the sex hormones testosterone and progesterone, have bone-building effects; and many other special molecules, called *growth factors,* stimulate individual bone cells to reproduce and/or to develop.

Parathormone: Parathormone's role is to keep the levels of calcium circulating in our blood and bathing all our cells from falling too low. When the parathyroid gland senses that the level of calcium is falling too low, it secretes parathormone, which stimulates the bones to release calcium, signals the kidneys to excrete less calcium in the urine, and stimulates the chemical conversion of vitamin D to its chemically active hormone form (see below).

Calcitonin: Calcitonin counters the effect of parathormone. If the calcium levels in the blood go too high—which can be damaging to cell function throughout the body—more calcitonin is excreted by the thyroid gland. This causes the bones to take up more calcium and form more bone, and the kidneys to release more calcium to be excreted through urinating.

Vitamin D: The many forms of vitamin D (which we now know to be a steroid hormone rather than a simple nutrient) help us to retain calcium in our bones and blood. We obtain vitamin D through our skin—a cholesterol precursor molecule in the skin is converted to one form of vitamin D by ultraviolet light—and in our diet. Vitamin D in our intestines serves to increase the amount of calcium taken out of our food and delivered into our bloodstream. Under the influence of parathormone, the kidney can convert vitamin D to at least two active forms, which in turn stimulates the kidney to hold on to more calcium and excrete less in the urine. At the bone level, vitamin D appears to be a stimulator of bone and cartilage formation, helping with the actual mineralization of the collagen that is first laid down in new bone; how it interacts with osteoblasts in part determines how much bone mineral is lost in the elderly.

Estrogen: Estrogen inhibits bone breakdown. This hormone may also stimulate bone formation, but how and by just how much is not yet clear. Estrogen's effect almost certainly occurs at many levels. Estrogen receptors are present on both osteoclasts and osteoblasts, suggesting that estrogen directly affects all phases of bone remodeling. It may indirectly promote bone formation as well, for it makes bone cells less responsive to parathormone, and more sensitive to calcitonin. Estrogen inhibits the production of certain molecules by osteoblasts, such as interleukin-6, a cytokine that causes bone breakdown by stimulating an increase in bone-resorbing osteoclasts. Estrogen also promotes total body calcium by decreasing the loss of calcium through the kidneys and by enhancing the absorption of calcium in the small intestine, helping vitamin D to do its work better.

NORMAL BONES TO OSTEOPENIA TO OSTEOPOROSIS

As women age, their bone remodeling becomes less efficient—more minerals are lost from the bones than are kept in the bones. There are many reasons for this, all revolving around calcium. The stronger the bone, the more mineral reserves are built up through a lifetime of adequate calcium in the diet and proper metabolism of that calcium by the bones, so the less likely it is that this natural event of calcium loss will cause a dangerously low state of bone calcification.

Osteoporosis doesn't strike suddenly. A gradual change in bone metabolism leads to a silent exodus of calcium, making the bones "thinner." This silent thinning, called *osteopenia,* does no obvious damage— osteopenic bones are still strong enough to do their job and function well.

When bone loss marches on because of a growing imbalance between the rates of bone breakdown and buildup, there is a net calcium loss out of bone (efflux). We gradually begin to see critical levels of bone weakening, orchestrated by the signals coming from the changing hormonal soup that bathes the bones as women age. Critical or "threshold" weakening means that the bones readily fracture and become deformed in response to ordinary stresses. Not only do these feeble bones have dangerously low levels of calcium, but their architectural structure is altered. The microscopic bony spicules, or tiny islands of calcified tissue, that make up the bone become malformed, so that the skeleton becomes even less sturdy, out of proportion to the loss of mass or of calcium. This makes osteoporotic bone less efficient in handling normal weight bearing. This severe bone weakening and structural deformity of the bony scaffold is called *osteoporosis.*

In its early stages, osteoporosis can go unnoticed; but it continues to worsen slowly and sometimes imperceptibly over many years. Thus, different degrees of osteoporosis can be defined by the extent of bone loss, the level of distorted architecture, and the fractures and compression that grossly distort the skeleton. The acute fractures and the visible reshaping of a woman's skeleton, which come later in this debilitating disease, and the associated chronic pain are the most troublesome consequences.

OSTEOPOROSIS OVER A WOMAN'S LIFETIME

Many of us, deep down, believe that osteoporosis is a disease of old women, that we are immune, and that, by the time we reach the age at which it might strike us, surely "they" will have found a cure for it. Though it's possible such a scenario could prove true, I wouldn't count on it now. Many women reading these pages are at this very moment losing precious bone they may never recover yet surely at some point will very much want to have back.

Women set the stage for their own susceptibility to osteoporosis, for throughout their lives the bone remodeling process can be either hampered or enhanced. Any loss of bone that occurs will have an effect determined by the baseline sturdiness of the bone at the time the loss starts. If you start with denser bones, the same loss, whenever it occurs, will produce less weakening than if you start with thinner bones. Thus, building sturdy and strong bones in youth protects you from falling into the fracture zone when you face those inevitable times of bone loss later in life. That's why men, who have denser bones throughout life, if faced with comparable bone loss for whatever reason, handle it better than women.

The skeleton of an adult woman is lighter and smaller than a man's, and her bony pelvic cavity is wider to accommodate childbearing. The angulation of her outstretched arms (called *carrying angles*) is different from men's, possibly reflecting her need to hold her baby. These specific shape differences are not surprising if one realizes that, virtually all her life, a woman's bones are affected by the course of her reproductive life. The periods of greatest skeletal activity and remodeling for a woman are at puberty, during pregnancy, and at menopause.

YOUNG GIRLS

Throughout a woman's childhood, she builds more bone than she loses—provided she takes in sufficient calcium to foster healthy bone growth. We are only beginning to realize that the buildup of bone density and mass in adolescent girls sets the stage for healthier bones in adulthood, influencing the risk of osteoporosis later in life. Women's bones are close to their densest at the end of puberty. Thus, the years of puberty are critical to a woman's bones; good nutrition, adequate calcium intake, and sensible exercise during this period are all mandatory for normal development of the bony scaffold that will last her a lifetime.

YOUNG WOMEN THROUGH MIDDLE AGE

From the teen years on into the mid-thirties, bone resorption and bone deposition are in close balance, with an edge toward buildup. Bone density increases through age thirty-five, at which age a woman has her peak lifetime bone mass.

Pregnancy is a critical time for a woman's bony skeleton. The growing fetus sucks up lots of calcium and minerals from the mother. If her calcium intake is not adequate to sustain the calcium needs of the developing fetus, Mom is expendable: her bones will give up calcium for the fetus. Sometimes acute maternal osteopenia occurs, and even osteoporosis, with bone fractures. (If a woman has had high exposure to lead earlier in life and does not take adequate calcium during pregnancy, the efflux of calcium carries with it the stored lead, and harms the fetus. A woman who suspects she has been exposed to lead in the past must be especially tuned to keeping her calcium levels up during pregnancy, to avoid disturbing the stored lead. Since lead is stored in bone, blood tests will not tell you about past lead exposure.)

Even if no problems surface during pregnancy, an inadequate calcium supply in those months can diminish bone strength and set the stage for osteoporosis thirty or forty years later.

Normally, starting at about age thirty-five, women start to lose bone mass slowly—at the rate of about 1 percent per year. Although bone is still being remodeled and calcium still flows into bone, the balance shifts and more bone is broken down than is built up. This slow loss of bone mass holds steady through menopause (normally till around age fifty), when the pace picks up dramatically.

As you can see, after a certain point it becomes more difficult to strengthen your bones; the easiest time to do so is when you are under thirty-five and natural buildup is still occurring.

AGES FIFTY TO SEVENTY

With menopause, a woman's risk for osteoporosis is greatly increased; the sudden depletion of estrogen (and perhaps other hormones, including progesterone and testosterone) leads to a bone loss of between 3 and 5 percent for a period of at least ten years after menopause. One reason for this is the increased loss of calcium in the urine, in response to low estrogen. There is also a small decrease in the ability of the intestines to absorb calcium. Lack of estrogen also promotes osteoclastic destruction of bone, an effect that cannot be overcome by just taking in more calcium.

Thus, before age sixty most women see more than 25 percent of loss of bone mass. After that age the loss slows, but by the time some women reach seventy their bone mass may be down as much as 50 percent from age thirty-five. By their mid-fifties, the bone mass of some women starts to fall below the fracture threshold (the level of bone mass, determined by researchers, below which your chance of getting a fracture rises dramatically, as measured by special bone-density-scanning techniques; see pages 432–33); by their mid-seventies, almost all women have fallen to that threshold level.

All these numbers underscore one important message: the sturdiness of a woman's bone structure and density of her bones at menopause in large part determine the extent to which she tolerates the inevitable "hit" of declining bone mass that is triggered by that change of life.

AGE SEVENTY AND BEYOND

After age seventy, even though the rate of bone loss proceeds more slowly, the structure of the remodeled bone becomes deficient. Vitamin-D-aided calcium absorption by the intestines becomes even less efficient. Other reasons for the slow but continuous loss of bone in these later years are the declining levels of certain androgenic hormones made by our adrenal glands—hormones that tend to build up bone and muscle. Also, as we move into our sixties and seventies we see a general decline in skeletal muscle mass and strength, which makes us even more frail and susceptible to falls and therefore to bone fractures.

OSTEOPOROTIC BONE FRACTURES

Most of us take our bones for granted, especially when we are young. Bone fractures in kids, often resulting from sporting accidents, are taken with light humor. Friends ceremoniously sign the cast; its removal is cause for celebration. But those are healthy young bones, and they mend quickly. The story is not so cute when the underlying architecture of the bone is damaged and the fracture is the symbol of a crumbling scaffold that will never again be restored.

Osteoporotic fractures can develop without much notice, or can occur dramatically. A compression fracture of the spinal vertebrae may arrive without symptoms, or may be marked by a sudden back pain, which can continue over many weeks and be excruciating, ultimately causing a loss of height and, over time, the development of a C-shaped spinal deformity known as a dowager's hump. Sometimes the first sign of osteoporosis is the more definitive broken wrist or hip, fractured by an impact that earlier in life would have caused no more than a bruise.

With severe osteoporosis, a fracture can be caused by slipping on a carpet at home, lifting a bag of groceries, being bumped too hard on the bus, coughing vigorously, or even turning over in bed. In these simple and seemingly mundane ways, approximately 15 percent of women in this country will sustain broken hips, about the same number will break their wrists, and more will fracture their spines.

Most osteoporotic fractures occur in the spongy trabecular bone, such as the ribs and the spine and near the joints of the long bones (such as the hip and the wrists), for it is in this part of the bone that the loss of minerals is most dramatic.

Fracture susceptibility can usually be predicted by just how much bone mass is present in any given bone—how *dense* the bone is, in terms of how much calcium it contains. Since women spend about half of their adult life hovering around the fracture threshold, and men rarely hit that threshold before the age of eighty, it is not at all surprising that fractures are more common in women.

RISK FACTORS
....

Some women are at greater hereditary risk for osteoporosis than others, and all of us face the concrete risks that the estrogen depletion of menopause and the weakened bone metabolism of age bring. None-theless, for each of us, the occurrence and course of osteoporosis are very much determined by our earlier lives and the kind of lifelong risks that we have exposed ourselves to. In brief, whether you realize your full genetically determined maximum bone mass, and therefore have a storehouse of calcium in your bones to draw upon when the inevitable leaching of calcium ensues, is determined very much by what you do or don't do throughout your lifetime.

MENOPAUSE

Menopause, at whatever age it occurs, is a critical turning point for a woman's bones. The most common form of osteoporosis, type I osteo-porosis, comes with menopause, occurring, as we've seen, because of the drop in estrogen. Although all women go through menopause and will experience bone loss at that time, only some will lose enough bone to cause them to lose strength and fracture. (Men, who produce high levels of testosterone virtually their entire lives, have continuous hor-monal protection for their bones and do not face this midlife bone crunch.)

AGE

Beyond age seventy, both men and women develop similar abnormalities in bone metabolism (including impaired calcium absorption and a de-crease in the conversion of vitamin D to its active form), which cause a slow loss of bone year by year. Age-related osteoporosis, type II, is associated with the thinning of both trabecular and cortical bone, leading to fractures of the hip and vertebrae.

Again, bone density studies show that, even with age-related loss of bone mass, the vast majority of men do not even begin to get close to the fracture threshold before their mid-eighties, and many have not lost sufficient bone mass to hit this level even by age one hundred. Be-cause women start out with less sturdy bones and lower bone density than men, they can tolerate the slow age-related bone loss far less. Given the combination of menopausal effects and age effects, virtually no woman reaches her eightieth birthday without having fallen below the fracture threshold.

GENES

Using twin studies, Dr. C. Conrad Johnston and his colleagues from Indiana University have shown that genes determine the maximum level of bone mass that an individual's skeleton can achieve. We've always known that your body type, which includes your skeleton—such as whether you are heavy-boned or light-boned—is hereditary, and we know that small, thin-boned women start out at greater risk for this disease. Osteoporosis runs in families, and if your grandmother, mother, or sister has been affected, you are more likely to suffer from it as well.

It has been suspected that the genetic control comes in part through calcium and vitamin D metabolism. This suspicion got strong support from a 1994 study from Australia that identified a single vitamin D receptor gene which correlates directly with bone mass. Studying families, including twins with different forms of the genes, Drs. John Eisman and Nigel Morrison and their colleagues at St. Vincent's Hospital in Sydney were able to predict differences in density of bone in the spine and femur of more than five hundred pre- and post-menopausal women based on the particular form of the vitamin D receptor gene they had inherited. Although this finding does not explain all types of osteoporosis, it does show that there are genetic factors contributing to variation in bone density among people and groups. It also points us toward a possible cause of osteoporosis—namely, a differing effect of vitamin D's interaction with the cells that regulate bone turnover, and ultimately, bone density.

Though your maximum bone mass is to a certain extent determined for you, the actions you choose to take determine whether or not you will achieve that maximum. It is quite possible that the maximum bone mass even of a woman who has inherited "light" bones is sufficient to protect her from osteoporosis, but she must take especially great care throughout her life to maintain that maximum mass.

RACE

Caucasian and Asian women are the most susceptible to osteoporosis (particularly fairer-skinned women from Northern Europe, the British Isles, and Japan). Black women are far less likely to develop osteoporosis, and throughout life generally have greater bone density. It has been estimated that white women over age sixty currently live with twice as many broken bones as black women.

A word of caution here, however. Although darker-skinned women have less risk, they still face this disease as they get older, and must assess their own personal vulnerability to it, including family history, diet, hormonal status, and exercise.

HORMONAL HISTORY

Young women who have amenorrhea or some types of abnormal menstrual cycles (such as having a shortened luteal phase; see page 101), or menstrual cycles without ovulation altogether, have been shown to develop bone loss. This is true also for those women who interrupt their normal menstrual cycles through excessive exercise. Women with menstrual abnormalities that prolong the luteal phase have increased bone density. Dr. Susan Thys-Jacobs and her colleagues from Columbia Presbyterian Medical Center in New York have recently shown that women with premenstrual syndrome (PMS) have a lower bone density than those without PMS, suggesting a relationship between PMS, bone loss, and abnormal calcium metabolism. (Some researchers claim that calcium supplements help symptoms of PMS.) As mentioned throughout this book, for postmenopausal women whether they have been on estrogen replacement therapy, and for how long, very much affects their osteoporosis risk.

ANOREXIA AND BULIMIA

We hear a lot about bulimia and anorexia nervosa, but we don't often hear about the toll these common problems can take on a woman's bones. For at least three reasons, chronic eating disorders set the stage for poor bone health in the years to come. First is the likely deficiency of calcium and vitamin D in the diet. Second is the amenorrhea that typically accompanies the starving state and leads to the loss of the protective effects of estrogen on bone. Finally, the state of increased stress these young women experience is invariably associated with increased levels of the steroid stress hormone cortisol, which causes bones to demineralize.

Anorexia and bulimia frequently continue for many years unrecognized and undetected, typically during a crucial age for the buildup of bone. As these problems erode a young woman's psychological well-being, they also silently erode the future health of her bones.

CIGARETTE SMOKING

Although we know a lot about the many hazards of smoking, one risk we don't hear much about is osteoporosis. Smoking decreases circulating levels of estrogen in premenopausal women and may affect the way estrogen functions in the body. Some research suggests that smoking decreases calcium absorption by directly affecting vitamin D metabolism. Chronic smokers also have earlier menopause—by as much as two years—and earlier menopause means more years of bone loss.

DIET AND NUTRITION

Intake of calcium and vitamin D is crucial to bone health throughout life, so obviously a generally imbalanced diet low in foods containing calcium is a risk factor for osteoporosis. A diet very high in fiber can impair calcium absorption, so that the body takes in less than is eaten. High-salt diets and carbonated drinks increase urinary excretion of calcium. Excessive caffeine decreases absorption of calcium by the gut and may also increase calcium loss in the urine. Dr. Robert Heaney and his group have shown that typical daily amounts of caffeine (two to three cups of coffee a day) cause little calcium loss in women, and even this may be compensated for by drinking an extra glass of milk per day—or café au lait.

ALCOHOL USE

Alcohol, in regular or excessive use, is toxic to bone. It impairs calcium and vitamin D absorption, and in the laboratory inhibits function of the bone-building cells, osteoblasts. Women who drink three alcoholic drinks per day are at greater risk for osteoporosis than those who drink less. Furthermore, women alcoholics are more likely to have osteoporosis, although this connection may be due in part to the poor diet, smoking, and limited exercise that often accompany alcoholism. There is also some information that moderate use of alcohol may be associated with loss of bone mass in older women. Thus, women who drink even occasionally should be sure they consume adequate calcium in their diets.

SEDENTARY LIFESTYLE

Being a couch potato is another risk factor for weak, osteoporotic bones. We know that bedridden patients of any age lose bone mass, an inadvertent negative consequence of old-fashioned medicine (which prescribed bed rest for almost any illness, sometimes for weeks on end). If your arm or leg is in a cast for several weeks, bone loss occurs. Women with sedentary lifestyles, getting little or no exercise, are also more likely to contract osteoporosis than those who engage in regular exercise and lead more physically active lives.

ABSENCE OF GRAVITY

Without the forces of gravity, our bones would eventually turn into rubber. Since astronauts who go into the weightless environment of space rapidly lose bone mass, in proportion to the length of time they spend in space, bone loss is one of the limiting factors for any long-term life for humans in space in the next century. Most of the bone loss American astronauts have encountered during short-term space flights has reversed itself when the astronauts returned to earth, but information from the Russian space program, where longer space flights were routine, suggests that there well may be a point of no return.

More and more women are going into space for weeks at a time. It remains to be seen what the long-term effects will be on these women's bone health, and whether or not they show more bone deterioration than men over time. Should women who are in the accelerated bone absorption phase of menopause avoid spending any time in space? We do not know, but if space stations or trips to Mars are in our future, this will be a crucial health issue to settle up front.

MEDICINES

Certain medicines can cause bone loss, in some cases severe enough to cause osteoporosis in men as well as women. One of the more common of such medications is steroid hormones, such as prednisone or cortisone, which decrease osteoblast function, decrease calcium absorption from the gut, and increase urinary excretion of calcium. Similar effects are seen with the anticoagulant heparin; certain diuretics; lithium, used in manic-depressive illness; and the antibiotic tetracycline. Some patients with epilepsy have been noted to develop abnormally low levels of vitamin D, suggesting that their medicines, such as dilantin, may also cause osteoporosis. Excess thyroid hormone, which is sometimes inappropriately ingested for weight control, will cause loss of bone mass. When any of these drugs are given for only a short time, there need be little concern. But if they are administered for years, or a lifetime, examining their effect on bone health becomes more of an issue.

A special note about thiazide diuretics, the gentle and inexpensive water pills (see page 405). They are one medicine that favors your bones. Thiazide diuretics have been shown to cause an *increase* in calcium retention by the body, unlike many other diuretics. Although no one is recommending that a woman take thiazide diuretics for bone health, perhaps they should be the diuretic of choice for any woman who needs them for her heart or blood pressure.

BODY WEIGHT

Thinness is a risk factor for osteoporosis, and increased body weight seems protective. It has been said that you can never be too thin or too rich. Very thin women, however, are at risk for osteoporosis as they get older, and the affliction does not make for a rich quality of life. This of course does not mean that obesity is good. The benefit of weight with regard to osteoporosis risk peaks at 10 percent over normal body weight.

RISK FACTOR MYTHS

For years medical folklore taught us that certain risk factors, like breast-feeding, being blond, or using antacids, predisposed women to osteoporosis. None of these findings have been borne out by large-scale studies.

DIAGNOSIS

Because so often the illness comes under no one domain of medical specialties, diagnosis of osteoporosis often falls between the cracks. Orthopedic surgeons are what we generally mean when we say "bone doctors," yet they mainly deal with broken bones and see women who are well along into their disease, with the first fracture. Rheumatologists specialize in joints but mainly focus on the autoimmune diseases, such as arthritis and lupus. Endocrinologists specialize in body metabolism in general and are often the ones who deal with osteoporosis, although the disease is more than an endocrine problem. Physical therapists and physiatrists deal with locomotion and any mobility impairment after osteoporosis has caused disability. To piece all this together, a woman needs a good generalist—an internist, a gynecologist, or a primary-care physician—who has experience in dealing with osteoporosis patients or can refer her to a specialist for ongoing care.

Diagnosis starts with a good history and physical examination. Complaints of bone pain, loss of height, or changes in posture are reviewed. Family history is important. Your doctor will routinely make a general assessment of long-term calcium intake and overall nutrition, and go over any and all medications. In the physical examination, your doctor will look at stature and carriage and spine curvature, and will measure your height for future reference. But most of these questions and maneuvers are part of any routine physical exam.

LABORATORY STUDIES

If your doctor suspects osteoporosis, he or she will ask you to undergo certain blood tests to measure the amount of calcium in your blood, your estrogen levels, and certain molecules such as osteocalcin (a marker of osteoblastic activity) and bone-specifric alkaline phosphatase (an enzyme that is part of bone building). Your physician may also test your thyroid and parathyroid functions, and vitamin D levels. Your urine will be tested, to see how much calcium is lost by the kidneys and to check the activity of bone turnover through urine levels of hydroxyproline and pyridinoline (molecules that come from the breakdown of bone).

None of the above tests provides, however, the crucial information for diagnosing osteoporosis—bone density. Bone density measurements can predict whether a woman is nearing a dangerous point in the weakening of her bone strength, and which women with osteoporosis are at greatest risk for developing fractures. Even a routine X ray of bone cannot detect osteoporosis until loss of bone mass exceeds 25 to 30 percent.

MEASURING BONE DENSITY—
A NEW MUST FOR ALL WOMEN

Definitive techniques are now available for measuring bone mass—and this recent technology stands to save hundreds of thousands of women from osteoporosis's most severe agonies. These technologies are not yet widely available or in general use—but I (and the National Osteoporosis Foundation) believe they must be made routine for all women, and soon, for both assessment and guidance in prevention and therapy. Bone density studies can detect osteopenia, and even the modest decreases that can heighten the risk of fracture. If a woman is prepared to take action in response to the findings, and to embark on such interventions as diet, perhaps hormone replacement, exercise, and other medications, I believe it is valuable to determine her bone density at a few critical points in her life. Just as we modify diet or medication in an individual patient in response to a blood pressure reading or cholesterol levels, we should do so in response to bone mineral content measures—before osteopenia has become osteoporosis, before osteoporosis has become a fracture.

Bone density measurements all involve radiological study of different parts of the skeleton (and as such are generally restricted to women past childbearing age). The tests are noninvasive, based on the simple principle that denser tissue absorbs more radiation than does less dense tissue. Trabecular bone is less dense than cortical bone; tests for osteoporosis most often study the vulnerable sites for fracture—namely, the spine, the hip, and the wrist.

The several different techniques to measure bone density vary mostly by the particular site of the skeleton measured, the radiation exposure, and the time and expense the study requires. All methods involve "absorptiometry"—that is, a measure of the amount of radiation taken up or absorbed by the bone being scanned.

Single photon absorptiometry (SPA): SPA was developed in the early 1960s by Drs. John Cameron and James Sorenson from the University of Wisconsin, as the first method to measure bone mineral density directly, and for years it was used mostly in research. It is still the easiest, cheapest, and most available. Because only a single beam of X ray is used, however, interference from other tissues creates problems, so the test is best applied to parts of the skeleton that have little surrounding tissue, such as the heel of the foot or the wrist. SPA does not tell you much about the hips or spine.

Dual photon absorptiometry (DPA): DPA was developed specifically to study the hips and spine. In this approach, low-dose gamma radiation is used, to measure the absorption of radiant energy and produce an image of the bone. This test measures total skeletal bone mass as well as providing targeted information at specific sites such as the spine and the hips. DPA does not allow for precise analysis of mineral content per gram of tissue, so that comparisons of studies taken over time are less reliable. The test takes about thirty minutes.

Quantitative computed tomography (QCT) involves CAT scanning, a technique that is widely used for all kinds of body imaging, not just bone. This test provides "slices" through layers of bone, producing a three-dimensional image of the bone and also allowing an assessment of total bone mass. QCT can distinguish cortical from trabecular bone and precisely image any bone in the body. Its major drawbacks are that it involves the most radiation exposure of all bone density procedures and is the most expensive.

Dual X-Ray Absorptiometry (DEXA) is now the state-of-the-art and preferred technique for bone density measurement. It is relatively inexpensive—about the same as a mammogram (one or two hundred dollars) and is becoming more widely available. In time it will likely supplant the other approaches. Among its advantages are the use of extremely low doses of radiation (a small fraction of the exposure of one chest X ray, and about equivalent to the exposure from an airplane trip from New York to California); its capacity to measure all needed sites, including the hips and spine; its rapidity (it takes only a few minutes to scan three or four sites); and its ability to produce clear images, diagnose early disease, and monitor the efficacy of treatment. Unfortunately, because the equipment is new, it is not available in all medical centers.

TREATMENT

The treatment of osteoporosis is dictated by how advanced the disease has become. The goals of treatment are threefold: to prevent more bone loss, hoping for some increase in bone mass as well; to treat the pain; and to devise lifestyle changes that will minimize fracture risk. The mother of all treatments has turned out to be—you guessed it— estrogen.

ESTROGEN

In the 1940s, the prominent Harvard physician Dr. Fuller Albright noted that young women who had undergone hysterectomy with ovary removal developed osteoporosis. He then surmised that these patients' calcium balance had been disturbed by the loss of ovarian hormones and could be restored by treating them with estrogen. Without any way to measure bone density, however, it was impossible to prove any treatment benefit, and estrogen treatment continued to be seen as just a way to keep women "feminine," not necessarily healthy.

Finally, in the late 1960s, a group of Scottish physicians including Drs. Robert Lindsay, David Hart, and Mark Aitken were able to provide more definitive proof. Using the then available bone density measurement (SPA) to study the effect of estrogen treatment on women who had had their ovaries removed and compare them with similar women not getting estrogen replacement, they were able to show that after five years of estrogen therapy the bone density was normal, while it fell dramatically in the nontreated group. At first, that observation didn't make much of an impact. But when, in 1980, the same treatment group was still free of fractures, vertebral compression, and loss of height, the news became hot. And since that time there has been a relentless stream of information coming from all over the world showing the treatment benefits of estrogen to women at risk for or suffering from osteoporosis.

Today, estrogen replacement therapy is the most effective way to interrupt the march of osteoporosis throughout our bones. Arresting or slowing the process of postmenopausal osteoporosis at any stage has benefit, at least up to age seventy-five.

Moreover, there is growing evidence that estrogen will also *increase* bone density—thereby, to some degree, reversing the forward motion of the disease. In recent studies, women up to age seventy-five who had osteoporosis associated with at least one bone fracture showed an increase in bone mineral density of the spine and extremities when treated with estrogen (either alone or in combination with progesterone) and a fracture rate approximately one-third lower compared to those not treated. Invariably, estrogen is most effective when combined with an adequate intake of calcium, which for postmenopausal women with osteoporosis should be at least 1,000 mg, and ideally 1,500 mg, per day. (The general belief is that calcium intake for all ages should not exceed 2,500 mg per day.)

The benefits of initiating estrogen treatment among women over eighty are not known, but most researchers are skeptical. This is the fastest-growing part of our population, however, and one that is often left out of clinical research. The truth is that we don't have the facts for them.

What must be remembered is that estrogen exerts its beneficial effect on the bone only while the hormone is being taken. Many women take estrogen for a short time to relieve the symptoms of menopause. If we women are to get the benefit for our bones (and hearts), estrogen must be taken long-term—a minimum of seven to ten years, studies have shown, but probably longer, since once the estrogen is stopped the bone mass starts to diminish just as at the time of menopause.

Unfortunately, long-term use entails risk: many clinical studies have shown that estrogen replacement therapy is associated with a small increase in the risk of breast cancer after ten years of use (see chapter 5). Weighing this against the risk of osteoporosis is tricky indeed, and must be based on your own personal health history and a thoughtful and informed discussion with your doctor. (For example, for a fair-skinned, thin-boned woman of Northern European extraction without a family history of breast cancer, the pluses for estrogen to protect bones are strong; for an athletic woman of African-American descent with a strong family history of breast cancer, the pluses are not so clear.)

We still don't know how to get the most bone-building benefit from estrogen with the least risk. We don't know, for example, which form of estrogen works most effectively: the patch or the pill; or which dosage, or in combination with which other hormones; or what schedule or regimen is best. (Some of this information will come with the PEPI trial and the Women's Health Initiative described on page 193.) All women, and their doctors, should be reevaluating regularly the decision to take estrogen, and in what form and dose, as new options and information become available.

CALCITONIN

Calcitonin is the only medication besides estrogen currently approved by the FDA for the prevention and treatment of osteoporosis. As it is commonly available (derived from salmon, or manufactured in a synthetic human form), calcitonin has its limits: it requires injection and is expensive. Unlike estrogen, calcitonin primarily affects bone directly, inhibiting the bone-destroying osteoclasts. There is reason to believe that calcitonin might augment estrogen's good effect on bone, and vice versa. Calcitonin, like estrogen, must be taken along with enough calcium supplementation to assure at least 1,500 mg of total daily calcium intake.

Calcitonin has another important but not fully understood effect: it decreases bone pain without having a narcotic effect on the brain. Bone pain is among the most difficult to treat, and spinal fractures can be excruciatingly painful and intractable. One theory of why calcitonin provides pain relief is that it locally activates the body's own natural opiates, the endorphins. Although the response is not universal, when it works calcitonin can be impressive and powerful.

Side effects include flushing, dizziness, nausea, and diarrhea, but its most distressing limitation is that it loses effectiveness after eighteen to twenty-four months, so that it cannot provide that decade or more of prevention needed after menopause, when bone loss is most rapid. We do not know why calcitonin self-destructs—perhaps because antibodies are developed to the commonly used salmon calcitonin, or because calcitonin receptors on bone sites become less sensitive to the extra stimulation of the hormone over time.

A calcitonin nasal spray is available in Europe and South America, but is not approved for use in the United States. Early clinical studies have shown that the nasal form of calcitonin may have fewer side effects than the injected medication, and it is surely easier for an older person to manage. An FDA panel approved the nasal spray in late 1994, but it is not yet released for general use by the FDA.

BISPHOSPHONATES: NOT YET FOR USE IN THE UNITED STATES

We have so little available in the way of treatment for existing osteoporosis that it seems to me a crime that a promising class of drugs, the *bisphosphonates* (or diphosphonates), are withheld from women in the United States. On the market abroad, these drugs are inexpensive and readily available worldwide. They work directly on bone to inhibit its breakdown, but also inhibit bone mineralization. Because they block calcium buildup in bones, they are given only intermittently—usually two weeks out of every three months. The bisphosphonates have been shown in many studies to increase bone density and also bone strength (but so far in the short term—that is, two years or less). Some have been demonstrated, in both the United States and Europe, to decrease the rate of fractures dramatically—including spinal fractures—in patients with known osteoporosis; in some studies, the fracture rate has been cut in half. The drugs are orally administered and engender very few side effects.

The best studied of these is *etidronate* (*Didronel*), which has been in use for some time for the treatment of other bone conditions and therefore is sold in the United States—but only for these other conditions. Similar drugs also not yet approved for treatment of osteoporosis include *pamidronate, tiludronate, alendronate,* and *clodronate.*

A new approach, called cyclical treatment, combines ediotronate with calcium and vitamin D in sequence. The treatment attempts to mimic the remodeling behavior of normal bones. Ediotronate is administered for two weeks to limit bone breakdown; then comes thirteen weeks of vitamin D (400 IU) and calcium (500 mg), matching the twelve- to thirteen-week period normally required for new bone to be laid down and mineralized. So far a few studies have been promising, and we need to look for further information.

The lingering concern in this country, which has led to regulatory

STUDIES TO WATCH FOR

On the horizon are different forms of bisphosphonates, which may resolve the concern about hampered bone mineralization. Clinical studies of one such agent, alendronate (Fosamax), *show that it inhibits bone resorption selectively without inhibiting bone mineralization, so that it can therefore be given continuously. Preliminary work suggests that this drug may remain effective beyond two years. On the market in Mexico and Europe, it is now in review in the United States.*

A major trial is being conducted at eleven clinical centers throughout the country, looking at Fosamax in women from fifty-five to eighty-nine years of age. Called the Fracture Intervention Trial (FIT), it is studying vertebral deformity and fracture rate in almost sixty-five hundred women, with a long follow-up period—approximately four years. The results of FIT, the largest treatment-controlled clinical trial ever undertaken for osteoporosis, are not likely to be available before 1997.

delay, is whether, in the long run, these drugs will block mineralization of any new bone that is forming and may lead to more, not fewer fractures. I personally find the delay troublesome. Since not all women can take estrogen or calcitonin, bisphosphonates offer great promise for women with established osteoporosis, like my mother-in-law. It seems to me a patient in her tenth decade should be given access to such drugs on an expedited basis. Whether to use them should be her and her doctor's choice. There are many other models of fast-tracking approvals—such as many AIDS drugs—because of personal and humanistic imperatives.

SODIUM FLUORIDE:
ALSO NOT IN THE UNITED STATES

Sodium fluoride is great for keeping teeth strong and sturdy and cavity-free. Why not use it to keep sturdy bones? Though it has never been approved for use here, this therapy is popular in Europe. Fluoride has been shown to bind to trabecular bone (within the spine in particular), stimulate new bone formation, and increase bone mass by as much as 30 to 35 percent. Sodium fluoride is not approved for use here, mainly because of a 1990 study done by the NIH that showed that sodium fluoride, even if it increased bone mass, did not decrease spinal fracture rate, and may have increased the fracture rate of long bones in the first year of use. From this study, researchers extrapolated that the benefit may come at the expense of cortical bone, and that the new bone may be denser but more brittle. Critics of the study, however, have pointed out that the dose of fluoride used was too high (75 mg or more per day), and given in the wrong form, and that at three years of use fracture rates *did* fall. Also, fluoride must be given with carefully monitored calcium treatment at high enough doses so that new bone growth in the spine does not come at the expense of calcium loss from the bones elsewhere in the body.

One recent study, published in 1994 by Dr. Charles Y. C. Pak and colleagues from the Southwestern Medical Center in Dallas, showed that using a *lower* dose of sodium fluoride (25 mg, slow release, twice a day) for twelve months followed by a two-month rest during which 800 mg of calcium is taken daily continuously is highly beneficial to bone: lower-dose sodium fluoride is associated with cutting the spinal fracture rate in half and increasing bone density by as much as 5 percent per year in postmenopausal women with osteoporosis. Their findings also suggest a small increase in hipbone density, and no adverse effect—that is, decrease in bone mass or increased fracture rate of the long bones. The lower doses of sodium fluoride are also associated with fewer side effects (those remaining include nausea and vomiting). This and other studies using fluoride consistently found that fracture rate invariably fell when bone mass increased, conforming to the likely benefit of this medication.

Despite the controversy in the United States, and the fact that this treatment is not FDA-approved (the medicine has no proprietary protection and is fairly inexpensive, so there are no great industrial champions to get it approved), sodium fluoride still has a following in Europe and among many bone researchers in this country. In the face of this enormous and growing public health need, I believe the NIH should take the lead and invest in getting the answers.

WEIGHT-BEARING EXERCISE: GRANDMOTHERS PUMPING IRON?

Bones are strengthened by exercise. Almost any kind of exercise that is weight-bearing—that is, working against the forces of gravity—will benefit bones (more about this on page 444). Weight-bearing exercise includes aerobics, bicycling, stair climbing, walking, jumping rope, or using exercise equipment graded for exercise level. All exercise should begin and end with some kind of stretching of the arms, legs, and back. As for swimming, although it may not be as effective as a weight-bearing exercise, I favor it, especially for women with osteoporosis. Because it is "low-impact," swimming is safe for those with more fragile bones and even a history of fractures, and is a good way to stretch and use large-muscle groups.

What has not been clear until very recently, however, is whether exercise is an independent treatment for rebuilding bone in postmenopausal women who have lost bone mass, or whether it serves only to prevent the disease from developing. Fortunately, there is growing evidence that, even for postmenopausal women with some bone deterioration, exercise can rebuild bone—it's not too late.

In a randomized study reported in December 1994 of sedentary women up to the age of seventy averaging ten years postmenopause (who had not been treated with hormone replacement therapy), one year of regular strength-training exercises unequivocally benefited bone. Drs. Miriam Nelson, Maria Fiatarone, and others from Tufts University showed that mineral bone density of both the hip and spine were *increased* among strength-trained women, as compared with their sedentary sisters, in whom bone density decreased over the same period. The exercise protocol included high-intensity dynamic exercise (contractions against resistance, with extensions and flexions of designed muscle groups) of the back, abdomen, hips, and knees, using sports health equipment for forty-five minutes twice a week, each session preceded by warm-up periods of five minutes of cycling and five minutes of stretching. Women were advised to increase calcium intake, and both exercise and nonexercise groups averaged about 1,000 mg of calcium per day; none were on estrogen replacement or other drugs known to increase bone mass. Also excluded were women with advanced osteoporosis, more than one crush fracture of the spine, or any fracture elsewhere in the body.

Over the one year of the study, the exercise group increased their bone density by about 1 percent, whereas the sedentary control group decreased their bone density by about 2.5 percent. Also, muscle strength and balance were increased dramatically in the exercise group, as was their overall physical activity. This particular study is important, since it tells us that, at least for women up to the age of seventy, regular weight-bearing exercise not only prevents further bone loss but actually builds up bone in those who have already faced postmenopausal bone loss and in some cases early osteoporotic spinal compression. It is important to remember, however, that other studies have shown that any gains are lost if exercise is stopped!

CALCIUM

The message is simple. If you are postmenopausal and not taking estrogens and invariably in the throes of some bone loss, you should be taking 1,500 mg of calcium per day, indefinitely. Although this will not by itself build up bone, it will help to diminish bone loss. If you are postmenopausal and taking estrogen, your calcium level should be at least 1,000 mg per day. (See page 443 for specific prevention recommendations.)

TREATING PATIENTS WITH PAST AND PRESENT OSTEOPOROTIC FRACTURES

The first step in treating any osteoporotic fracture is to prevent it from happening in the first place. To this end, treatment of osteoporosis must include counseling about avoiding situations that are apt to lead to fractures. You should be clearly advised on how to prevent falls by eliminating any risks in your local environment, such as poor lighting, slippery floors, or poorly secured rugs. Installing railings or other hand supports and arranging furniture to eliminate obstacles are simple bone-saving actions.

Avoiding fractures also means eliminating activities that might overstress fragile bones, including the seemingly simple tasks of daily living such as lifting a mattress or vacuuming or going out on an icy sidewalk. It means, if you're slim, wearing hip pads when you venture out on uncarpeted terrain. It means employing good sense in identifying and rejecting exercise or recreational activities that present high risk for bone damage. And it does *not* mean being sedentary, but might just mean substituting swimming for skiing, or walking in the temperature-controlled and well-lit shopping mall rather than jogging on the sidewalk in your neighborhood. I think all postmenopausal women need to be sensitive to these precautions and reconsider them year by year. How far you need take them depends on your age, your risk factors, and an assessment of your own bone health as determined by your doctor.

If a fracture develops, the goal at the outset is to fix it so that locomotion is restored. Of all the fracture risks a woman faces, broken hips are the worst, often requiring a major operation with pinning or hip replacement, and a long convalescence in which the patient is bedridden—and thus potentially losing bone. Full recovery is seen in only half of the women who suffer osteoporotic hip fracture; some end up in long-term care or with markedly reduced mobility.

Compression fractures of the spine are treated with pain medication and bed rest for about two weeks. Even when healed, the distortion in back structure is a source of chronic pain, all too often requiring chronic medication. Wrist fractures are set in casts and take about six weeks to heal. They usually heal well and allow good recovery of hand use.

Any fracture in a postmenopausal woman is a red flag that she may well have osteoporosis, and this underlying condition must be addressed. As more therapies come along with the promise of restoring bone density and preventing future fractures, it behooves any doctor to think in terms of future prevention as well as treatment when confronted with an osteoporotic fracture—and any woman to take quick and clear preventive action.

STUDIES TO WATCH FOR

The National Institute of Aging and the National Institute of Arthritis and Metabolic Diseases of the NIH have recently initiated a major clinical research effort focusing on understanding and treating osteoporosis in people sixty-five and over. Called STOP/IT, Sites Testing Osteoporosis Prevention Intervention Treatments, the program includes separate interventions tested at different sites around the country. One site is looking at the effect of different kinds of exercise on hipbone density and fracture rate. Another is analyzing the impact of vitamin D and calcium; another is evaluating estrogen and progesterone in older women; and yet another is looking at testosterone replacement in older men in nursing homes who are testosterone-deficient. Also being studied are the fundamental mechanisms that lead to bone loss, and factors that are unique to the elderly population with regard to responding to treatments. Results from STOP/IT will be available by 1996.

The Women's Health Initiative (see page 10) will also provide a vast amount of information about osteoporosis in women fifty and beyond from a broad spectrum of socioeconomic, ethnic, and racial groups. This study will look at the effects of diet, exercise, hormone replacement therapy, and vitamin D and calcium supplements on the development of osteoporosis. Why some women are especially susceptible and others seem uniquely resistant will also be explored. The large number of patients, representing a cross section of American women, will provide invaluable information on risk profiles for women of different backgrounds, along with more specific information on risks and benefits of different interventions in different populations. The WHI will lay the groundwork for molecular and genetic studies that may eventually target more specifically the patients most likely to be helped by selected treatments.

PREVENTION

Prevention of osteoporosis is a lifelong task, in our and our daughters' hands. Since in its early phase osteoporosis is silent, every young woman should take steps to ensure her bone health. Although it is far easier to think about osteoporosis when we reach midlife and start feeling some creaks in our bones, we must capture the interest and imagination of young girls and young women. The message to all is simple but demands interest, initiative, and personal engagement: diet, exercise, and hormones make up the formula for the prevention of osteoporosis.

ESTROGEN

Although it is as a means of treating, not preventing, osteoporosis that estrogen therapy has been heralded, there is now unequivocal evidence that estrogen can in fact prevent the disease. Numerous studies have shown that women undergoing hormone replacement therapy after menopause markedly decrease their chances of getting a bone fracture. According to one study, the chance of getting a compression fracture of the spine—the major culprit in spinal deformities—could be reduced by 90 percent with HRT. Another study documented the fact that the combination of estrogen and progesterone is as effective as estrogen alone, also substantially reducing the chance of getting a broken hip. Remember, however, that, as in treatment, such beneficial effects are seen only if the estrogenic hormone is taken for close to ten years and in a dose of 0.625 mg/day.

CALCIUM AND VITAMIN D

Most American women, regardless of age, have a calcium-deficient diet. Young girls and adult women average somewhere between 400 and 600 mg of calcium intake per day, when in reality a woman should consume at least 1,000 mg of calcium per day, and as she goes through menopause and beyond (and when pregnant or nursing) her intake should increase to about 1,500 mg. Our entrenched pattern of eating was based on a prevailing attitude that extra calcium was only for kids with developing bones. We now know better.

Since it is very hard to consume this much calcium in a regular adult diet—it would take five glasses of milk or three to four yogurts per day—supplements make sense. Moreover, several studies have now shown that taking supplemental calcium of 1,000 mg over and above what is already in the diet slows bone loss in the hips, extremities, and the spine. The effectiveness of calcium intake may be increased by also taking vitamin D supplements of 400–800 IU per day, for vitamin D improves absorption of calcium by the body. (Again, we do not recommend exceeding 2,500 mg of calcium per day, but it would in any case be difficult to ingest this amount on a regular basis.)

The kind of calcium that one ingests is also important. It should meet USP standards as indicated by a mark that is on the label. Calcium carbonate is generally preferred, since it dissolves the most readily (and is also less costly, because the amount of calcium per tablet is higher). Calcium citrate malate is another form of calcium considered by some experts like Dr. Beth Dawson-Hughes to be as good as or better than calcium carbonate as a supplement for postmenopausal women.

One easy way to get calcium is to take Tums antacid tablets (TUMS-500), but chronic use of any antacid can disrupt your own level of stomach acid. Another option is to take two tablets of OS-Cal 500 per day or calcium-fortified orange juice in which one eight-ounce glass gives you about 300 mg. It is best to take the calcium in divided doses over the course of the day, if possible, but absorption seems to be the best when calcium is taken at night, before bed, so that is the preferred time. Since bone-building activity peaks in the night, that is when you want to have plenty of calcium available.

One should not forget, however, that supplements are just that— supplements to your diet. You should be sure to include in your regular diet a variety of foods naturally rich in calcium, including skim milk, with 300 mg of calcium per 8-ounce glass; yogurt, with more than 400 mg per 8 ounces; and mozzarella and ricotta cheese, which provide about 200 mg per ounce. Canned sardines with bones, broccoli, turnips, collards, tofu, and almonds are all rich in calcium as well as other healthful nutrients. Most important of all, regardless of the source, you should do a tally from time to time of how much calcium you are ingesting daily; if it is not adequate, make a change.

WEIGHT-BEARING EXERCISE

Our bones are designed to bear weight—the weight of gravity, and of motion against gravity, such as walking, running, or climbing. The research is compelling—we must do what our bodies are meant to do. Weight-bearing exercise is essential to bone health.

Exercise is important to the health and strength of bones of both premenopausal and postmenopausal women. Exercise plus calcium will decrease bone weakening, and exercise also maintains muscle tone, important to balance and the prevention of falls. Exercise is just now being shown actually to strengthen bones in postmenopausal women (see page 439).

What do I mean by exercise? Blessedly, moderate, sensible exercise that any woman can manage will do the trick. A proven prescription is a weight-bearing activity in the range of thirty to sixty minutes three times a week. That might be walking three miles three times a week or a little over a mile a day every day. Dancing, jumping rope, walking up stairs, taking aerobics classes, and using exercise equipment and arm and leg weights all fit the bill. And don't forget to involve your arms in whatever exercise you choose.

An exercise program should always be combined with attention to daily calcium intake. Exercise must be sustained, becoming a lifestyle, a habit. If we stop exercising, bone mass returns to where it was before a pattern of exercise was started, and loss of bone resumes at the preexercise level (anywhere between 1 and 4 percent per year, depending on age). Continued moderate exercise maintains the benefit. Varying the actual type of exercise—walking one week, bicycling the next, dancing another—can break the monotony that often leads to a resumption of sedentary ways for all of us.

For women who are unable to take estrogen replacement therapy, combining calcium and exercise becomes a must, particularly during the decade following menopause. The ideal is, however, to combine all three—*estrogen, diet,* and *exercise*—if at all possible.

OSTEOPOROSIS NEEDS A STRONG RESEARCH FUTURE

Certainly we've come a long way in what we know about osteoporosis: at least the medical world now recognizes it as a disease deserving attention, and not just an inevitable part of aging. But we must learn more, so we have the tools with which to insist that the medical and lay worlds both recognize it as a disease worth treating and preventing. Among the areas crying out for future study are:

- *Progesterone and testosterone.* We need more information on progesterone and testosterone to prevent and treat osteoporosis. Though we don't know for sure, progesterone may have an independent value in promoting bone health; it may also enhance or prolong estrogen's effects on bones. Testosterone is now being explored for the treatment of osteoporosis in men. Testosterone levels in women also drop with menopause, but whether testosterone is beneficial to bone health in women is unclear.

- *Estrogen alternatives.* For women who cannot take estrogen, estrogenlike hormones are a potential alternative. We must learn more about synthetic hormones like tamoxifen, which may well offer the bone-building benefits of estrogen without the coinciding risk of breast cancer (see page 197). Studies now under way will provide definitive information as to whether tamoxifen protects against spinal fractures in healthy women in their postmenopausal years. Other estrogenlike compounds are also being developed. Raloxifene, for instance, is similar to tamoxifen but has no uterine-stimulatory effect, thereby decreasing the risk of endometrial cancer carried by estrogen or tamoxifen use.

- *The challenge of rebuilding bone.* The single most needed breakthrough for the treatment of the millions of women with osteoporosis is the discovery of a concrete, failsafe means of rebuilding bone once it has been lost, and once the body's own rebuilding ability has peaked. Besides learning more about the bisphosphonates and fluoride, we need to pursue other approaches, such as finding growth factors targeted at bone-forming cells. Such devices would also be invaluable to accelerate bone healing after a fracture, which would dramatically decrease the morbidity associated with bone breaks in older women. In this context, *the sodium fluoride controversy must be settled.*

- *Vitamin D.* We must expand our knowledge about vitamin D and calcium metabolism and associated hormones like parathyroid hormone that affect bone calcification. The metabolically active form of vitamin D, calcitriol or 1,25 dihydroxy vitamin D, does stimulate bone formation but is difficult to regulate and sometimes can cause life-threatening elevations in blood calcium.

- *Bone density screening.* We must determine the most cost-effective way to screen women for osteopenia and osteoporosis. Although we are shying away from any new technology these days, and haggling over which tests should be covered by insurance, commonsense application of a technology like DEXA could in the long run be highly cost-effective. Not all women are at risk for osteoporosis, and risk stratification would allow more targeted preventive strategies as well as more precise risk-benefit evaluations of selective interventions. *We need to answer the simple question: why not use DEXA as we do mammograms once women turn fifty? It makes great sense to me.*

QUESTIONS FOR YOUR DOCTOR

Those suffering from osteoporosis or who have a loved one enduring the disease need no reminder of the toll it takes. Knowledge is your best ally—don't hesitate to demand the following of your health professional.

- Discuss with your doctor whether osteoporosis or the signs and symptoms of it have run in your family. Height and weight are routine parts of a physical examination, and you should periodically review your height measurements over time with your physician. If you change physicians, be sure to get copies of your records for your own safekeeping; it is helpful to have long-standing records of such information.
- Review all your medications regularly with your doctor. Are you taking any medications that can cause loss of calcium? If you are prescribed a diuretic, what about a thiazide? (Thiazides are not only beneficial for calcium retention but inexpensive too.)
- Review your diet with your doctor. Estimate how much calcium you take in per day. Should you take calcium supplements? Which ones?
- What about an exercise program? What bone-strengthening exercises are safe and right for you considering your age and present bone and muscle status?
- Should you have bone density studies, and if so when? Does your doctor have access to DEXA? If not, is it available elsewhere in your community?
- You will surely discuss estrogen replacement therapy once you have reached menopause. How do you factor in your personal risk for osteoporosis in your personal risk-benefit analysis? A bone density measurement may be indicated at this juncture. Ask about the latest results coming from the PEPI trial and the Women's Health Initiative.
- What do you need to know about your daily activities if you have osteoporosis? How should you change your living situation and habits to protect against falls, fractures, injuries?

- If you have osteoporosis, periodically ask for an update on the newer agents that are becoming available to treat osteoporosis.
- Ask your doctor if he has any advice to your daughters.

WHAT WOMEN CAN DO PERSONALLY AND POLITICALLY

Much needs to be done to increase public awareness of osteoporosis, to lift it out of the realm of some faraway problem curving old women's spines and into focus as a reality in the future of every woman. Currently, about 20 percent of American women have osteoporosis, and the number is growing. That must sound an alarm in our homes and our communities: this health problem of concern to all women won't go away.

We can raise the public consciousness through local newspaper, TV, and radio stories and through public service announcements. Such announcements have taught everyone that smoking causes cancer and heart disease; how many know that it leads to fragile bones? Public polls have shown that few women of any age know or care much about osteoporosis, and black and Hispanic women believe they are immune. Organizations like the National Osteoporosis Foundation, dedicated to public education, need support and visibility just as much as the American Heart Association and the American Cancer Society do.

Even though osteoporosis shows up later in life, the final outcome is in part determined by what young girls do when they are in their teens. Our public education and public health programs, however, rarely address this problem to the young audience. We must call for education on osteoporosis in our grade schools and high schools to influence young girls to attend to their bone health. Write or speak to your local school board about putting this in the curriculum.

Perhaps the reason this disease so often falls outside the policy maker's radar screen of major health problems is that it typically affects women when they have become socially isolated at home or entrenched in a nursing home, unable to stand tall and too frail to fight. We may see some seventy-five or eighty-year-old statesmen on Capitol Hill or even in the White House, but rarely do they have dowager humps, or risk wrist fractures as they lower the gavel in their exercise of power. We must get their attention by writing and calling—relentlessly.

Osteoporosis currently commands a large part of the NASA life science budget. It is ironic that a few men's rubbery bones in space have captured so much more attention than millions of women's broken bones on earth. Write to NASA and to your local congressmen about how the NASA research can be applied to women on earth. Stress the need for osteoporosis research to become a greater priority within the NIH.

Also, put pressure on the FDA to expedite the review processes for treatments of established osteoporosis—particularly the inexpensive ones, such as sodium fluoride, which may not have corporate champions.

Each one of us must recognize that the human cost of osteoporosis is every bit as great as that of cancer or heart disease. If we take into account fear of falling, depression, social isolation, intractable pain, and the certain knowledge of a bleak outlook for tomorrow, the human suffering is as intense as in any mortal illness. But the diagnosis is not so dramatic, and the sympathy factor from friends and family is somehow less. Each of us must change her own thinking about this.

Regardless of age, a woman's perspective on osteoporosis very much becomes her perspective on tomorrow. The perspective needs to be that we all are likely to live into our eighties or nineties, or even reach one hundred. With osteoporosis, unlike so many other illnesses, we can not only prevent the disease but also have a great opportunity to cure those who are already afflicted.

I have not given up on that kind of help for Nonie. Fully expecting her to pass her hundredth birthday, I predict she will celebrate the year 2000 with denser bones, a gift of the new bone-building agents just now on the horizon.

ELEVEN

ALZHEIMER'S DISEASE
The Endless Night

Without memory there is no experience.

— WILLIAM HARVEY,
  ENGLISH PHYSICIAN, 1651

I enjoy thinking about what our lives in the future will be like. I imagine a spring day in the year 2040. The air will be clearer. The tobacco industry will have joined the buggy whip industry. Many of the diseases we know and fear today will exist only in tales told to grandchildren: cystic fibrosis will be cured by the inhalation of an aerosol carrying a crippled common cold virus linked to a normal CF gene; AIDS will have gone the way of smallpox; cancers will no longer spread throughout the body. A loaf of bread may cost ten dollars, but most of us will think no more of that than we do of the cost of bread today.

On such a day, I will be in the tenth decade of my life. My daughters, Bartlett and Marie, will be in or approaching their sixties. We will gather for lunch and one of us, reminiscing about our life in Cleveland in the nineties, will realize that she cannot recall the names of the two golden retrievers who frolic outside my window as I write this.

A cloud creeps into my daydream. I wonder: Will we laugh at this small lapse of memory? Or will we shudder, as so many women do today, at the slightest hint that a seemingly insignificant mind slip might be the first whisper of Alzheimer's disease? I hope with all my heart our reaction will be the former, that Alzheimer's too will have gone the way of polio. I fear, though, that too many families, in the spring days of forty or fifty years from now, will still come to know the dark and terrible night of Alzheimer's, the disease that robs us of our very selves. For without memory, there can be no experience, and without experience there is no existence.

ALZHEIMER'S: THE DISEASE OF OUR FUTURE

In this final chapter, I will outline what is known and suspected about this dreadful disease. I hope what you'll take from the chapter, though, is the sense that everything about this illness is uncertain; we all must make our voices heard so that Alzheimer's research is among our nation's highest health priorities and becomes as visible in the next decades as the war on cancer has been in the last.

The prevalence of Alzheimer's is increasing at an alarming rate, particularly in women. You might assume that there are more people with Alzheimer's each year simply because, with our population boom and greater longevity, we find more older people in our society. After all, the U.S. Senate's Special Committee on Aging estimates that by the year 2010, 25 percent of the population will be over fifty-five years old.

This disease, however, appears to be increasing faster than our population is aging, and we don't know why. In a 1985 report on aging, the National Institutes of Health estimated that there were 2.5 million cases of Alzheimer's disease in the United States. They also noted that this number was ten times larger than the 1975 estimates. By 1993, only seven years later, both the NIH and its Institute on Aging were estimating that 4 million Americans had Alzheimer's and that 250,000 new cases were being diagnosed every year. Others felt that those estimates were on the low side, that as many as 300,000 and 400,000 new cases are diagnosed annually. Almost everyone involved with these studies admits that the estimates are conservative. It is possible, even probable, that the numbers are much worse, in part because of our new awareness of the disease. On that gentle spring day I and my daughters hope to enjoy in the year 2040, it is not at all unreasonable to assume that perhaps 20 million or more Americans will then be afflicted with Alzheimer's.

The aging of our general population cuts twice. It both increases the number of elderly and it reduces the number of people who will be paying for their care and caring for them. Dr. Robert Binstock of Case

Western Reserve University calls this "apocalyptic demography," for Alzheimer's brings with it potentially backbreaking costs. Today's estimated cost of professional home care or nursing home care for each Alzheimer's victim is about fifty thousand dollars a year—a current grand total of around sixty billion dollars a year in medical costs, nursing care, and lost productivity from the sufferers (and not including the value of unpaid caregivers). If no advances against this disease are made, these costs will skyrocket as America moves into the twenty-first century. It is not beyond the imagination to assume that, with costs reaching well into the trillions, my daughters may be devoting one-third of their earnings to paying for the care of the nation's elderly—before they even get to caring for their own children.

Dollars measure only a small part of the cost of Alzheimer's. No other malady, not AIDS or even that disease called war, holds greater potential for crippling our nation and others in the developed world. AIDS and war take the young; Alzheimer's takes the old. While the young create culture and push societies forward, it is the old who preserve culture and provide stability, which ensures that societies survive the push.

WOMEN BEAR THE BURDEN

Two-thirds of these elderly victims will be women, for women currently live about eight years longer than do men, making them vulnerable to this late-onset disease. But what is long life without memory, without contribution to the world?

As the caregivers in our society, women bear the burden of Alzheimer's in another way as well. Most elderly women are still younger than their husbands; if an elderly husband is stricken with Alzheimer's, generally his wife will continue his care herself. (If, however, it's the wife who gets the disease, her husband, who is apt to be older, is more likely to place her in a nursing home or other institution to ensure adequate care.)

Most often the care of an Alzheimer's parent falls directly on the shoulders of her daughter or daughter-in-law. This responsibility harbors severe psychological and medical consequences. The National Institute on Aging notes that women caring for a relative with Alzheimer's face a "triple jeopardy." They must cope with the physical and emotional stress and with the devastating financial burden. Often the very individual they care for is openly hostile to their efforts. It is not unusual for a caregiver to feel abandoned, not only by the one she cares for but by her entire family.

The medical literature frequently refers to the caregiver as "the second patient." Studies show that Alzheimer's caregivers have reported reduced immune system function; at least a third of family members caring for Alzheimer's patients will suffer clinical depression during the course of their loved one's illness. There are no numbers that show how many caregivers and families are economically and psychologically destroyed by Alzheimer's. One can only imagine. And that insight alone should spur us into doing something now.

WHAT WE DON'T KNOW, AND WHY

Despite the obvious urgency of this illness, it is the disease we know least about and, considering the magnitude of its human cost, the disease for which research efforts are most seriously underfunded and public awareness most wanting (although former president Ronald Reagan's late 1994 announcement that he is stricken with the illness may change all that). The position it holds in current medical knowledge is, in many ways, similar to where stroke or cancer was thirty years ago—virtually in the Dark Ages. We don't know if Alzheimer's is caused by virus or a toxin; we don't know what triggers it or how to treat it; we can't prevent it from happening or even reliably slow it down, once it starts down its destructive course. We have only vague ideas as to who is at risk—and, unbelievable as it sounds, we can't even be absolutely sure someone has had this disease until after she's dead.

I think one of the reasons Alzheimer's has failed to generate national concern is that it is still so new to us, and I find great hope in that fact. The expanding problem of Alzheimer's has arisen in large part because of our successes. Until very recently, few of us lived long enough to be threatened by this disease. Over the past half century, our life expectancies have shot upward, thanks to the explosion in knowledge of treatment and prevention of so many other once deadly diseases, from measles to polio to heart attacks and even stroke.

Although Alzheimer's disease was named after Dr. Alois Alzheimer, who early in this century first recognized the havoc it wrought on the brain, no one, doctor or layperson, used the name commonly until very recently. I was taught about senility in med school and learned to use the term *presenile dementia* for people who seemed to lose memory and function uncommonly early. Senility was seen as a natural part of getting old, not as a symptom of a disease. Even had we suspected a disease, we had few tools or techniques to begin to examine it where it occurred, deep within the cells of the brain.

The disease itself hides from us. Its approach is subtle, difficult to recognize and long in coming. A slip of the mind, such as forgetting where the car keys are or not remembering someone's name, could be an innocent lapse. These momentary lags are common to daily life at every age and become even more so in mid-life. But this is also how Alzheimer's begins, and it can take as long as five years for Alzheimer's to interfere enough with day-to-day functions to prompt a trip to the doctor.

But there is another, perhaps understandable but less forgivable reason that Alzheimer's has not gotten the priority and attention it deserves. Our culture does not value its elderly. It is natural for our hearts to be broken when we hear of young parents taken from their children by diseases such as cancer or heart disease. But too many of us feel the elderly have outlived their useful years and are bound for eventual senility anyway.

The truth is that senility doesn't exist. Unless they have a debilitating disease such as Alzheimer's, our elderly can be as valuable and productive in society as can our young. It is up to us to reinforce this notion in ourselves and in our children. How we confront Alzheimer's disease will in part determine how we find ourselves treated in that distant year of 2040.

Altering society's vision of its elderly is of course not an easy thing for any individual to do. Speaking up for those elderly is another matter. Alzheimer's is invisible partly because victims have few advocates. They can't speak for themselves as can survivors of breast cancer or heart attacks. You won't see a powerful Alzheimer's lobby storming Washington; you don't even see its victims anywhere in your everyday life. Few reminders show us that this disease exists. We must become those reminders ourselves.

Our challenge is to apply to this scourge the same passion and effort that inspired the phenomenal medical successes of our times. Just as polio, influenza, heart disease, and the yet-without-cure AIDS characterize this century, Alzheimer's may well characterize the next. Let's take a close look at what we do know about this mysterious disease so that for our sake and our children's, we can take informed action to make sure it is a century of triumph.

THE SYMPTOMS OF ALZHEIMER'S

Alzheimer's disease is the most common form of what is called *dementia,* itself a symptom of a state of generally diminished higher brain function with loss of intellect and an apathetic emotional state. Many types of dementia are reversible, such as those caused by low thyroid hormone levels, certain B vitamin deficiencies, chronic alcoholism with combined nutritional deficiencies, an inflammation (*encephalitis*) caused by an acute viral infection of the brain, or even a brain tumor. Even the dementia brought on by the second most common origin of memory loss in the elderly, the mini-strokes discussed on page 383, can sometimes be reversed.

The diagnosis of Alzheimer's is a last resort, because the dementia is often well along before a diagnosis can accurately be made and because it is the cause a physician wants least to find. When dementia is caused by Alzheimer's, it is not reversible. It is a permanent and progressive impairment linked to a gradual destruction of brain tissue.

Alzheimer's attacks the higher and most developed part of our brain, the cerebrum, which controls thought, reason, self-awareness, creativity, conscience, emotional feelings, and intelligence. The deterioration of these faculties corresponds to progressive loss of brain tissue, the degeneration and death of brain cells, and a gradual shrinking of the brain. As the brain dwindles, so do memories developed over a lifetime. In his famous "All the world's a stage" soliloquy, Shakespeare characterizes the seventh, final stage of life as one of "childish treble" and "oblivion," "sans teeth, sans eyes, sans taste, sans everything." Though he wrote this at the midpoint of his career, around the age of thirty-six, Shakespeare must have met a few unfortunate souls who had Alzheimer's even back then at the end of the sixteenth century.

For an accountant or a teacher or an actress who must memorize her lines, the mental impairment is going to be noticed sooner than is the same impairment in a person less reliant on her mental skills in day-to-day life. Virtually all sufferers will fall into one of three stages of severity—loosely called early, intermediate, and advanced Alzheimer's—based on the extent of memory loss and behavioral abnormalities. These three stages are useful to measure an illness that runs such a long and drawn-out course, but they can overlap, and are far from precise.

Stage 1: Alzheimer's devours memories occasionally at first, then consistently. In a healthy person, absentmindedness is an occasional lapse, an amusing foible. In the person with undiagnosed Alzheimer's, the absentmindedness begins as an irritation and becomes a serious handicap. She will eventually forget her keys and glasses every time she puts them down. She will sit in the car and wonder why she is there. She will stand in front of the stove trying to think of why the burner is on. She may have trouble sleeping and inadvertently aggravate her mental impairment through overusing sleeping medication. This early stage of Alzheimer's can last anywhere from one to five years.

Stage 2: In this middle stage of the disease, which can also last several years, tasks such as cooking or driving a car become too organizationally complex for the mind to handle. Everyday objects such as books, sugar bowls, medicine, and purses are now continually misplaced; the Alzheimer's sufferer begins to believe a secret force is hiding or stealing these common things, since she has no memory of moving them. The terms for everyday objects elude her. A pencil is called a "writing thing," or a fork, a "food sticker." She forgets names and faces even of those closest to her, such as her husband or children, distressing the entire family. She may become increasingly paranoid or undergo personality changes that are subtle at first, then increasingly disturbing. The once buoyant woman who laughed at the antics of her grandchildren becomes irritable, suspicious, perhaps openly hostile or uncharacteristically indifferent. She may inexplicably burst into anger or profanity; her personality may become so distorted that she'll require tranquilizers or other psychiatric medication, which she can no longer be allowed to take without supervision; she may be among the third of all Alzheimer's victims who become severely depressed. She may have threatening hallucinations or see visions of children or old friends in an empty room. She will be increasingly restless and agitated and may exhibit a symptom called *sundowning*: wandering about throughout the night, disrupting others' sleep and getting into mischief. She may be increasingly interested in sex; she will probably become indifferent about eating, dressing, and bathing. Her movements may slow down—a symptom called *bradykinesia*—so that she looks as if she is trying to move through thick syrup.

Stage 3: In the final, tragic stage, which can go on for many years, her ability to initiate any movement wanes and disappears. She forgets how to eat and may sleep only during the day. She has no control over her bladder or bowels and must be in diapers continually. She may fix on a specific word or phrase and repeat it endlessly (called *echolalia*) or lose all ability to speak (*mutism*). In the advanced stages of the disease, psychotic behavior with frank delusions or hallucinations may get worse. Death often comes mercifully, in the form of pneumonia, an unchecked urinary infection, other incidental infections, or a fall that breaks a hip. For many families, death comes as deliverance. They cannot be faulted for that reaction.

WHAT IS MEMORY? THE STRUCTURE OF THE HEALTHY BRAIN

Our hope for understanding and ultimately preventing or treating Alzheimer's lies in demystifying the last of the human body's major mysteries: the brain. We know so little about the way our brains work, so little about how memory functions. Any of the aspects of the brain discussed below (starting on page 459) could hold the key to unlocking the memories so coldly denied us by Alzheimer's.

Memory may well be the most amazing of all of our human faculties. In a split second, it links together our primitive reactions, sophisticated reasoning, and innate talents. We are only just beginning to learn about the complex neurochemical, cellular, and genetic mechanisms that underlie memory, and the acquisition and storage of memory (learning).

Memory has different patterns. Some of our memories are fleeting, others last a lifetime. *Short-term memory* is the memory that holds life's events only briefly. It is the memory that keeps the pizza shop's telephone number in our heads long enough to dial the telephone. It is the memory of where we put our glasses, set down the newspaper; it is remembering the noon lunch date. Short-term memory gets us through the day. When evening comes and the bedcovers are pulled up, the mind dumps these memories because they are no longer necessary. For instance, you might remember what you had for lunch today, but do you remember what you had for lunch on July 23, 1993, or even last Wednesday? Do you need to?

Committing something to *long-term memory* takes something extra. It occurs naturally when the event that will be remembered has a particular emotional charge to it, the cliché being our memories of where we were the day we learned President John F. Kennedy was shot. We can best force an experience into our long-term memories when we can relate it to something we already know, a very conscious and sometimes grueling process.

Within our brains, long-term memory involves more elaborate processing than does short-term memory in order to be permanently committed into the "hard drive" of our memory bank. Everything we remember gets processed through a control center deep within our brains, in an area called the *hippocampus*—a part of our brain that has no contact with the outside world. Stimulation must reach it through our senses and through other parts of the brain, so that by the time an experience is processed into memory by the hippocampus, it is far removed from the actual event and totally at the mercy of the accurate functioning of this incredible processing center. I've said that emotionally charged events tend to be remembered in the long term; interestingly, the hippocampus is located in the limbic system, which is also the seat of all our emotions.

Signals converge upon the hippocampus from all over the brain through a complex web of nerve cells and neurotransmitters (see page 285). Each highly specialized cell in the brain, primarily cells called *neurons* and *glial cells,* has a message to convey either to or from the hippocampus, as we continually store memories and then recall them. (Even as I type this sentence, I'm both remembering and storing an incredible amount of information more powerfully than any computer. I must remember how to spell, how to read, basic grammar, what I know about the brain, what I must research, what I've just written, what I'm about to write, how my computer works, how to type—and on and on.)

Simply put, neurons support thought and glia support neurons. While we don't know much about the glial cells, we are learning more and more, and I suspect we will find their function extends beyond the purpose we now attribute to them—holding up the neurons as a sort of glue or scaffolding would.

Most of the brain cells called neurons look something like an octopus, with each neuron having a long tentacle (*axon*); sprouting from the tentacle in every direction are thousands of short arms (*dendrites*). Axons weave throughout the cells in the brain, connecting areas that are fairly remote geographically—for example, from the vision center in the back of your brain to the hippocampus in the middle of your brain, from the motor cortex on the top of the cerebrum to the depths of the hypothalamus.

When I was in medical school, we were taught that the brain held a fixed amount of nerves and interconnections, dealt us at birth and wearing down as we age. We now know that dendrites sprout and grow as we learn. I'll say that again—*the nerve cells in our brain are constantly changing, growing as we grow intellectually throughout our lives.* At any age, we can grow our brainpower through learning, through committing experience and knowledge into our long-term memories. This discovery is truly a blockbuster, and we'll look further at its practical impact later in this chapter.

Electrical pulses race through these axons and dendrites, carrying their messages from the outside world to the inner. In order for the message to reach its destination, a crucial chemical element comes into play: the neurotransmitter. Neurotransmitters act as processors or connectors. Without them, the electrical impulses carried by the brain cells would reach a dead end on the tip of each axon or dendrite. The cells would have no way of communicating; the octopus tendrils can wave and wave, but no message would be conveyed. The major neurotransmitter system allowing us to remember is called the acetylcholine system (to a lesser degree, the noradrenaline and serotonin systems are also involved).

If the flow of electrical impulses is impeded, or if a series of neurons does not have enough stored neurotransmitters to communicate the message from one neuron to another, the thought peters out, the memory of birthdays past fades, and the glasses remain lost. In this fashion, Alzheimer's robs us of our past.

CAUSES OF ALZHEIMER'S: MANY POSSIBILITIES, NO CERTAINTIES

We don't know what causes Alzheimer's, but we do have some important leads. We are certain that the problem is biological, not psychological. We are almost as certain that it is not caused by a virus but instead is some type of dysfunction in our fundamental cellular processes, in the same way that cancer is caused by unnatural cell growth. And many researchers believe that Alzheimer's victims may be born with a genetic tendency for the cells to misfire in this way.

WHERE THERE IS ALZHEIMER'S, THERE IS AMYLOID

In the brain of an Alzheimer's patient, something slowly clogs up and destroys the vital impulse-sending neurons, blocking our memories from reaching or exiting the control center called the hippocampus. Fibers form and creep through the axons and dendrites, thin fibers that slowly bunch up into dense bundles and finally, insidiously, destroy the entire neuron, just as Alzheimer's itself eventually and unstoppably steals our memories and identities.

We now know that this "something," first recognized by Dr. Alzheimer almost one hundred years ago, is a type of molecule called *amyloid,* or more exactly, the *amyloid beta protein.* The terms *amyloid plaques* and *neurofibrillary tangles* are commonly used to describe the abnormalities associated with this molecule run amok in a brain stricken with Alzheimer's. Parts of the precursor molecule of amyloid is neurotoxic. The presence of some amyloid deposits in the brain by no means implies that you'll automatically get the disease. But people who have Alzheimer's have abundant buildups of amyloid, in the cells of the hippocampus and scattered elsewhere throughout the brain.

As in just about everything else having to do with Alzheimer's, we know little more about amyloid itself beyond the fact that it exists. We don't know its function in a healthy body, and we certainly don't know what causes it to accumulate in the brain, although we do have some theories (see below). Amyloid is beyond doubt the biological hallmark of Alzheimer's. It is the primary abnormal finding in an Alzheimer's brain. But we still cannot say that amyloid "causes" the disease; it may simply be a marker that deposits itself after something else causes the initial damage. Once the amyloid is there, though, we have no doubt that it exacerbates the disease manyfold; amyloid clumps are toxic to the circuitry of our minds and memories.

THE CAUSE OF THE CAUSE? OUR GENES

There are actually about ten different forms of amyloid proteins, most made from chemical building blocks called *precursor proteins.* All these forms of amyloid in general seem to be soluble and therefore can circulate in the blood without doing damage. In an Alzheimer's patient, though, one type of amyloid (the amyloid beta we discussed) forms deposits in the brain—perhaps because, for some of us, a genetic mutation or a combination of mutations causes this normally soluble protein to become insoluble and deposit or because something triggers its precursor protein to be produced in excessive amounts, leading again to increased deposits. Researchers have identified abnormalities in genes that are known to be important in producing or processing the amyloid protein. The more we know about these possible genetic causes, the more we can learn who may be at risk and, more important, the better we can understand the underlying molecular mechanisms and find a way to fix the defect.

Chromosomes 21 and 14

Victims of one form of hereditary early Alzheimer's, which strikes before middle age, have genetic mutations on chromosome 21, the same chromosome that is defective in people with Down's syndrome. Down's patients do produce an excess amount of the amyloid precursor protein and have a dramatically increased incidence of early-onset Alzheimer's. This discovery clearly links amyloid to Alzheimer's, but testing for abnormalities on chromosome 21 has no utility in the general elderly population, as the mutations appear specific only to those with this rare early-onset form of the disease.

In this same population of younger victims, several different research groups have found an abnormality in chromosome 14 even more frequently than on chromosome 21, suggesting that many different genes play a role in the metabolic derangement that converges to form Alzheimer's.

Apolipoprotein E and Chromosome 19

An exciting finding in our understanding of Alzheimer's that may ultimately have application in its treatment was first marked by Japanese scientists years ago and only recently confirmed by scientists at Duke University. Chromosome 19 carries the gene for apolipoprotein (ApoE), a lipoprotein that by definition floats through the blood carrying around cholesterol and helping the body metabolize lipids (the fatty molecules we've discussed on page 34). ApoE attaches to amyloid and, depending on the ApoE form, makes the amyloid more or less soluble in the blood.

The ApoE2, ApoE3, and "J" forms of ApoE may in fact protect us from Alzheimer's by influencing the amyloid to remain soluble. ApoE4 is a genetic variant that tends to stabilize the amyloid protein when it binds to it and therefore gives it the opportunity to accumulate and form the destructive plaques of Alzheimer's, rather than being destroyed by the body's enzymes as it normally would be while circulating in the blood. The Alzheimer's risk is either the presence of ApoE4 or the absence of the protective ApoE3—or a combination of both.

Some researchers estimate that perhaps a third of us carry the gene that produces ApoE4. By carrying this gene, our risk for getting Alzheimer's may be as much as eight times greater than without the gene. Genes come in pairs, and the more copies of the gene any one of us possesses, the greater the risk—by far. For example, one study suggests that if a person has a double dose of the ApoE4 gene (i.e., she received the same gene from both parents), she faces a 90 percent chance of getting the disease if she lives past eighty.

These findings have not been confirmed—but if they are, they hold the promise of our being able both to test for those facing a high risk of Alzheimer's and, more important, to design targeted therapy aimed at blocking the binding of ApoE4 to amyloid. Such treatment could prevent the amyloid from being deposited in the cells and stop Alzheimer's from occurring. The tests and the treatment are a way off.

NOT BY AMYLOID OR GENES ALONE: OTHER POSSIBLE CAUSES

While amyloid deposits are always found in the brains of Alzheimer's victims, large quantities of amyloid in the blood don't necessarily mean you will get the disease. For example, while patients with Down's syndrome produce substantially higher levels of amyloid than people without Down's, only half of patients with these high levels develop Alzheimer's. Half don't.

These types of findings lead researchers to believe that other causes contribute to Alzheimer's.

NEUROTRANSMITTERS

As we've seen, neurotransmitters in our brains keep our memories jumping from nerve cell to nerve cell, in and out of our consciousness on demand. Alzheimer's patients have deficiencies in a host of neurotransmitters, but most particularly acetylcholine. Although many researchers believe that the decrease in these transmitters is a result, not a cause, of the cell death in Alzheimer's, these deficiencies may have important therapeutic implications.

INFLAMMATION

Perhaps cells are not dying from the inside out. Perhaps, once the amyloid deposits begin to form, the annihilation of the neurons is accelerated from the outside by an overzealous immune system.

Our immune systems are comprised of a host of different cells and compounds that roam the body like an army on patrol. Part scavenger, part killer, immune system cells respond to anything deemed to be foreign to the body—such as bacteria, viruses, toxins, and cellular debris—by causing destructive inflammation. As long as the threat is present, the cells remain active and chronic inflammation, which can destroy healthy and diseased cells alike, becomes established.

Alternatively, it's possible that the inflammation comes first, with the immune system cells themselves producing proteins that contribute to amyloid deposits. This scenario is in fact what does sometimes occur elsewhere in the body (with a slightly different form of amyloid than the brain's damaging amyloid beta protein), as when chronic inflammatory diseases such as rheumatoid arthritis or chronic tuberculosis strike.

DEFICIENCIES AND TOXINS IN THE DIET

Some suspect that excesses of certain minerals may exacerbate Alzheimer's. Alzheimer's sufferers have been shown to be deficient in the antioxidants—vitamins E, C, and A—and this area is currently being studied. In the course of normal metabolism, there is a buildup of "oxidation" by-products, which are toxic to cells and tissues; the antioxidants normally prevent the buildup of these damaging free oxygen radicals (see page 45).

Aluminum is the dietary factor that has come under the closest scrutiny, but the evidence is quite inconsistent. Increased amounts of aluminum have been found associated with amyloid plaques in the brains of people with Alzheimer's, and one Great Britain study linked increased levels of aluminum in drinking water from different water supplies to a greater incidence of Alzheimer's. But other studies have failed to show more Alzheimer's among those who work in aluminum smelting plants or in those who chronically consume antacids containing aluminum. The general consensus among Alzheimer's researchers is that a cause-effect link between aluminum and the disease is simply too far a stretch.

Zinc is another metal that has just recently emerged as having a possible tie to Alzheimer's. Unlike aluminum, zinc is a trace element that is important to our body's functions (see page 50). But too high a level of zinc may accelerate or precipitate amyloid plaque formation in the brain by causing the harmless amyloid dissolved in the fluids bathing the brain to clump together into a large mass and then deposit in brain tissue. For the most part, this research is still at a test tube level. However, there are reports that giving zinc supplements to patients who already have Alzheimer's, with the hope of helping them by testing various food supplements, actually caused acute deterioration in their mental function. For now, the most advice I would give is not to take zinc supplements but do keep an eye on this information as it emerges from the research laboratory.

RISK FACTORS

While no one can say with any certainty what causes Alzheimer's, we do know that the following are clear risk factors for the disease. While none are guarantees that you will be stricken, falling into any of the categories below increases your odds.

FAMILY HISTORY

The clearest risk factor for Alzheimer's is heredity. Twenty-five to 30 percent of those with the disease have had a blood relative who also succumbed to Alzheimer's. Of course, there is nothing anyone can do about her family history, but I see the indisputable genetic component as a positive aspect of the problem. If we know a problem is genetically based, we have moved a step forward toward identifying the precise genetic defect that has caused it; with a cause pinpointed, we are en route to a treatment or even a cure.

AGE

Yes, the older you are the more likely you are to encounter Alzheimer's, but aging by no means makes the disease inevitable. This risk factor does reinforce one certainty: Alzheimer's is only going to increase in frequency as our overall population ages. According to the Office of Technology Assessment, the risk of dementia in the population younger than sixty-five is less than 1 percent. Between the ages of sixty-five and seventy-five, the risk doubles. After age seventy-five, the risk suddenly rises to 7 percent and after passing one's eighty-fifth birthday, one in four Americans is estimated to have Alzheimer's. Some experts claim an even gloomier picture: that the disease will strike close to 20 percent of the population after the age of seventy-five and almost half of those over the age of eighty-five. If these figures are correct, and every other person in their mid-eighties and beyond will be demented, we should qualify our wish for long life: "May you have long life only if it's without Alzheimer's."

HEAD TRAUMA

People with a history of head trauma also have a disproportionate occurrence of Alzheimer's (and Parkinson's disease) later in life. This dementia, sometimes called being "punch drunk," is occasionally seen in the type of recurrent head trauma suffered by boxers and in people who have suffered concussions in accidents. Such head traumas do result in at least temporary inflammation and swelling of the brain. As we've seen above, many theorists suspect there is a connection between brain inflammation and Alzheimer's. Perhaps such chronic inflammation predisposes the amyloid to deposit, or perhaps the simple loss of neurons that these injuries cause can deplete the brain reserves.

FEMALE GENDER

There are studies performed across many countries that suggest that women are at an increased risk for Alzheimer's, above and beyond the obvious extra risk of simply living longer into the Alzheimer's-prone years than do men. Although we cannot do anything about our gender, the observation has already pointed researchers toward studying gender differences, specifically hormones, that might explain our different susceptibility and perhaps lead to a viable preventive strategy.

EDUCATIONAL LEVEL

Finally, a risk factor we can do something about. Lack of education has been shown to correlate with a greater chance of developing dementia later in life in different societies and many parts of the world (the United States, Sweden, Italy, France, Finland, Israel, China). Why this is we don't yet know—it may be because education stimulates the growth of new cells in the brain or, it may mean that those who have had a better education are more apt to keep their brains active as they age—but it raises some highly provocative questions about the ability of our environment to shape and protect our brains. This fact is both fascinating and extremely encouraging.

NO DIAGNOSIS, LITTLE TREATMENT, LESS PREVENTION

There isn't much we can do about Alzheimer's now—except learn all we can. We know a bit more than we did a few years ago. We must understand more about diagnosis so we can treat early; we must find the answers to treatment and prevention so we can live happily.

DIAGNOSING ALZHEIMER'S

At present we have no positive test that confirms Alzheimer's. In the later stages, a fairly accurate diagnosis can be guessed at. The symptoms, as we've discussed, become quite obvious. But a guess is not a diagnosis, and we can be absolutely certain only after the victim has died and pathologists have studied her brain.

As soon as you suspect Alzheimer's in yourself, you will in all likelihood seek the help of your doctor. If your doctor concurs with your suspicion or notices symptoms himself, he will recommend that you meet with a neurologist or possibly a "geriatrician," a doctor who specializes in the diseases of the elderly.

A doctor will diagnose Alzheimer's only after determining that a change in mental function is truly dementia as defined in the handbook of neurologic and psychiatric disorders, DSM-IV (see page 312); the handbook states basically that dementia involves progressive deterioration in one or more areas of thinking, plus a loss of memory. The physician then exhausts all other possible causes of a patient's decline. If you tell your physician you suspect that a family member, say, your mother, has Alzheimer's, the doctor will obtain a detailed medical history from both you and your mother, asking questions about nutrition, alcohol and substance abuse, diabetes, thyroid disease, past TIAs (see page 382), depression, and social environment, as well as about medications your mother may be taking, such as sleeping pills, antidepressants, or barbiturates. The physician will also conduct a complete neurological exam, including some kind of formal and systematic test using a series of questions and simple tasks (see sidebar, page 469). A sample of spinal fluid will be tapped from the base of the spine and examined for signs of infection or tumor. Sometimes a brain wave test (an EEG) is also obtained. A blood test will help eliminate the possibility of thyroid disease, B_{12} deficiency, uremia, advanced liver disease, or a history of syphilis—all of which can have dementia as a symptom. Even if all these tests come out negative, I would still go the next step and order a CAT scan or MRI to make sure there wasn't a brain tumor. (Late in Alzheimer's, one of these advanced tests can show the shrinkage of brain tissue that indicates Alzheimer's, but early in the disease—"early" meaning five to ten long years—CAT scans may well show nothing unusual.)

Once all other likely suspects are eliminated, as the dementia continues to worsen and Alzheimer's is indicated, usually your physician will suggest a specially trained social worker or occupational therapist to evaluate your mother's daily activities, to help sort out the stage of the disease and make recommendations about longer-term care.

TREATMENT

Of course, the greatest tragedy of Alzheimer's is that even when a diagnosis (as definitive as is possible at this time) is made, we still have no effective way of treating it. We are not without strong possibilities, though, on both the medical and the environmental fronts.

MEDICATION

None of the drugs below fit the category of a breakthrough treatment for Alzheimer's. On the other hand, none seem to do any real harm, and one medication in particular, tacrine (and others like it), does offer a history of modest success and hope for the future.

We've seen that our memories require neurotransmitters in order for messages to make the leap from dendrite to dendrite; without the neurotransmitters, particularly acetylcholine, memories get stuck and never reach our consciousness. The most promising drugs currently available are those that protect acetylcholine so that it can carry out its crucial communications work.

Tacrine (Cognex) is such an agent. It stops the enzyme *acetylcholinesterase* from breaking down acetylcholine and thereby allows

STUDY TO WATCH FOR

Dozens of researchers are currently hunting for a definitive, inexpensive, noninvasive diagnostic test for Alzheimer's. Even if we're not close to a cure, such a test could help prevent missed diagnoses of other diseases—if, for example, a simple test comes back negative, a physician would intensify his search for a curable cause of the dementia that prompted the test.

Researchers at Harvard Medical School led by Drs. Leonard F. M. Scinto and Huntington Potter just released a provocative study. They found (in a sample too small to be definitive) that the pupils of Alzheimer's patients become significantly more dilated than the norm when a weak solution of topicamide (a common drug used by optometrists to dilate the pupil) is dropped into their eyes. The drops work by inhibiting acetylcholine, and theorists suspect that Alzheimer's sufferers show this hypersensitivity to the drops because their acetylcholine is already diminished. The doctors found that nineteen of twenty people with Alzheimer's showed this increased reaction, and thirty of thirty-two people without Alzheimer's did not. Based on this tiny sample, a major pharmaceutical company has already obtained marketing rights on the eye drops and test measurements.

Additionally, Dr. Daniel Alkon of the NIH has devised a simple laboratory skin test for the disease—not yet available to the public. He and his colleagues noted that certain potassium channels in the brain cells of Alzheimer's patients were either closed or missing. They reasoned that if Alzheimer's does this to brain cells, it might have the same effect on cells elsewhere in an Alzheimer's victim's body; they therefore conducted tests on samples of olfactory neurons (similar to brain cells in structure, these are the cells in the nose that sense odors) and samples of cells called fibroblasts, which are found in skin. Dr. Alkon found that the potassium channels in these cells, too, were indeed abnormal. We are awaiting further verification of this as a definitive and specific early test for Alzheimer's.

TESTING FOR DEMENTIA

Developed by Dr. Marshall Folstein and his colleagues at Johns Hopkins in the seventies, the Folstein Mini–Mental State Exam below is now one of the many useful and rapid neurological exams your physician may use to assess a patient's mental functioning and distinguish between true dementia and other mental states such as depression. It tests orientation, attention span, recall, and language. (Some of the questions do presuppose a minimal level of baseline literacy.) This is not meant to be a home test but rather an example of the kinds of straightforward questions and tasks your doctor will use in a mental status evaluation.

MINI–MENTAL EXAM

TASK	SCORE
• What is the year, season, month, and day?	5
• Where are you: state, city, place?	5
• Name three unrelated objects and then have the patient repeat them until she has learned all three.	3
• Ask the patient to spell *"world"* backwards or do serial sevens backwards from thirty-five.	5
• Ask the patient to recall the three objects repeated above.	3
• Hold up a common object—a pencil, ring, watch, glass— and ask its name.	2
• Have the patient repeat, "No ifs, ands, or buts."	1
• Have the patient follow a three-stage command (example: Take a paper in your right hand, fold it in half, and lay it on the floor).	3
• Have the patient read and obey a written simple command, such as "Close your eyes," then do it.	1
• Have the patient write a sentence.	1

TASK	SCORE
• Have the patient copy a geometric design you have drawn on a piece of paper.	1

Source: Adapted from M. F. Folstein, S. E. Folstein, and P. R. McHugh, " 'Mini-mental state': A practical method for grading the cognitive state of patients for the clinician," *Journal of Psychiatric Research* 12 (1975): 189–198. Used with permission.

A perfect score on this test is 30; "normal" is 27 to 30; people suffering from depression generally score in the 20 to 30 range; and those with dementia score under 20, averaging about 10. If a patient does poorly on this simple test, it does not necessarily mean Alzheimer's, but it signals the need to find out the cause of the dementia.

more acetylcholine to accumulate in the gaps between neurons. This way, it (presumably) maximizes the capacity of surviving neurons to compensate for those that have been lost in patients with mild to moderate Alzheimer's. Note that it does nothing to slow the progress of the disease itself or to reverse the damage that has already been done.

Tacrine can and has improved cognitive function in Alzheimer's victims—for a time. In one recent study, 42 percent of the people taking tacrine showed some objective improvement in intellectual function (compared to 20 percent who showed improvement with a placebo). The results with tacrine are unpredictable, but give encouragement to other lines of study that focus on treating Alzheimer's through enhancing levels of acetylcholine in the brain. In fact, the results of the tacrine trials have spurred on a broad research effort to find even more powerful neurotransmitter-affecting drugs. There are several other acetylcholine-enhancing agents now under investigation.

Tacrine was just approved by the FDA in 1993, despite the fact that its benefits are neither clear nor dramatic. Because there is a veritable absence of anything else even half as well studied for this tragic disease, I think it was a wise move—provided that false hope is not given to anyone and that research continues on newer and better drug strategies.

Also approved by the FDA is the drug Hydergine, a mixture of compounds called ergoloid mesylates, that has been in use a long time. We know next to nothing about this drug, and its impact is entirely equivocal. Some studies in animals indicate it might stimulate the metabolism of the brain, make more proteins, and enhance the function of certain neurotransmitters, but many neurologists feel strongly that it is of no use whatsoever. Even modest successes in medications are nonetheless encouraging—and are far more than we had on the table even twenty years ago.

We have a long way to go in developing new drugs for Alzheimer's. The ideal drug would keep amyloid from building up in the first place. With the clear relationship between amyloid and Alzheimer's, finding a chemical that can block its accumulation in neurons would be one of the most obvious approaches to moving forward in curing the disease. At the very least, if we can block amyloid protein from depositing, we will learn with certainty whether the protein plays a role in causing or enabling the disease to progress; at best, if amyloid is in fact causal, an amyloid blocker could conquer the disease. Drug companies and laboratories have been hunting such a blocker for years, but as yet have been unsuccessful.

SUPPORTIVE SURROUNDINGS

The fact that there is no cure or proven therapy for Alzheimer's does not mean that all therapeutic efforts should be abandoned when the disease is diagnosed. To the contrary; quality of life still matters. As patient or as caretaker, you must pay attention to hygiene, routines for daily living, exercise, nutrition, and human companionship. Physical exercise, for example, contributes to a more cheerful outlook and healthy appetite. Meals balanced with nutrients and vitamins will help, whether or not the antioxidant vitamins (see page 45) will ultimately be found to prevent or delay the progress of this illness. Keeping your loved one in a bright, mentally stimulating environment surely enhances the quality of her life.

The environment must be tailored to a person with Alzheimer's. For example, early in the course of the illness, the Alzheimer's victim struggles with conscious recollection of past events. Strategies like lists, cues, and notes help the patient function within her environment. As the disease progresses, however, a deterioration in attention, concentration, and reasoning sets in, at which point the patient starts to rely on memory systems that do not depend on conscious recall but are the result of experiences or repetitive practice—such as getting dressed. At this stage, an excellent facility would provide cues to encourage the use of old learned behavioral routines. For example, having her own familiar surroundings—bed, chest of drawers, pictures, the bathroom fixed up as she is accustomed to—reduces the incidence of poor hygiene or other abnormal behaviors.

Such actions also help to prevent another aspect of Alzheimer's called *excess disability*. Initially, most Alzheimer's patients have a reasonable idea of what the future holds. Understandably, this can be horribly depressing. The temptation to brood on lost tomorrows is great. It contributes to the sort of depression in which health fails and the patient suffers more infectious diseases and falls (see page 294). Depression, in turn, can make her cognitive losses seem worse than they really are.

FAMILY SUPPORT

The burden of Alzheimer's affects the entire family—and the reaction of the family has a huge impact on the health of the victim. Because of this, everyone in the family, including children, should know something about the nature of the disease. All should be prepared for the stresses and labors that lie ahead, be warned against innocently cruel comments about the Alzheimer's patient's failings, and bolster themselves against the frustration of wondering exactly who this loved one has become. Don't hesitate to find a local Alzheimer's support group (through your physician or hospital), which can provide the latest information on research progress and developing therapies as well as some much-needed emotional support.

LONG-TERM CARE AND SPECIAL CARE FACILITIES

There is a point in virtually all cases when the care of the Alzheimer's patient becomes too much for any family to handle, and your loved one will have to be moved to a special care facility. While there are a growing number of facilities with areas designed expressly for the care of Alzheimer's patients, you may encounter difficulty in finding one near you. Most nursing homes and other facilities have been designed to meet the needs of the elderly of the past many decades, when most were suffering from physical disability rather than Alzheimer's. Many of these facilities resemble hospital wards. They are often sterile, characterless, and—with the exception of a few inexpensive prints hanging on the walls—devoid of the warm, mentally stimulating environment required by Alzheimer's patients. The staffs of these facilities, although they are highly dedicated and excellently trained to provide medical and physical therapy, are not always experienced in the techniques required to deal with the many dimensions of Alzheimer's. As we look to the future, this is changing, but if it is not changing quickly enough to meet your needs, speak out to push the change!

PREVENTION

You can't prevent Alzheimer's by keeping your blood pressure down, sticking to a low-fat diet, taking medication, or with certainty by any other means. Prevention can mitigate risks for virtually every other human disease, but with Alzheimer's the major risk factors—aging and family history—are completely beyond our control.

However, we may not be completely helpless. There are some measures—medication and otherwise—that can be taken across our life span that do no harm and *might* well confer some preventive benefits.

ANTI-INFLAMMATORY DRUGS

Based on the assumption that inflammation in the brain at least exacerbates Alzheimer's, Dr. John Breitner of Duke University recently conducted a provocative study that showed that chronic users of anti-inflammatory drugs such as ibuprofen, naproxen, and piroxicam (for conditions such as arthritis) had a markedly lower chance of developing Alzheimer's. Observing fifty pairs of twins where one of the pair had extensively used anti-inflammatory drugs and the other had not, Breitner learned that the users had a fourfold lower chance of getting Alzheimer's or they were more likely to get it later than the twin nonuser. (Unfortunately, the study did not have adequate information on aspirin, the most common of all the over-the-counter anti-inflammatory drugs—and the one I use!)

The most provocative findings in his Duke study showed that the benefit of anti-inflammatory drugs was most marked among women and the elderly—and was not statistically significant among male twins. These findings not only once again reinforce a gender dimension to Alzheimer's but also suggest that specific treatments tailored to women must be sought in a focused and aggressive manner. They also encourage researchers to continue to pursue the inflammation theory as a cause or contributor to Alzheimer's. Clear-cut findings in this area could open a variety of avenues of prevention and therapy, perhaps involving drugs already approved and on the market for other diseases.

The results of this study have been received with caution by the medical community, and I would not urge anyone to run out and take an ibuprofen a day on the basis of these findings. But I would encourage us all to keep alert and aware of this potentially simple preventive measure.

ESTROGEN

Another preventive measure about which I am optimistic is hormone replacement therapy (see page 194). We have seen several very exciting reports that HRT both improves cognition in Alzheimer's patients and is associated with a decreased incidence of the disease to begin with. Estrogen, like tacrine, may increase the level of acetylcholine in the brain. In animal models, estrogen also promotes the growth of brain cell connectors (dendrites) and thereby enhances the transmission of signals from one nerve cell to another—and may well be able to create additional memory capacity. I strongly believe this possibility merits aggressive study; in the meantime, add these findings to the potential benefits column as you assess whether or not you'll choose HRT after menopause.

EDUCATION

An education when you're young prevents you from the tragedy of dementia when you're old. The higher the education level, the lower the risk for the Alzheimer's that develops later in life. We've seen this association of education to health before in this book, but the relationships were far more circuitous. An educated person is simply more likely to have learned about good preventive nutrition somewhere along the line, for example, and therefore won't be as likely to eat the very high fat diet that leads to atherosclerosis. With Alzheimer's, the connection seems to be direct and physiological. As we've seen, when you learn, your dendrites grow, your brain reserves increase, and you form neuronal connections that may well buffer against a certain amount of brain cell loss.

According to Robert Katzman from the University of California, San Diego, those without Alzheimer's have roughly twice the educational attainment as those with Alzheimer's. A high school education versus only elementary school is associated with a delayed onset of Alzheimer's by four to five years.

This crucial information is something we must somehow get through to our children—and to those controlling the education of our nation's children. Just as we should urge teenage girls to build up bone reserves to protect against osteoporosis, we should instill in our children the importance of building up brain reserves to protect against Alzheimer's.

EXERCISING THE MIND

Education as a preventive measure for Alzheimer's does not stop when you are young; it lasts a lifetime. It seems there is a direct, physiological link between using your brain and not losing your brain. Continuously challenging yourself with new ideas, tasks, and efforts *at every age* stimulates neuronal growth and interconnections—which means that you have a functionally bigger and better brain. The strategy of creating synapses as preventive therapy cannot be overemphasized and may well be the most sound preventive focus well beyond all others. Exercise your brain! Pay formal attention to clearly planned mental exercise, particularly if you are in a situation where your mind is not challenged daily. There is some evidence that doing mental work, including actively reminiscing about the past, improves cognition for the elderly in general. But other mental efforts surely work as well: crossword puzzles; playing bridge; reading, analyzing, and discussing with someone what is in the newspaper; joining a reading circle; writing letters with thought and care; helping a grandchild with her homework. I look at my ninety-four-year-old mother-in-law who may have weak bones but who has a sturdy, vibrant mind. Almost daily, she writes beautifully thought-out letters—a dying art—in her Victorian script; she quotes poetry, she reads and discusses at least one good book a week, she knows current events sometimes better than I do, she plays bridge with her younger friends, and she is very much involved with family activities.

I'm convinced that this kind of mental exercising can be preventive and can play a role in delaying the symptoms of early Alzheimer's. Diana F. McGowin, who has early-onset Alzheimer's, wrote her moving book about the disease, *Living in the Labyrinth*, as an effort of mental stimulation. She certainly believes that the exercise slowed her decline. Clearly more work must be done to see if her optimism is valid hope for others; in the meantime, I suggest you read her book. Or any book. Take a class, face that computer, learn something new. You may be saving your brain.

QUESTIONS FOR YOUR DOCTOR

If another family member has been touched by Alzheimer's, consider the preventive measures discussed in this chapter. Additionally, because this disease carries with it such stigma and so much ignorance, you must take particular care to ask pointed questions of your medical professionals.

• In your first consultation regarding memory problems for yourself or a family member, ask: What is your doctor's experience in dealing with Alzheimer's? What is the likelihood that these memory problems mean dementia? How will she go about making the diagnosis? Can she provide you with a detailed plan of her diagnosis? If not, why doesn't she feel such a plan is needed? Has she ruled out all reversible forms of cognitive impairment, including depression? (Before dementia is fully diagnosed, ask about having a CAT scan or an MRI performed and what might be looked for.)

• If Alzheimer's is the diagnosis, ask about the qualifications, skills, and costs of a social worker or occupational therapist. Ask about a nutritionist to recommend vitamin supplements and general nutrition. Find out about home health care services in your community. What extended care facility does your doctor recommend and why?

• If you find you or a family member needs an extended care facility, visit many and ask if they have special programs for Alzheimer's patients. What are they? How do they train their staff? What type of nutrition do they provide, and who oversees the diet? How do they monitor their patients' nutrition? What type of mental exercise do they encourage? What type of physical activities? How often do they interact with the patients? What is their philosophy of medication? Maximal sedation or minimal?

• Ask your doctor what groups or organizations offer support to Alzheimer's patients and their families. Regularly ask about new developments in Alzheimer's research.

• Inquire about your community to see if it has the facilities needed by Alzheimer's patients. Ask about local research programs and research investments. What is your doctor doing, personally, to actively encourage Alzheimer's research? (After all, you want your physician invested in curing this illness, too.)

WHAT WOMEN CAN DO
PERSONALLY AND POLITICALLY

The magnitude of the pending crisis is slowly, I believe, waking our entire society to the impact of Alzheimer's. Research into every aspect of the disease is proceeding, sped by new biotechnological tools. Men and women who design, staff, and manage nursing facilities are recognizing the need for more stimulating and therapeutic environments. But we are not doing nearly enough. It is critical that societal, political, and commercial organizations become aware of the scope of the burden that will descend on us and direct more funds and human talent both toward aiding today's victims and researching the means of preventing and treating a future large-scale crisis in our society.

Society is a dynamic enterprise, with shifting fads, values, and mores. As a society, we need to seriously rethink how we deal with the elderly. The buzzword of concern for the elderly today—at least in the political arena—is Social Security. This is not enough concern; throwing small amounts of their own hard-earned money at our future elderly population does little to demonstrate true respect or even to ensure an adequate quality of life. The far bigger issue is how society, and each one of us in that society, values our elderly as individuals. Right now we still encourage "retirement," a socially engineered fantasy prompted by the Industrial Revolution and sold to the public in a time when there were more young than old in society and when few people lived to retirement age, anyway. The concept of retirement for healthy people seems deeply flawed to me: why discard the elderly's brains and talents? Mental exercise and working at some task—perhaps with reduced hours—within a social structure of companionship, challenge, and reward may well delay the onset of Alzheimer's; as a society today, we encourage just the opposite.

Additionally, the burdens placed on the Alzheimer's caregiver would not be so heavy if we lived in a world that accepted, accommodated, and embraced the needs of the frail elderly in the same way we seem willing to accommodate the frail young. These social issues need thorough airing and heightened attention, and soon.

I think it would be wise for each person concerned about making change in the way we view Alzheimer's to take a cue from those so actively involved in combating AIDS. As a group of interested and concerned citizens, AIDS activists mounted one of the most impressive political campaigns of this century to ensure that research into the disease was not only properly funded but properly directed toward sophisticated scientific involovement. The lessons to be learned from this activism seem particularly applicable to the complex disease of Alzheimer's. For Alzheimer's, the only hope lies in funded and focused science, at both the basic and clinical level.

I advise you to call and write your representatives and senators, the White House and the statehouse, first asking what each is doing for the elderly with Alzheimer's (so you are assured a response) and then giving your own views. Encourage your friends to do the same. Join and influence one of the most effective advocacy groups for the elderly, the American Association of Retired Persons. The AARP needs to address this issue forcefully and make it one of its highest priorities for political and social action.

Note your own tendency to shy away from people you may encounter who show signs of "senility." Reassess your thinking anytime you may dismiss the elderly, Alzheimer's victim or not. Remember, the baby boom is aging; we will ourselves produce the biggest boom in elderly in the history of the world. Twenty or thirty or forty years from now, it may be you who sits invisibly on that park bench—unless we all work hard to ferret out our own biases and prevent them from getting in the way of what could be some very enriching relationships with today's elderly people. Take a lesson from my friend Harry Lever's thirteen-year-old son, who volunteered to play the piano in a home for the elderly every week, and try to instill such respect and values in your own children—and in yourself.

It is lunchtime in the year 2040. My daughters and I are laughing. There is a pause in the conversation. Then Marie says, "Oh, Mom. Of course we remember! Their names were Augustus and Maxstead—Gus and Max. They were such neat dogs. Remember?"

"Yes, girls," I intend to reply. "I remember them well."

A PERSONAL EPILOGUE

If I try to be like him, who will be like me?

— A N O N Y M O U S ,
J E W I S H   W I S D O M ,   *1 9 9 4*

In the opening pages of this book I suggested that you view our journey together as the beginning of your own personal and lifelong quest for your best health and for excellent health care. To ease your travels I've urged you to ask questions of your physicians, to fight for adequate health care in your community, and to insist that resources be provided and attention paid to women's health issues in all levels of government and industry. I've stressed how important it is to encourage your daughters to learn about their health needs, and above all for you to continue to learn as much as you can about your body and about the medical advances being made every day, and the political forces that either aid or impede those developments.

We now both close this book, and I wish you Godspeed: may you find your life voyages safe and enlightening. As I leave you with my visions and wishes for your future health care, I can tell you that I see no more effective way to traverse safely the path of good health than with a suitcase packed full of education.

Knowledge, it is said, is power. I believe this with all my heart. And as we move more and more deeply into the information age, the playing field between men and women is leveling: it is the brain, and not the brawn, that will prevail. Women *as* women will contribute fully in the marketplace of the future, driven by ideas and intelligence. Education is a route to power accessible to all women as never before: use it. For us and our daughters, controlling our health in the future means getting smarter. Most of the cures and remedies of the future will have their heaviest impact on women, for it's women who live longer and are most beset by chronic debilitating diseases. Medical technology is rushing forward into territories that demand understanding from us, for they raise as many ethical questions as they provide medical miracles. To protect ourselves, to make wise choices, and to take advantage of what the future holds, we must have a clear sense of the complexities of medicine and health care of the future.

Yet, while women have more of a stake than ever, science and medicine are still viewed, in our schools and in our attitudes, as masculine fields of endeavor. As long as we allow this to go on, we deny ourselves access to our most powerful weapon. The best legacy we can leave our daughters is a lust for learning. Education, with a strong dose of science, will serve our daughters better than any trust fund. I say this from observation and experience.

A BRIEF LOOK BACK

It is not hyperbole to say that modern medicine has transformed our lives and our expectations about life in an amazingly short time—since the 1950s. For me, and for at least some of you, the 1950s were only a short time ago. I was a teenager growing up a few blocks away from the Queensborough Bridge in Astoria, a tidy, mostly Italian immigrant New York City neighborhood. Living over my parents' small business, I prided myself on my homemade clothes and my prowess with books, and believed in my heart that I was the luckiest kid in the world.

A sense of buoyancy radiated from those cracked concrete sidewalks and asphalt shingled row houses on the block where I lived, even though most of the people who lived on it (including my parents) hadn't graduated from high school. That buoyancy arose from an abiding faith in the American dream and in the dignity and worth of the individual human spirit—and the power of education to bring opportunity. Every little child in every little house would have the chance to do better than his or her parents. The formula was simple: all we had to do was work hard, study hard, follow the rules, and, of course, honor our parents. And it worked: not just for Mike and Vi Healy's four girls but for Tony and Rose Macchiarulo's three and the many other families that worked and lived next door to each other.

The fifties weren't simply a time of youthful optimism when struggle was somehow accepted as necessary, and being an immigrant with big dreams was a badge of honor. On a national scale, the economy was expanding, our country was prosperous, we had peace at home, and, with the Marshall Plan, we were rebuilding Europe after World War II. President Franklin Roosevelt declared that after the war our nation would direct the power of science and technology, which was so successful in winning the war, toward civilian goals. Roosevelt— perhaps because he knew the suffering of chronic debilitating disease—singled out medicine above all as the national pursuit to bring maximum benefit to the lives of all Americans. To achieve the common good, the next war was to be the war on human disease.

What was medicine like back then in the glorious fifties when we embarked on this American crusade? In truth, it was in the dark ages. Medicine was not very expensive but it was also not so glorious. We were in the midst of an epidemic of heart attacks and sudden death among middle-aged men that we didn't understand. Cancer was an unspeakable, incurable disease. Those with severe mental illness and the elderly with dementia were seen as hopelessly insane. I used to look down on a mysterious edifice perched on a little island one could see from a distance while crossing the Queensborough Bridge—it was called the Hospital for the Incurably Ill. I imagined it to be a scary place, an Alcatraz for the sick and discarded.

The sick *were* often discarded back then. Not because we did not value them but rather because we did not have the means to help them. There was no heart surgery to make blue babies pink, to treat deformed or damaged heart valves. We did not have cardiac pacemakers, artificial hips or knees, kidney dialysis or organ transplantation. We had no effective treatments for high blood pressure, no chemotherapy or radiation treatment for cancer. Penicillin was a miracle breakthrough of the war years, but essentially the only available antibiotic. Rheumatic fever was still rampant among our children.

I vividly remember summer fears of polio. More than once the health officials closed the public swimming pool in our neighborhood because of the risk of the crippling disease. I recall the fear in all the moms each time their child had a summer fever or sore throat. And there was Louie who once lived next door to us and who got polio; he survived but was left paralyzed. How far we have come in medicine these many years from the glorious fifties!

It was also a time when women were not welcome in medicine. Medical schools had their unstated quotas. Not only was it hard to find a woman doctor, but many women and most men would not dream of going to one. Were it not for my father's bold and unabiding statement that his girls "could do anything; even be doctors," and of course *he* would go to a woman doctor, "if she were smart," I'm not sure I would be writing this book. His visions were out of the mainstream, bucking the currents of a time when men were so thoroughly the norm that when it came to seeking a place in medicine, M.D.-employment ads after World War II did not hesitate to state: "Women need not apply."

AND TODAY

One must look in awe at what has happened in less than half a century. Medical innovation has revolutionized our lives. We take for granted many of the cures and the treatments. We now can cure many cancers, and treat virtually all. We have dramatically decreased mortality from heart disease and stroke. Polio is no longer a summer dirge of our inner cities. Those past successes have only increased our expectations for doing better and doing it faster.

By choice, medicine and medical research in this country have become a spending priority. As a nation, we spend a trillion dollars a year on our health. To sustain the advances in medicine and to cure the illnesses of tomorrow we invest about 11 billion dollars in biomedical research through the National Institutes of Health, and another 11 to 12 billion dollars through private sector research by industry. This massive investment in medical care and innovation is part of that sustained strategic commitment to health made some fifty years ago. And that commitment is why we lead the world in advanced health care, but also why it is so expensive.

Our success since the fifties has created the very problems we are struggling with in our health care system today: great medicine, with even greater expectations for the future, but at great financial cost. We have been striving to produce the best at whatever cost. Modern medicine has changed our *expectations* of life, as much as quality of life and length of life. As one wag noted aptly: In most countries, people view death as inevitable. Americans see it as an option.

Why does America spend so much for health research and health care? My diagnosis is that the belief that every individual matters is deeply rooted in the American psyche, even our political heritage. It is this belief that has propelled women over the past several decades to rectify the imbalances that they have seen by making critical strides, in work, in family, and in health.

Let me tell you a story that illustrated this to me. Some time ago I saw a report on CNN about a mental hospital for children and adolescents in Moscow shortly after the breakup of the Soviet Union. Under glasnost, cameras were allowed in to film docile kids lining up to get their heavy doses of tranquilizers and other drugs three times a day. The head of the hospital acknowledged that most of these children were there for relatively minor behavioral infractions that we might call being a teenager: infractions like running away from home, not going to school, or sniffing glue. Very few had medically defined psychiatric illness. The reporter asked the head of the hospital, who was critical of the practice, how this could have been tolerated. He replied, "You must understand that in our system of government we do not value the individual—only the group. Our practices do not harm the group." In the United States we take for granted the fact that we place as much value on the rights and well-being of the individual as of the group.

Disease and death do not happen to a nation, they happen to individuals one-by-one, as men and as women. One cannot trample on the rights, choices, and privacy of individual women or men when it comes to their only real possessions—their mind and their body. The challenge for us all today is to change what needs to be changed in our American system that has served us well, without doing it harm. And as a people we must not forget the vital need to sustain the critical path of innovation and discovery for the patients of tomorrow.

AND TOMORROW . . .

As we look to the next century, it is easy to predict the profound transformations of our world by discoveries in biology and medicine. No human disease should be safe from extinction or radical control. Genetically engineered cancer vaccines hold the promise of destroying even the most advanced and spreading tumors of the breast or ovary. Reconstituting the human immune system will allow AIDS victims to live with their disease. Learning how to destroy human viruses lurking within living human cells will bring us cures for HIV, hepatitis, human papilloma virus, many tumors, and even, at long last, the common cold. The dread Alzheimer's disease will be understood and prevented or cured—to our own benefit and for the sake of our children.

We are on the brink of discovering more adventurous and promising—and frightening—means of altering our own bodies than any alchemist ever dreamed. The powers of molecular and structural biology and biotechnology know no bounds. We are currently deciphering the human genome, the complex genetic code that makes us the individuals we are, from the color of our hair to the specific reasons the intricate systems of our bodies can founder. We have already discovered the genes that indicate cystic fibrosis and colon and breast cancer. We are learning about the gene or genes that contribute to heart disease, osteoporosis, and Alzheimer's disease; and next it will be the DNA molecules that make one vulnerable to depression or schizophrenia. With each discovery comes the understanding needed to detect the disease; the ability to delay and to cure it are generally not far behind. And women with their special vulnerabilities will be the great beneficiaries.

But even as all the advances are under way in the science of life, we are beginning to see the question life raises about science. Allegories from *Faust* to *Frankenstein* to *Jurassic Park* caution us against reaching too far, against attempting to interfere with our innate limitations. As these immensely popular morality tales illustrate, science and religion are not at all distinct, and these lines will become even more blurred as we become able to actually alter our own genes. What we can do versus what we morally should do are the questions that will dog our medical advances into the foreseeable future. I believe strongly in pursuing these advances. I do not believe experimentation that is fully informed from all angles—environmental impact, emotional ramifications, long-term effect on individuals and communities, as well as potential for increased scientific knowledge—can be destructive as long as our ethical center is firmly grounded.

For example, genetic testing will allow us to detect traits long before they are realized. Traits for alcoholism as well as heart disease, for depression or violence as well as for cancer may be discernible in a fetus. How much do we want to know? How much control do we want to have? And who should wield the power? Who should even know? Do you really want to know if you are harboring the gene for Alzheimer's disease when you are an otherwise healthy and happy hard-working woman making your way through life, particularly when that gene predicts only the possibility, not the certainty, of the disease? And what about your privacy: what happens if your friends find out, or your employer, or your spouse or prospective spouse, or your children? These problems may seem far off, but believe me, they are not.

This explosion of knowledge in biology and medicine is changing not only the nature of healing, but also the society in which we live. We are seeing large shifts in demography, with an aging population living longer and becoming progressively more female. The meaning of life and death is being reexamined. Extending life will be easier than deciding when not to; new diseases will emerge as people survive the old ones; and we will come face-to-face with a whole new realm of ethical and legal dilemmas.

In all this, your own attention will make the difference. On a very personal level, the more you know about your own health issues, the greater the likelihood that you will stay healthy. Should a health crisis arise, you will be prepared to meet it head-on if you understand it. Any medical procedure becomes far less threatening if you understand the medical jargon, or if you have the wherewithal and conviction to insist on answers to all your questions.

By the same token, the larger societal issues become simpler when you understand their intricacies. And you must. For science to flourish and all our dreams to be realized, we must insist that ethics and public interest become companions to science wherever it goes. The greater community must engage these issues, not just those of us in medicine, but all of us who will be touched by it and the power of the life sciences.

This exciting, yet somewhat frightening, medical future will require a generation of informed leadership to tap deeply into the talents of women. It will take persistence and discipline. It will take knowing what you stand for, not just what you stand against, to make the choices critical to keeping this future on course. It will require making it your own way with persistence, with discipline, with confidence, and with courage. It will require activism. It will require that the third wave of feminine leadership lead men as well as women.

And as we think about this third wave, let us not forget the first. This book is finished in the year of the seventy-fifth anniversary of women's securing the right to vote in America, itself a culmination of a movement started by women in parlors and convention halls almost seventy-five years before that. At the Seneca Falls Women's Rights Convention in 1848, women astounded the world with their Declaration of Sentiments and Resolutions, which took the Declaration of Independence further than anyone had dared interpret it: "We hold these truths to be self-evident, that all men and women are created equal; that they are endowed by their Creator with certain inalienable rights; that among these are life, liberty, and the pursuit of happiness."

One immutable fact tha t has not changed, nor will it change in the years ahead, is that for women to pursue happiness, they must pursue health; and they must do so not just like men, but as women, proudly.

SOURCES

I intend this book to be a conversation about your health rather than a textbook of medicine. You have in each chapter my analysis of the myriad new and old information about the critical health issues facing women. To reference every new or old observation would be of little value to the general reader. Nonetheless, should you want to delve further into any of the issues discussed, I have provided here a range of references from the technical and scientific to the more general and also the popular when I have called upon them in my chapter. Remember also that the nature of science and medicine is that it is an evolving story, which will change many times in the years ahead. Having a framework for digesting the new information is critical even as that framework expands in the future. And when you hear about new information that seems to contradict the old, and it is relevant to your health, think about it, ask about it, read about it, and understand that this is the way knowledge grows and gets better for you.

The following books and articles deal with the subjects I have discussed in each chapter. The books can be found in good libraries or acquired through interlibrary loans. However, a number of the medical and scientific articles are available only in hospital medical libraries. Some hospitals open these to the public and those that do not will provide photocopies of the articles to physicians who request them. If you are personally unable to acquire specific articles, ask your doctor to help you obtain them. Such requests should not be troubling to your doctor and have the added benefit of opening a dialogue between the two of you.

Although I have tried to avoid articles that are research oriented or scientifically dense, some material comes heavily laden with medical terminology. Do not be put off by this. For the most part, it is only the necessary jargon of the profession. You need not look up the definition of every term. It is more important to identify the general thrust of the article and discuss it with your doctor. He or she will fill in the blanks.

As I put together this list, I do so with a sense of just how exciting and powerful medical knowledge is. I am already looking forward to writing the next edition of this book in about six or seven years to compare how far we go in promoting women's health in that measured period of time. I am optimistic that with your interest and support and pressure on the system to keep the work going, it will be a great story to tell.

GENERAL REFERENCES

American Medical Association Encyclopedia of Medicine. New York: Random House, 1989. (Excellent general encyclopedia that gives you clear definitions of terms and health issues as a first place to start.)

Drug Evaluations Annual. Chicago: American Medical Association, 1993. (A large and technical reference book used by health professionals that gives practical and current information on approved drugs and their use.)

Isselbacher, K. J., E. Braunwald, J. Wilson, J. B. Martin, A. S. Fauci, and D. L. Kasper, eds. *Harrison's Principles of Internal Medicine.* New York: McGraw-Hill, 1994. (Also in 1995, a brief guide based on the larger textbook was published. Technical, detailed, and authoritative.)

The Journal of Women's Health. B. Healy, ed. New York: Mary Ann Liebert Publishers. (A journal for physicians with some review and perspective pieces of general interest to the public.)

Macklis, R. M., M. E. Mendelsohn, and G. M. Mudge, Jr. *Introduction to Clinical Medicine: A Student to Student Manual.* Boston: Little, Brown, 1994. (A brief medical students' guide, which is in parts somewhat technical for the lay reader.)

Meir, G. *My Life.* New York: Putnam, 1975.

National Institutes of Health. Office of the Director. Office of Research on Women's Health. 1992. *Report of the National Institutes of Health: Opportunities for Research on Women's Health.* NIH Publication no. 92-3457.

The PDR Family Guide to Prescription Drugs. Montvale, NJ: Medical Economics Data, 1993.

Ravitch, D., ed. *The American Reader: Words That Moved a Nation.* New York: HarperCollins, 1990.

Safire, W. *Lend Me Your Ears: Great Speeches in History.* New York: W. W. Norton, 1992. (Important collection of speeches from all times; includes the words of Queen Elizabeth I, Louis Pasteur, Justice Oliver Wendell Holmes, Elizabeth Cady Stanton, Susan B. Anthony, Senator Margaret Chase Smith, and many others, some quoted throughout my book.)

Safire, W., and Safire L., eds. *Words of Wisdom: More Good Advice.* New York: Simon & Schuster, 1989.

The World Book Health and Medical Annual. Chicago: World Book, 1994. (Annual that covers general medical topics in a review format each year, and includes many features relevant to women's health. An interesting and relevant read for the entire family.)

GENERAL SOURCES

American Medical Association
515 North State Street
Chicago, IL 60610
312/464-5000

American Osteopathic Association
142 East Ontario Street
Chicago, IL 60611
312/280-5800

Association for Women in Science (AWIS)
1522 K Street N.W., Suite 820
Washington, DC 20005
202/408-0742

National Health Information Center
800/336-4797
(The Center provides data on 1,000 organizations that provide health information. Also check with your local hospital or nearby medical school. Many have women's health centers that contain current information for the general public on a wide range of health issues.)

National Institutes of Health
National Institute of Child Health and Human Development
Bldg. 31, Room 2A03
9000 Rockville Pike
Bethesda, MD 20892
301/496-5133

National Institutes of Health
Office of Alternative Medicine (OAM)
6120 Executive Blvd.
Executive Plaza South, Suite 450
Rockville, MD 20892-9904

301/402-2466 (completely automated menu)
Fax 301/402-4741

National Institutes of Health
Office of Research on Women's Health
Bldg. 1, Room 201
9000 Rockville Pike
Bethesda, MD 20892-0161
301/402-1770

National Institutes of Health
Women's Health Initiative
Federal Bldg., Room 6A09
9000 Rockville Pike
Bethesda, MD 20892
800/54-WOMEN (800/549-6636)

National Library of Medicine
8600 Rockville Pike
Bethesda, MD 20894
301/496-6308

National Medical Association
1012 Tenth Street N.W.
Washington, DC 20001
202/347-1895
Fax 202/842-3293

Society for the Advancement of Women's Health Research
1920 L Street N.W.
Washington, DC 20036
202/223-7009

CHAPTER 2—NUTRITION: WOMEN'S WORK BECOMES WOMEN'S HEALTH

Books

Brody, J. E. *Jane Brody's Nutrition Book: A Lifetime Guide to Good Eating for Better Health and Weight Control.* New York: Bantam Books, 1987.

Griffin, G. C., and W. P. Castelli. *Good Fat, Bad Fat: How to Lower Your Cholesterol & Beat the Odds of a Heart Attack.* Tucson: Fisher Books, 1989.

Grundy, S., and M. Winston, eds. *The American Heart Association Low Fat, Low Cholesterol Cookbook.* New York: Times Books/Random House, 1989.

National Research Council. *Diet and Health: Implications for Reducing Chronic Disease Risk.* Washington, D.C.: National Academy Press, 1989.

Shils, M. E., J. A. Olson, and M. Shike, eds. *Modern Nutrition in Health and Disease.* Philadelphia: Lea & Febiger, 1994.

Tufts University Diet and Nutrition Letter. New subscription information: P.O. Box 10948, Des Moines, IA 50940. (Tel. 1-800-288-8387).

U.S. Department of Agriculture and U.S. Department of Health and Human Services. 1990. *Nutrition and Your Health: Dietary Guidelines for Americans.* Washington, D.C.: U.S. Government Printing Office. Publication no. 232.

U.S. Department of Health and Human Services. 1988. *The Surgeon General's Report on Nutrition and Health: Summary and Recommendations.* DHSS Publication no. 88-50211. (Available from the U.S. Government Printing Office, Washington, D.C. 20402, 202/512-0000; or Superintendent of Documents, 202/512-1800.)

Williams S. R. *Essentials of Nutrition and Diet Therapy.* St. Louis: Times Mirror/Mosby College Publications, 1994.

Wotecki, C. E., and P. T. Thomas, eds. *Eat for life: The Food and Nutrition Board's Guide to Reducing Your Risk of Chronic Disease.* New York: Harper-Perennial, 1993.

Articles

Danford, D. E., and S. Fletcher. Methods of voluntary weight loss and control. National Institutes of Health Technology Assessment Conference. *Annals of Internal Medicine* 119: 641–770 (1993).

Danford, D. E., and M. G. Stephenson. Healthy People 2000: Development of nutritional objectives. *Journal of the American Dietetic Association* 91(12): 1517–1519 (Dec. 1991).

Gizis, F. C. Nutrition in women across the life span. *Nursing Clinics of North America* 27(4): 971–92 (Dec. 1992).

Hankin, J. H. Role of nutrition in women's health: Diet and breast cancer. *Journal of the American Dietetic Association* 93(9): 994–999 (Sept. 1993).

Johnson, K., and E. W. Kligman. Preventive nutrition: An "optimal" diet for older adults. *Geriatrics* 47(10): 56–60 (Oct. 1992); and Preventive nutrition: Disease-specific dietary interventions for older adults. *Geriatrics* 47(11): 39–40, 45–49 (Nov. 1992).

Keen, C. L., and S. Zidenberg-Cherr. Should vitamin-mineral supplements be recommended for all women with childbearing potential? *American Journal of Clinical Nutrition* 59(2 Suppl): 532S–538S; discussion 538S–539S (Feb. 1994).

Olson, C. M. Promoting positive nutritional practices during pregnancy and lactation. *American Journal of Clinical Nutrition* 59(2 Suppl): 525S–530S; discussion 530S–531S (Feb. 1994).

Sources

American Dietetic Association
216 West Jackson Boulevard, Suite 800
Chicago, IL 60606
312/899-0040

ADA Consumer Nutrition Hot Line
800/366-1655

Food and Drug Administration
5600 Fishers Lane
Rockville, MD 20857
301/443-2410

National Institute of Diabetes and Digestive and Kidney Diseases (NIDDK)
Office of Nutrition Research
National Institutes of Health
Bldg. 31, Room 9A04
31 Center Drive—MSC 2560
Bethesda, MD 20892-2560
301/496-3583

National Institutes of Health
National Institute of Child Health and Human Development
Bldg. 31, Room 2A03
9000 Rockville Pike
Bethesda, MD 20892
301/496-5133

United States Department of Agriculture
14th Street and Independence Avenue S.W.
Washington, DC 20250
202/720-2791
Also: Meat and Poultry Hotline
800/535-4555

CHAPTER 3—REPRODUCTIVE LIFE: POWER AND VULNERABILITY

Books

Love and Sexuality:

Beauvoir, S. de. *The Second Sex.* New York: Bantam, 1961. Reprint. New York: Random House, 1989.

Buss, D. *Evolution of Desire.* New York: HarperCollins, 1994.

Fromm, E. *The Art of Loving.* New York: HarperCollins, 1989.

Hite, S. *The Hite Report: A Nationwide Study of Female Sexuality.* New York: Macmillan, 1976. Reprint. New York: Dell, 1987.

Huxley, A. *Brave New World.* New York: Harper & Row, 1969.

Masters, W., and V. Johnson. *Human Sexual Response.* Boston: Little, Brown, 1966.

Maurois, A. *Seven Faces of Love.* New York: Didier, 1944.

Michael, R. T., J. H. Gagnon, E. O. Laumann, and G. Kolata. *Sex in America: A Definitive Survey.* Boston: Little, Brown, 1994.

Tennov, D. *Love and Limerence. The Experience of Being in Love.* New York: Scarborough Books/Stein and Day, 1980.

Contraception:

Blank, Robert H. *Fertility Control: New Techniques, New Policy Issues.* Westport, Conn.: Greenwood Press, 1991.

Chesler, E. *Woman of Valor: Margaret Sanger and the Birth Control Movement in America.* New York: Anchor Books/Doubleday, 1993.

Garrow, David J. *Liberty and Sexuality. The Right to Privacy and the Making of Roe v. Wade 1923–1973.* New York: Macmillan, 1994.

Harlap, S., K. Kost, and J. D. Forrest. *Preventing Pregnancy, Protecting Health.* New York: Alan Guttmacher Institute, 1991.

Marrs, R. P. *Assisted Reproductive Technologies.* Cambridge, Mass.: Blackwell Scientific Publications, Inc., 1993.

Sanger, M. *Woman and the New Race.* New York: Brentano, 1920.

Shoupe, E. D., and F. P. Haseltine, eds. *Contraception.* New York: Springer-Verlag, 1993.

Conception and Infertility:

Corson, Stephen L. *Conquering Infertility: A Guide for Couples.* Rev. ed. Englewood Cliffs, NJ: Prentice-Hall/Simon & Schuster, 1991.

Menning, B. E. *Infertility: A Guide for the Childless Couple.* New York: Prentice-Hall, 1988.

Office of Technology Assessment. *Infertility: Medical and Social Choices.* Washington, D.C.: U.S. Government Printing Office, 1988.

Pregnancy and Childbirth:

American Academy of Pediatrics' Committee on Fetus & Newborn, Staff, and American College of Obstetricians and Gynecologists' Committee on Obstetrics, Maternal & Fetal Medicine Staff. *Guidelines for Perinatal Care.* Elk Grove Village, IL: American Academy of Pediatrics, 1992.

Bean, C. A. *Methods of Childbirth: A Classic Work for Today's Woman.* New York: Wm. Morrow, 1990.

Cherry, S. H. *Understanding Pregnancy and Childbirth.* New York: Maxwell Macmillan International, 1992.

Creasy, R. K., and R. Resnick, eds. *Material-Fetal Medicine: Principles and Practice.* 3d ed. Philadelphia: W. B. Saunders, 1993. (A major medical text that covers the breadth of reproductive medicine, including contraception and childbirth.)

Eisenberg, A., H. Murkoff, and S. Hathaway. *What to Expect When You're Expecting.* New York: Workman, 1991. (Excellent!)

Gilstrap, L. C., and B. B. Little. *Drugs and Pregnancy.* New York: Elsevier, 1992.

Institute of Medicine. *Nutrition During Pregnancy and Lactation: An Implementation Guide.* Washington, D.C.: National Academy Press, 1992.

Articles

General:

Dennis, R. Cultural change and the reproductive cycle. *Social Science & Medicine.* 34(5): 485–489 (Mar. 1992).

Fredricsson, B., and H. Gilljam. Smoking and reproduction. Short and long-term effects and benefits of smoking cessation. *Acta Obstetricia et Gynecologica Scandinavica* 71(8): 580–592 (Dec. 1992).

Meyer, W. R., E. F. Pierce, and V. L. Katz. The effect of exercise on reproductive function and pregnancy. *Current Opinion in Obstetrics and Gynecology* 6(3): 293–299 (Jun. 1994).

Prior, J. C., Y. M. Vigna, and D. W. McKay. Reproduction for the athletic woman: New understandings of physiology and management. *Sports Medicine* 14(3): 190–199 (Sept. 1992).

Rausch, J. L., and B. L. Parry. Treatment of premenstrual mood symptoms. *Psychiatric Clinics of North America* 16(4): 829–839 (Dec. 1993).

Rosenfield, R. L. Puberty and its disorders in girls. *Endocrinology and Metabolism Clinics of North America* 20(1): 15–42 (Mar. 1991); and Menstrual disorders in adolescence. *Endocrinology and Metabolism Clinics of North America* 22(3): 491–505 (Sept. 1993).

Senanayake, P. Women's reproductive health: Challenges for the 1990s. *Advances in Contraception* 7(2–3): 129–136 (June–Sept. 1991).

Infertility:

Agarwal, S. K., and A. F. Haney. Does recommending timed intercourse really help the infertile couple? *Obstetrics and Gynecology* 84(2): 307–10 (Aug. 1994).

Davis, K. M., and J. A. Rock. Endometriosis. *Current Opinion in Obstetrics and Gynecology* 4(2): 229–237 (Apr. 1992).

Healy, D. L., A. O. Trounson, and A. N. Andersen. Female infertility: Causes and treatment. *Lancet* 343(8912): 1539–1544 (Jun. 18, 1994).

Murphy, A. A. and P. Z. Castellano. RU486: Pharmacology and potential use in the treatment of endometriosis and leiomyomata uteri. *Current Opinion in Obstetrics and Gynecology* 6(3): 269–278 (Jun. 1994).

Younger, J. B. Endometriosis. *Current Opinion in Obstetrics and Gynecology* 5(3): 333–339 (Jun. 1993).

In Vitro Fertilization:

Cohen, J., G. Schattman, M. Suzman, A. Adler, M. Alikani, and Z. Rosenwaks. Micromanipulating human gametes. *Reproduction, Fertility & Development* 6(1): 69–81; discussion 81–83 (1994).

Cohen, J., B. E. Talansky, A. Adler, M. Alikani, and Z. Rosenwaks. Controversies and opinions in clinical microsurgical fertilization. *Journal of Assisted Reproduction & Genetics* 9(2): 94–96 (Apr. 1992).

Harvey, J. C. Ethical issues and controversies in assisted reproductive technologies. *Current Opinion in Obstetrics & Gynecology* 4(5): 750–755 (Oct. 1992).

Healy, B. Egg donors for hire: A medical dilemma in search of solutions, not college students. *Journal of Women's Health* 4 (2): in press (1995).

Moghissi, K. S., and R. Leach. Future directions in reproductive medicine. *Archives of Pathology and Laboratory Medicine* 116(4): 436–441 (Apr. 1992).

Penzias, A. S. and A. H. DeCherney. Clinical Review 55: Advances in clinical in vitro fertilization. *Journal of Clinical Endocrinology & Metabolism* 78(3): 503–508 (Mar. 1994).

Wasserman, D., and Wachbroit R. The technology, law, and ethics of in vitro fertilization, gamete donation, and surrogate motherhood. *Clinics in Laboratory Medicine* 12(3): 429–448 (Sept. 1992).

Contraception:

Aldhous, P. A booster for contraceptive vaccines. *Science* 266:1484–1486 (1994).

Alexander, C. S., and B. Guyer. Adolescent pregnancy: Occurrence and consequences. *Pediatric Annals* 22(2): 85–88 (Feb. 1993).

Burkman, R. T., Jr. Noncontraceptive effects of hormonal contraceptives: Bone mass, sexually transmitted disease and pelvic inflammatory disease, cardiovascular disease, menstrual function, and future fertility. *American Journal of Obstetrics & Gynecology* 170(5 pt. 2): 1569–1575 (May 1994).

Darney, P. D. Hormonal implants: Contraception for a new century. *American Journal of Obstetrics & Gynecology* 170(5 pt. 2): 1536–1543 (May 1994).

Davis, A. J. The role of hormonal contraception in adolescents. *American Journal of Obstetrics & Gynecology* 170(5 pt. 2): 1581–1585 (May 1994).

Forrest, J. D. Epidemiology of unintended pregnancy and contraceptive use. *American Journal of Obstetrics & Gynecology* 170(5 pt. 2): 1485–1489 (May 1994).

McGregor, J. A., and H. A. Hammill. Contraception and sexually transmitted diseases: Interactions and opportunities. *American Journal of Obstetrics & Gynecology* 168(6 pt. 2): 2033–2041 (Jun. 1993).

Sulak, P. J. The career woman and contraceptive use. *International Journal of Fertility* 36 (Suppl 2): 90–97; discussion 97–100 (1991).

Sulak, P. J., and A. F. Haney. Unwanted pregnancies: Understanding contraceptive use and benefits in adolescents and older women. *American Journal of Obstetrics & Gynecology* 168(6 pt. 2): 2042–2048 (Jun. 1993).

Abortion:

Adler, N. E., H. P. David, B. N. Major, S. H. Roth, N. F. Russo, and G. E. Wyatt. Psychological factors in abortion: A review. *American Psychologist* 47(10): 1194–1204 (Oct. 1992).

Blumenthal, P. D. Abortion: epidemiology, safety, and technique. *Current Opinion in Obstetrics and Gynecology* 4(4): 506–512 (Aug. 1992).

DiPierri, D. RU 486, mifepristone: A review of a controversial drug. *Nursing Practitioner* 19(6): 59–61 (Jun. 1994).

Weiss, B. D. RU 486: The progesterone antagonist. *Archives of Family Medicine* 2(1): 63–69; discussion 70 (Jan. 1993).

Pregnancy:

Hanft, R. S. New reproductive genetics: Political issues. *Clinical Obstetrics and Gynecology* 36(3): 598–604 (Sept. 1993).

Olson, C. M. Promoting positive nutritional practices during pregnancy and lactation. *American Journal of Clinical Nutrition* 59(2 Suppl): 525S–530S; discussion 530S–531S (Feb. 1994).

Stovall, T. G., D. D. Bradham, F. W. Ling, and M. Naughton. Cost of treatment of ectopic pregnancy: Single-dose methotrexate versus surgical treatment. *Journal of Women's Health* 3(6): 445–450 (1994).

Wang, I. Y., and I. S. Fraser. Reproductive function and contraception in the postpartum period. *Obstetrical and Gynecological Survey* 49(1): 56–63 (Jan. 1994).

Wertz, D. C. Ethical and legal implications of the new genetics: Issues for discussion. *Social Science and Medicine* 35(4): 495–505 (Aug. 1992).

Wertz, D. C., D. H. Fanos, and P. R. Reilly. Genetic testing for children and adolescents: Who decides? *Journal of the American Medical Association* 272(11): 875–881 (Sept. 1994).

Sources

American College of Obstetricians and Gynecologists
409 12th Street S.W.
Washington, DC 20024
(202) 638-5577

American Society of Reproductive Medicine
1209 Montgomery Highway
Birmingham, AL 35216
(205) 978-5000
Fax 205/978-2005

The Alan Guttmacher Institute
111 Fifth Avenue
New York, NY 10003
212/254-5656
Fax 212/254-9891

CHAPTER 4—SEXUALLY TRANSMITTED DISEASES: THE SILENT PLAGUE

Books

Holmes, King K., Per-Anders Mardh, P. Frederick Sparling, Paul J. Wiesner, eds. *Sexually Transmitted Diseases*. New York: McGraw-Hill, 1990.

Articles

Centers for Disease Control and Prevention. 1993. Sexually transmitted diseases treatment guidelines. *Morbidity and Mortality Weekly Report*. (MMWR) 42 (RR 14) 50–61.

Edlin, B. R., K. L. Irwin, S. Faruque, and others. Intersecting epidemics: Crack cocaine use and HIV infection among inner-city young adults. *New England Journal of Medicine* 331: 1422–1427 (Nov. 1994).

McGregor, J. A., J. I. French, and N. E. Spencer. Prevention of sexually transmitted diseases in women. *Obstetrics and Gynecology Clinics of North America* 16: 697–702 (1989).

McGregor, J. A., and H. A. Hammill. Contraception and sexually transmitted diseases: Interactions and opportunities. *American Journal of Obstetrics & Gynecology* 168(2): 2033–2041 (Jun. 1993).

McNeeley, S. G., Jr. Pelvic inflammatory disease. *Current Opinion in Obstetrics and Gynecology* 4(5): 682–686 (Oct. 1992).

Peaceman, A. M., and B. Gonik. Sexually transmitted viral disease in women. *Postgraduate Medicine* 89(2): 133–140 (Feb. 1, 1991).

Seidman, S. N., and R. O. Rieder. A review of sexual behavior in the United States. *American Journal of Psychiatry* 151(3): 330–341 (Mar. 1994).

Talashek M. L., A. M. Richy, and H. Epping. Sexually transmitted diseases in the elderly—issues and recommendations. *Journal of Gerontological Nursing.* 16(4): 33–40 (Apr. 1990).

Tichy, A. M., and M. L. Talashek. Older women: Sexually transmitted diseases and acquired immunodeficiency syndrome. *Nursing Clinics of North America* 27(4): 937–949 (Dec. 1992).

Vail-Smith, K., and D. M. White. Risk level, knowledge, and preventive behavior for human papilloma viruses among sexually active college women. *Journal of American College Health* 40(5): 227–230 (Mar. 1992).

Sources

Centers for Disease Control and Prevention (CDC)
Division of STD Prevention (all divisions)
1600 Clifton Road, N.E.
Atlanta, Georgia 30333
404/639-3311

CDC National AIDS Hotline
(This is a confidential 24-hour-a-day, 7-day-a-week operation—they are open even on holidays. Note special numbers.)
800/342-AIDS (342-2437)
For hearing impaired and deaf communities: 800/243-7889 (TTY/TDD)
For Spanish speakers: 800/344-7432

CDC National Sexually Transmitted Disease Hotline
800/227-8922

National Institute of Allergy and Infectious Disease
Bldg. 31, Room 7A03
9000 Rockville Pike
Bethesda, Maryland 20892-0161
(301) 496-5717

CHAPTER 5—MENOPAUSE:
THE NEW PRIME TIME

Books

Beard, M. K., and L. R. Curtis. *Menopause and the Years Ahead.* Tucson: Fisher Books, 1991.

Greenwood, S. *Menopause, Naturally: Preparing for the Second Half of Life.* Volcano, Calif.: Volcano Press, 1992.

Greer, G. *The Change: Women, Aging, and the Menopause.* New York: Knopf, 1992. Reprint. New York: Fawcett, 1993.

Sheehy, G. *The Silent Passage: Menopause.* New York: Pocket Books/Simon & Schuster, 1993.

Sitruk-Ware, R., and W. H. Utian, eds. *The Menopause and Hormonal Replacement Therapy.* New York: Marcel Dekker, 1991.

U.S. Congress. Office of Technology Assessment. *The Menopause, Hormone Therapy, and Women's Health: A Background Paper.* Washington, D.C.: U.S. Government Printing Office, May 1992.

Wells, R. G., and M. C. Wells. *Menopause & Mid-Life.* Wheaton, Ill.: Tyndale House Publishers, 1990.

Articles

Bachmann, G. A. The changes before "the change": Strategies for the transition to the menopause. *Postgraduate Medicine* 95(4): 113–115, 119–121, 124 (Mar. 1994).

Bachmann, G. A. Sexual function in the perimenopause. *Obstetrics & Gynecology Clinics of North America* 20(2): 379–389 (Jun. 1993).

Belchetz, P. E. Hormonal treatment of postmenopausal women. *New England Journal of Medicine* 330(15): 1062–1071 (Apr. 14, 1994).

Fishbein, E. G. Women at midlife: The transition to menopause. *Nursing Clinics of North America* 27(4): 951–957 (Dec. 1992).

Griffing, G. T., and S. H. Allen. Estrogen replacement therapy at menopause: How benefits outweigh risks. *Postgraduate Medicine* 96(5): 131–140 (Oct. 1994).

Haseltine, F. P. Postmenopausal motherhood: Will hysterectomy rates drop? *Journal of Women's Health* 3: 83–84 (Apr. 1994).

Healy, B. PEPI in perspective: Good answers spawn pressing questions. *Journal of the American Medical Association* 273:240–241 (1995).

McCraw, R. K. Psychosexual changes associated with the perimenopausal period. *Journal of Nurse-Midwifery* 36(1): 17–24 (Jan.–Feb. 1991).

Van Hall, E. V., M. Verdel, and J. Van Der Velden. "Perimenopausal" complaints in women and men: A comparative study. *Journal of Women's Health* 3: 45–50 (1994).

The Writing Group for the PEPI Trial. Effects of estrogen or estrogen/progestin regimens on heart disease risk factors in postmenopausal women: The Postmenopausal Estrogen/Progestin Interventions (PEPI) trial. *Journal of the American Medical Association* 273: 199–208 (1995).

Zubialde, J. P., F. Lawler, and N. Clemenson. Estimated gains in life expectancy with use of postmenopausal estrogen therapy: A decision analysis. *Journal of Family Practice* 36(3): 271–280 (Mar. 1993).

Sources

American College of Obstetricians and Gynecologists (ACOG)
409 12th Street S.W.
Washington, DC 20024
202/638-5577

National Institute on Aging
9000 Rockville Pike
Bethesda, MD 20892
800/222-2225 (Information Center)

North American Menopause Society
2074 Abington Road
Cleveland, OH 44106
216/884-3334

Older Women's League
666 11th Street N.W.
Washington, DC 20001
202/783-6686

CHAPTER 6—CANCER: HURRY FOR A CURE

Books

DeVita, V. T., S. Hellman, S. A. Rosenberg, eds. *Cancer: Principles and Practice of Oncology.* Philadelphia: J.B. Lippincott, 1993.

Gee, E. *The Light Around the Dark.* New York: The Center for Human Caring / National League for Nursing Press, 1992.

Holleb, A. I., and others, eds. *American Cancer Society's Complete Book of Cancer: Prevention, Detection, Rehabilitation, Cure.* Garden City, NY: Doubleday, 1986.

Houts, P. S., A. M. Nezu, C. M. Nezu, J. A. Bucher, and A. Lipton. *American College of Physicians Home Care Guide for Cancer: How to Care for Family and Friends at Home*. Philadelphia: American College of Physicians, 1994.

Kushner, R. *Alternatives. New Developments in the War on Breast Cancer*. Cambridge, Mass: The Kensington Press, 1984. Originally published as *Why Me?*

Love, S. M., with K. Lindsey. *Dr. Susan Love's Breast Book*. 1990. Reprint. Reading, Mass.: Addison-Wesley, 1991.

McKay, J., and N. Hirano. *The Chemotherapy Survival Guide*. Oakland, Calif: New Harbinger Publications, 1993.

Morra, M. E. *Triumph: Getting Back to Normal When You Have Cancer*. New York: Avon, 1990.

Radner, G. *It's Always Something*. New York: Avon Books, 1989.

Schindler, L. R. *A Health Guide for All Women: Understanding Breast Cancer*. Bethesda: National Institutes of Health. National Cancer Institute, 1993. Shipping list no. 93-3536.

Tannock, I. F. and R. P. Hill. *The Basic Science of Oncology*. New York: McGraw-Hill, 1992.

Articles

General:

Culotta, E., and D. Koshland, Jr. p53 sweeps through cancer research. *Science* 262: 1958–1960 (Dec. 1993); see also 264: 1658 (Apr. 1994).

Drucker, B. J., H. J. Mamon, and T. M. Roberts. Oncogenes, growth factors, and signal transduction. *New England Journal of Medicine* 321: 1383–1391 (1989).

Markman, M. Realistic goals of cancer therapy: Effective and humane care. *Cleveland Clinic Journal of Medicine* 61: 468–472 (1994).

Breast Cancer:

ACOG Committee Opinion. Committee on Gynecologic Practice Number 135—April 1994. Estrogen replacement therapy in women with previously treated breast cancer. *International Journal of Gynaecology & Obstetrics* 45(2): 184–188 (May 1994).

Clark, G. M. The biology of breast cancer in older women. *Journal of Gerontology* 47 (special issue): 19–23 (Nov. 1992).

Dowden, R. V., and R. J. Yetman. Mastectomy with immediate reconstruction: Issues and answers. *Cleveland Clinic Journal of Medicine* 59(5): 499–503 (Sep.–Oct. 1992).

Early Breast Cancer Trialists' Collaborative Group. Systemic treatment of early breast cancer by hormonal, cytotoxic, or immune therapy: 133 randomised trials involving 31,000 recurrences and 24,000 deaths among 75,000 women. *Lancet* 339(8784): 1–15 (Jan. 4, 1992).

Eberlein, T. J. Current management of carcinoma of the breast. *Annals of Surgery* 220(2): 121–136 (Aug. 1994).

Elledge, R. M., G. M. Clark, G. C. Chamness, and C. K. Osborne. Tumor biologic factors and breast cancer prognosis among white, Hispanic, and black women in the United States. *Journal of the National Cancer Institute* 86(9): 705–712 (May 4, 1994).

Futreal, P. A., Q. Liu, D. Shattuck-Eidens, and others. BRCA 1 mutations in primary breast and ovarian cancers. *Science* 266: 120–122 (1994).

Healy, B. Mammograms—Your breasts, your choice. *The Wall Street Journal.* December 28, 1993.

Henderson, I. C. Adjuvant systemic therapy for early breast cancer. *Cancer* 74 (1 Suppl): 401–409 (Jul. 1, 1994).

Heys, S. D., J. M. Eremin, T. K. Sarkar, A. W. Hutcheon, A. Ah-See, and O. Eremin. Role of multimodality therapy in the management of locally advanced carcinoma of the breast. *Journal of the American College of Surgery* 179(4): 493–504 (Oct. 1994).

Hilakivi-Clarke, L. J. Rowland, R. Clarke, and M. E. Lippman. Psychosocial factors in the development and progression of breast cancer. *Breast Cancer Research and Treatment* 29(2): 141–160 (Feb. 1994).

Hortobagyi, G. N. Multidisciplinary management of advanced primary and metastatic breast cancer. *Cancer* 74(1 Suppl): 416–423 (Jul. 1, 1994).

Kerlikowske, K., D. Grady, S. M. Rubin, and others. Efficacy of screening mammography. *Journal of the American Medical Association* 273: 149–154 (1995).

Marchant, D. J. Estrogen-replacement therapy after breast cancer: Risks versus benefits. *Cancer* 71(6 Suppl): 2169–2176 (Mar. 15, 1993).

Meropol, N. J., B. A. Overmoyer, and E. A. Stadmauer. High-dose chemotherapy with autologous stem-cell support for breast cancer. *Oncology* 6:53–60, 63–64 (1992).

Morrow, M. Breast disease in elderly women. *Surgical Clinics of North America* 74(1): 145–161 (Feb. 1994).

Pierce, L. J. and E. Glatstein. Postmastectomy radiotherapy in the management of operable breast cancer. *Cancer* 74(1 Suppl): 477–485 (Jul. 1, 1994).

Pisansky, T. M., M. Y. Halyard, A. L. Weaver, and others. Breast conservation therapy for invasive breast cancer: A review of prior trials and the Mayo Clinic experience. *Mayo Clinic Proceedings* 69(6): 515–524 (Jun. 1994).

Report of the Council on Scientific Affairs. Management of patients with node-negative breast cancer. *Archives of Internal Medicine* 153(1): 58–67 (Jan. 11, 1993).

Winer, E. P. Quality-of-life research in patients with breast cancer. *Cancer* 74 (1 Suppl): 410–415 (Jul. 1, 1994).

Wong, K., I. C. Henderson. Management of metastatic breast cancer. *World Journal of Surgery* 18(1): 98–111 (Jan.–Feb. 1994).

Endometrial Cancer:

Austin, H., C. Drews, and E. E. Partridge. A case-control study of endometrial cancer in relation to cigarette smoking, serum estrogen levels, and alcohol use. *American Journal of Obstetrics & Gynecology* 169(5): 1086–1091 (Nov. 1993).

Creasman, W. T. Adenocarcinoma of the uterine corpus. *Current Opinion in Obstetrics and Gynecology* 5(1): 80–83 (Feb. 1993).

Van Leeuwen, F. E., J. Benraadt, J. W. Coebergh, and others. Risk of endometrial cancer after tamoxifen treatment of breast cancer. *Lancet* 343(8895): 448–452 (Feb. 19, 1994).

Ovarian Cancer:

Bookman, M. A., and R. F. Ozols. Future directions for paclitaxel (TAXOL) in the treatment of ovarian cancer. *Seminars in Oncology Nursing* 9(4 Suppl 2): 21–29 (Nov. 1993).

Byrne, A. and D. N. Carney. Cancer in the elderly. *Current Problems in Cancer* 17(3): 145–218 (May–Jun. 1993).

Cannistra, S. A. Cancer of the ovary. *New England Journal of Medicine* 329(21): 1550–1559 (Nov. 18, 1993).

Gershenson, D. M. Update on malignant ovarian germ cell tumors. *Cancer* 71(4 Suppl): 1581–1590 (Feb. 15, 1993).

Mann, W. J. Diagnosis and management of epithelial cancer of the ovary. *American Family Physician* 49(3): 613–618 (Feb. 15, 1994).

Markman, M. Ovarian cancer update: Management challenges and advances. *Cleveland Clinic Journal of Medicine* 61(1): 51–58 (1994).

Nason, F. G., and B. E. Nelson. Estrogen and progesterone in breast and gynecologic cancers: Etiology, therapeutic role, and hormone replacement. *Obstetrics and Gynecological Clinics of North America* 21(2): 245–270 (Jun. 1994).

NIH develops consensus statement on ovarian cancer. *American Family Physician* 50(1): 213–216 (Jul. 1994).

Ozols, R. F. Treatment of ovarian cancer: Current status. *Seminars in Oncology* 21(2 Suppl 2): 1–9 (Apr. 1994).

Soper, J. T. Management of early-stage epithelial ovarian cancer. *Clinics in Obstetrics and Gynecology* 37(2): 423–438 (Jun. 1994).

Spitzer, G., W. Velasquez, F. R. Dunphy, and V. Spencer. Autologous bone marrow transplantation in solid tumors. *Current Opinion in Oncology* 4(2): 272–278 (Apr. 1992).

Lung Cancer:

Edell, E. S., D. A. Cortese, and J. C. McDougall. Ancillary therapies in the management of lung cancer: Photodynamic therapy, laser therapy, and endobronchial prosthetic devices. *Mayo Clinic Proceedings* 68(7): 685–690 (Jul. 1993).

Green, M. R. New adjuvant strategies for the management of resectable non-small-cell lung cancer. *Chest* 103(4 Suppl): 352S–355S (Apr. 1993).

Hansen, H. H. Management of small-cell cancer of the lung. *Lancet* 339(8797): 846–849 (Apr. 4, 1992).

Jett, J. R. Current treatment of unresectable lung cancer. *Mayo Clinic Proceedings* 68(6): 603–611 (Jun. 1993).

Souhami, R. Lung cancer. *British Medical Journal* 304(6837): 1298–1301 (May 16, 1992).

Colon Cancer:

Giovannucci, E., G. A. Colditz, M. J. Stampfer, and others. A prospective study of cigarette smoking and risk of colorectal adenoma and colorectal cancer in U.S. women. *Journal of the National Cancer Institute* 86(3): 192–199 (1994).

Giovannucci, E., M. J. Stampfer, G. A. Colditz, and others. Folate, methionine, and alcohol intake and risk of colorectal adenoma. *Journal of the National Cancer Institute* 85(11): 875–884 (Jun. 2, 1993).

Heys, S. D., T. J. O'Hanrahan, J. Brittenden, and O. Eremin. Colorectal cancer in young patients: A review of the literature. *European Journal of Surgical Oncology* 20(3): 225–231 (Jun. 1994).

Lipkin, M., and H. Newmark. Effects of added dietary calcium on colonic epithelial proliferation in subjects at high risk for familial colonic cancer. *New England Journal of Medicine* 313: 1381–1384 (1985).

Mandel, J. S., J. H. Bond, T.R. Church, and others. Reduction in the mortality for colorectal cancer by screening for occult blood. *New England Journal of Medicine* 328: 1365–1371 (1993).

Vogelstein, B., E. F. Fearon, S. R. Hamilton, and others. Genetic alterations during colorectal tumor development. *New England Journal of Medicine* 319: 525–532 (1988).

Skin Cancer:

Ackerman, A. B. A critique of an N.I.H. consensus development conference about "early" melanoma. *American Journal of Dermatopathology* 15(1): 52–58 (Feb. 1993).

Black, H. S., J. A. Herd, L.H. Goldberg, and others. Effect of a low-fat diet on the incidence of actinic keratosis. *New England Journal of Medicine* 330(18): 1272–1275 (May 5, 1994).

NIH consensus conference. Diagnosis and treatment of early melanoma. *Journal of the American Medical Association* 268(10): 1314–1319 (1992).

Vargo, N. L. Basal and squamous cell carcinomas: An overview. *Seminars in Oncology Nursing* 7(1): 13–25 (Feb. 1991).

Weinstock, M. A., G. A. Colditz, W. C. Willett, and others. Melanoma and the sun: The effect of swimsuits and a "healthy" tan on the risk of nonfamilial malignant melanoma in women. *American Journal of Epidemiology* 134(5): 462–470 (1991).

Weinstock, M. A., G. A. Colditz, W. C. Willett, and others. Nonfamilial cutaneous melanoma incidence in women associated with sun exposure before 20 years of age. *Pediatrics* 84(2): 199–204 (1989).

Sources

American Academy of Dermatology
930 Meacham Road
Schaumburg, IL 60172
708/330-0230
Fax 708/330-0050

American Cancer Society
National Office
1599 Clifton Road N.E.
Atlanta, GA 30329
404/320-3333
Fax 404/325-2217

American Gastroenterological Association
7910 Woodmont Avenue
Bethesda, MD 20814
301/654-2055

American Lung Association
1740 Broadway
New York, NY 10019
212/315-8700
Fax 212/265-5642

National Cancer Institute
Bethesda, MD 20205
301/496-5583
1-800-4-CANCER (NCI Cancer Information Service Hotline)

Susan G. Komen Foundation
Komen Alliance Clinical Breast Center
3500 Gaston Avenue
Dallas, TX 75246
214/820-2430

CHAPTER 7—DEPRESSION AND ANXIETY: LIVING WITHOUT JOY

Books

Becker, J., and A. Kleinman, eds. *Psychosocial Aspects of Depression*. Hillsdale, N.J.: Lawrence Erlbaum Associates, 1991.

Daffron, C. *Edna St. Vincent Millay*. New York: Chelsea House Publishers, 1989.

Diagnostic and Statistical Manual of Mental Disorders. 4th ed. (DSM-IV). Washington, D.C.: American Psychiatric Association, 1994.

Flach, F., ed. *Affective Disorders*. New York: Norton, 1988.

Gould, J. *The Poet and Her Book: A Biography of Edna St. Vincent Millay*. New York: Dodd, Mead, 1969.

Greist, J. H., and J. W. Jefferson. *Depression and Its Treatment*. Washington, D.C.: American Psychiatric Press, 1992.

Halmi, K. A., ed. *Psychobiology and Treatment of Anorexia Nervosa and Bulimina Nervosa*. Washington, D.C.: American Psychiatric Press, 1992.

Horney, K. *Feminine Psychology*. New York: W. W. Norton, 1967.

Jones, E. *The Life and Works of Sigmund Freud*. 3 parts. New York: Basic Books, 1953–1957.

Kagan, J. *The Nature of the Child*. New York: Basic Books, HarperCollins, 1994. (Superb look at temperament and personality development in the child.)

Katon, W. *Panic Disorder in the Medical Setting*. U.S. Department of Health and Human Services. National Institute of Mental Health. 1989. Washington, D.C.: U.S. Government Printing Office, DHHS Publication, no. 89–1629.

Kramer, P. *Listening to Prozac: A Psychiatrist Explores Antidepressant Drugs and the Remaking of the Self*. New York: Viking, 1993.

McGrath, E., ed. *Women and Depression: Risk Factors and Treatment Issues*. Final Report of the American Psychological Association's National Task Force on Women and Depression. Washington, D.C.: American Psychological Association, 1990.

Millay, Edna St. Vincent. *Collected Poems*. New York: Harper & Row, 1956.

Montagu, A. *The Natural Superiority of Women*. New York: Collier Books/Maxwell Macmillan International, 1992. Originally published by Macmillan, 1954.

Paykel, E. S., ed. *Handbook of Affective Disorders*. 2nd ed. New York and London: The Guilford Press, 1992.

Rosenthal, Norman E. *Seasons of the Mind: Why You Get the Winter Blues & What You Can Do About It*. New York: Guilford Press, 1993.

Articles

Blumenthal, S. Women and depression. *Journal of Women's Health* 3(6): 467–479 (1994).

Coleman, P. M. Depression during the female climacteric period. *Journal of Advanced Nursing* 18(10): 1540–1546 (Oct. 1993).

Gonsalves, L., J. Domb, and G. Gidwani. Depression, chronic fatigue, and the premenstrual syndrome. *Primary Care* 18(2): 369–380 (Jun. 1991).

Gregg, R. Choice as a double-edged sword: Information, guilt and mother-blaming in a high-tech age. *Women and Health* 20(3): 53–73 (1993).

Hauenstein, E. J. Young women and depression: Origin, outcome, and nursing care. *Nursing Clinics of North America* 26(3): 601–612 (Sept. 1991).

Kendler, K. S., M. C. Neale, R. C. Kessler, A. C. Heath, and L. J. Eaves. A population-based twin study of major depression in women: The impact of varying definitions of illness. *Archives of General Psychiatry* 49: 257–266 (1992).

NIH Consensus Conference. Diagnosis and treatment of depression in late life. *Journal of the American Medical Association* 268: 1018–1024 (Aug. 1992).

Notman, M. T., and C. C. Nadelson. Personality development and psychopathology. *Journal of Women's Health* 3(6): 459–466 (1994).

Tesar, G. E. Assessing depression in medical patients. *Cleveland Clinic Journal of Medicine* 61: 174–175 (1994).

Tesar, G. E., and J. F. Rosenbaum. Recognition and treatment of panic disorder. *Advances in Internal Medicine* 38: 123–149 (1993).

Wollersheim, J. P. Depression, women, and the workplace. *Occupational Medicine* 8(4): 787–795 (Oct.–Dec. 1993).

Yonkers, K. A. Panic disorders in women. *Journal of Women's Health* 3(6): 481–486 (1994).

Sources

American Academy of Psychoanalysis
170 E. 77th Street
New York, NY 10023
212/475-7980

American Psychiatric Association
1400 K Street N.W.
Washington, DC 20005
202/682-6000
Fax 202/682-6114

National Alliance for the Mentally Ill (NAMI)
2101 Wilson Blvd.
Arlington, VA 22203-3754
800/950-6264 or 703/524-7600

National Depressive and Manic Depressive Association
730 Franklin Street
Chicago, IL 60610
312/624-0049

National Institute of Mental Health
5600 Fisher Lane
Rockville, MD 20857
301/443-4513

CHAPTER 8—HEART DISEASE: A WOMAN'S PROFILE

Books

Pashkow, F. C., and C. Libov. *The Woman's Heart Book: The Complete Guide to Keeping Your Heart Healthy and What to Do If Things Go Wrong.* New York: Dutton/Penguin, 1993.

Schlant, R. C. et al. *Hurst the Heart.* 8th ed. New York: Healthcare Management Group/McGraw-Hill, 1993.

Topol, E. J., ed. *Textbook of Interventional Cardiology.* Philadelphia: W. B. Saunders, 1994.

Weiner, F. *Recovering at Home with a Heart Condition: A Practical Guide for You and Your Family.* New York: Body Press/Perigee, 1994.

Articles

Barry, P. Coronary artery disease in older women. *Geriatrics* 48(Suppl 1): 4–8 (Jun. 1993).

Dec, G. W., and V. Fuster. Medical progress: Idiopathic dilated cardiomyopathy. *New England Journal of Medicine* 331:1564–1575 (Dec. 1994).

Eaker, E. D., J. Pinsky, and W. P. Castelli. Myocardial infarction and coronary death among women: Psychosocial predictors from a 20-year follow-up of women in the Framingham Study. *American Journal of Epidemiology* 135(8): 854–864 (Apr. 15, 1992).

Eaker, E. D., J. H. Chesebro, F. M. Sacks, and others. Cardiovascular disease in women. *Circulation* 88(4 pt. 1): 1999–2009 (Oct. 1993).

Eysmann, S. B., and P. S. Douglas. Reperfusion and revascularization strategies for coronary artery disease in women. *Journal of the American Medical Association* 268(14): 1903–1907 (Oct. 14, 1992).

Forman, D. E., and J. Y. Wei. MI: Making therapeutic choices when the options are unclear. *Geriatrics* 48(7): 32–38, 43–45 (Jul. 1993).

Gore, J. M., and J. E. Dalen. Cardiovascular disease. *Journal of the American Medical Association* 271(1): 1660–1661 (Jun. 1, 1994).

The GUSTO Investigators. An international randomized trial comparing four thrombolytic strategies for acute myocardial infarction. *New England Journal of Medicine* 329(10): 673–682 (Sep. 2, 1993).

Kostis, J. B., A. C. Wilson, K. O'Dowd, and others. Sex differences in the management and long-term outcome of acute myocardial infarction: A statewide study. MIDAS Study Group. Myocardial Infarction Data Acquisition System. *Circulation* 90(4): 1715–1730 (Oct. 1994).

Krummel, D., T. D. Etherton, S. Peterson, and P. M. Kris-Etherton. Effects of exercise on plasma lipids and lipoproteins of women. *Proceedings of the Society for Experimental Biology and Medicine.* 204(2): 123–137 (Nov. 1993).

Morris, D. L., S. B. Kritchevsky, and C. E. Davis. Serum carotenoids and coronary heart disease: The Lipid Research Clinics' coronary primary prevention trial and follow-up study. *Journal of the American Medical Association* 272: 1439–1441 (1994). (All male study.)

Ness, R. B., I. Cosmatos, and K. M. Flegal. Gravidity and serum lipids among Hispanic women in the Hispanic Health and Nutrition Examination Survey. *Journal of Women's Health* 4(2): in press (1995).

Robinson, K., E. Mayer, and W. Jacobsen. Homocysteine and coronary artery disease. *Cleveland Clinic Journal of Medicine* 61:438–450 (1994).

Topol, E. J., R. M. Califf. Thrombolytic therapy for elderly patients. *New England Journal of Medicine* 327(1): 45–47 (Jul. 2, 1992).

Weintraub, W. S., N. K. Wenger, A. S. Kosinski, and others. Percutaneous transluminal coronary angioplasty in women compared with men. *Journal of the American College of Cardiology* 24(1): 81–90 (Jul. 1994).

Pamphlet

Cleveland Clinic Foundation. *How to Choose a Doctor and Hospital If You Have Coronary Artery Disease.* For copies, contact John Clough, M.D., Director, Health Affairs, The Cleveland Clinic Foundation, 9500 Euclid Avenue, Cleveland, OH 44195.

Sources

American College of Cardiology
9111 Old Georgetown Road
Bethesda, MD 20814
301/897-5400

American Heart Association
National Center
7272 Greenville Avenue

Dallas, TX 75231
214/373-6300
Fax 214/706-1341
Note: 800/AHA-USA1 (800/242-8721)—this toll-free number will get you in touch
with the AHA office nearest to you.

National Institutes of Health
National Heart, Lung and Blood Institute
4733 Bethesda Avenue, Suite 530
Bethesda, MD 20814
301/951-3260

CHAPTER 9—STROKE: THE ENDLESS DAY

Books

American Heart Association. *Heart and Stroke Facts.* Dallas, Tex.: 1994. (Up-
dated yearly.)

Dunkle, R. E., and J. W. Schmidley, eds. *Stroke in the Elderly: New Issues in Diagnosis, Treatment and Rehabilitation.* New York: Springer Publishing, 1987.

Gordon, W. A. *Advances in Stroke Rehabilitation.* Stoneham, Mass: Butterworth-
Heinemann/Reed International Books, 1993.

Kasell, P., ed. *The Best of the Stroke Connection.* Golden Valley, Minn.: Courage
Press, 1990.

Singleton, L. *The Black Health Library Guide to Stroke.* New York: Henry Holt,
1993.

Toole, J. F. *Cerebrovascular Disorders.* 4th ed. New York: Raven Press, 1990.

Articles

Amarenco, P., A. Cohen, C. Tzourio, and others. Atherosclerotic disease of the
aortic arch and the risk of ischemic stroke. *New England Journal of Medicine*
331: 1474–1479 (Dec. 1994); and accompanying editorial by J. P. Kistler. The
risk of embolic stroke, 1517–1519.

Couch, J. R. Antiplatelet therapy in the treatment of cerebrovascular disease. *Clinical Cardiology* 16(10): 703–710 (Oct. 1993).

Covinsky, K. E., L. Goldman, E. F. Cook, and others for the SUPPORT Investigators. The impact of serious illness on patients and families. *Journal of the
American Medical Association* 272(23): 1839–1844 (December 21, 1994).

Dalen, J. E. Atrial fibrillation: Reducing stroke risk with low-dose anticoagulation. *Geriatrics* 49(5): 24–26, 29–32 (May 1994). (This is an article on long-
term warfarin.)

Davis, P. Stroke in women. *Current Opinion in Neurology* 7(1): 36–40 (Feb. 1994).

Downhill, J. E., Jr., and R. G. Robinson. Longitudinal assessment of depression and cognitive impairments following stroke. *Journal of Nervous & Mental Disease* 182(8): 425–431 (Aug. 1994).

Dyken, M. L. Controversies in stroke: Past and present—The Willis Lecture. *Stroke* 24:1251–1258 (1993).

Eaker, E. D., J. H. Chesebro, F. M. Sacks, and others. Cardiovascular disease in women. *Circulation* 88(4 pt. 1): 1999–2009 (Oct. 1993).

Grady, D., S. M. Rubin, D. B. Petitti, and others. Hormone therapy to prevent disease and prolong life in postmenopausal women. *Annals of Internal Medicine* 117(12): 1016–1037 (Dec. 15, 1992).

Hachinski, V. C. Stroke and hypertension and its prevention. *American Journal of Hypertension* 4(2 pt. 2): 118S–120S (Feb. 1991).

Higa, M., and Z. Davanipour. Smoking and stroke. *Neuroepidemiology* 10(4): 211–222 (1991).

Kaira, L. Does age affect benefits of stroke unit rehabilitation? *Stroke* 25(2): 346–351 (Feb. 1994).

Kittner, S. J., R. J. McCarter, R. W. Sherwin, and others. Black-white differences in stroke risk among young adults. *Stroke* 24(12 Suppl): I13–I15; discussion I20–I21 (Dec. 1993).

Lindeberg, S., and B. Lundh. Apparent absence of stroke and ischemic heart disease in a traditional Melanesian island: A clinical study in Kitava. *Journal of Internal Medicine* 233: 269–275 (1993).

Lindestrom, E., B. Gudrun, and J. Nyboe. Lifestyle factors and risk of cerebrovascular disease in women. The Copenhagen City Heart Study. *Stroke* 24: 1468–1472 (1993).

McAnally, L. E., C. R. Corn, and S. F. Hamilton. Aspirin for the prevention of vascular death in women. *Annals of Pharmacotherapy* 26(12): 1530–1534 (Dec. 1992).

Meade, T. W. and A. Berra. Hormone replacement therapy and cardiovascular disease. *British Medical Bulletin* 48(2): 276–308 (Apr. 1992).

Palmer, A. J., C. J. Bulpitt, A. E. Fletcher, and others. Relation between blood pressure and stroke mortality. *Hypertension* 20(5): 601–605 (Nov. 1992).

Pearson, M. L., K. L. Kahn, E. R. Harrison, and others. Differences in quality of care for hospitalized elderly men and women. *Journal of the American Medical Association* 268(14): 1883–1889 (Oct. 14, 1992).

Pamphlet

Cleveland Clinic Foundation. *Stroke: Are You at High Risk?* (one in the series of pamphlets *How to Choose a Doctor and Hospital . . .*). For copies, contact John Clough, M.D., Director, Health Affairs, The Cleveland Clinic Foundation, 9500 Euclid Avenue, Cleveland, OH 44195.

Sources

American Heart Association
National Center
7272 Greenville Avenue
Dallas, TX 75231
214/373-6300
Fax 214/706-1341
Note: 800/AHA-USA1 (800/242-8721)—this toll-free number will get you in
touch with the AHA office nearest to you.

American Physical Therapy Association
1111 N. Fairfax Street
Alexandria, VA 22314
703/684-2782

National Easter Seal Society
70 East Lake Street
Chicago, IL 60601
800/221-6827

National Institutes of Health
National Institute of Neurological Disorders and Stroke (NINDS)
Bldg. 31, Room 8A54
9000 Rockville Pike
Bethesda, MD 20892-2540
800/352-9424 or 301/496-5751

National Stroke Association
300 East Hampden Avenue
Englewood, CO 80110
800/367-1990 or 303/771-1700

The Stroke Foundation, Inc.
898 Park Avenue
New York, NY 10021
212/734-3461

CHAPTER 10—OSTEOPOROSIS: FRAGILE BONES

Books

Kamen, B., and S. Kamen. *Osteoporosis: What It Is, How to Prevent It, How to Stop It*. New York: Pinnacle Books, 1984.

Perry, H. M. III, J. E. Morley, and M. C. Rodney, eds. *Aging and Musculoskeletal Disorders*. New York: Springer Publishing, 1993.

U.S. Congress. Senate. Committee on Labor and Human Resources. Subcommittee on Aging. *Osteoporosis: Hearing before the Subcommittee on Aging of the Committee on Labor and Human Resources: On reviewing the diagnosis and treatment of osteoporosis*. 99th Cong. 1st sess., June 10, 1985. Washington, D.C.: U.S. Government Printing Office, 1985.

U.S. Congress. Office of Technology Assessment. *Public Information About Osteoporosis: What's Available and What's Needed?* Washington D.C.: U.S. Government Printing Office, July 1994. Publ. no. 052-003-01381-9.

U.S. Food and Drug Administration: National Conference on Women's Health Series. 1987. *A Special Topic Conference: Osteoporosis*. Washington, D.C.: U.S. Government Printing Office. Shipping list no. 87-638-p.

Articles

Allen, S. H. Primary osteoporosis: Methods to combat bone loss that accompanies aging. *Postgraduate Medicine* 93(8): 43–46, 49–50, 53–55 (Jun. 1993).

Baran, D. T. Magnitude and determinants of premenopausal bone loss. *Osteoporosis International* 4 (Suppl 1): 31–34 (1994).

Belchetz, P. E. Hormonal treatment of postmenopausal women. *New England Journal of Medicine* 330(15): 1062–1071 (Apr. 14, 1994).

Craik, R. L. Disability following hip fracture. *Physical Therapy* 74(5): 387–398 (May 1994).

Felson, D. T., Y. Shang, M. T. Hannan, and others. The effect of postmenopausal estrogen therapy on bone density in elderly women. *New England Journal of Medicine* 329: 1141–1146 (1993).

Gambrell, R. D., Jr. Update on hormone replacement therapy. *American Family Physician* 46(5 Suppl): 87S–96S (Nov. 1992).

Harris, S. S., and B. Dawson-Hughes. Caffeine and bone loss in healthy postmenopausal women. *American Journal of Clinical Nutrition* 60(4): 573–578 (Oct. 1994).

Johnson, K., and E. W. Kligman. Preventive nutrition: Disease-specific dietary interventions for older adults. *Geriatrics* 47(11): 39–40, 45–49 (Nov. 1992); and Preventive nutrition: An "optimal" diet for older adults. *Geriatrics* 47(10): 56–60 (Oct. 1992).

Johnston, C. D., C. W. Slemenda, and J. L. Melton III. Clinical use of bone densitometry. *New England Journal of Medicine* 374:1105–1109 (1991).

Krall, E. A., and B. Dawson-Hughes. Smoking and bone loss among postmenopausal women. *Journal of Bone and Mineral Research* 6: 331–338 (1991).

Licata, A. A. Prevention and osteoporosis management. *Cleveland Clinic Journal of Medicine* 61: 451–460 (1994).

McNeeley, S. G., Jr., J. S. Schinfeld, T. G. Stovall, F. W. Ling, and B. H. Buxton. Prevention of osteoporosis by medroxyprogesterone acetate in postmenopausal women. *International Journal of Gynaecology & Obstetrics* 34: 3253–3256 (Mar. 1991).

Meunier, P. J., M. C. Chapuy, M. E. Arlot, P. D. Delmas, and F. Duboeuf. Can we stop bone loss and prevent hip fractures in the elderly? *Osteoporosis International* 4 (Suppl 1): 71–76 (1994).

Morrison, N. A., J. C. Qi, A. Tikita, and others. Predictions of bone density from vitamin D receptor alleles. *Nature* 367: 284–287 (1994).

Nelson, M. E., M. A. Fiatarone, C. M. Morgani, and others. Effect of high-intensity strength training on multiple risk factors for osteoporotic fractures: A randomized controlled trial. *Journal of the American Medical Association* 272: 1909–1914 (1994).

NIH Consensus Development on optimal calcium intake. *Journal of the American Medical Association* 272: 1942–1948 (1994).

Odell, W. D., and H. Heath. 3d. Osteoporosis: Pathophysiology, prevention, diagnosis, and treatment. *Disease-a-Month* 39(11): 789–867 (Nov. 1993).

Putukian, M. The female triad: Eating disorders, amenorrhea, and osteoporosis. *Medical Clinics of North America* 78(2): 345–356 (Mar. 1994).

Riggs, B. L. Overview of osteoporosis. *Western Journal of Medicine* 154(1): 63–77 (Jan. 1991).

Slemenda, C. W., J. C. Christian, C. J. Williams, and others. Genetic determinants of bone mass in adult women. *Journal of Bone Mineral Research* 6: 561–567 (1991).

Wardlaw, G. M. Putting osteoporosis in perspective. *Journal of the American Dietetic Association* 93(9): 1000–1006 (Sep. 1993).

Sources

National Institute of Arthritis and Musculoskeletal and Skin Diseases
Bldg. 31, Room 4C05
9000 Rockville Pike
Bethesda, MD 20892
301/496-8188

National Institute on Aging
Information Center
P.O. Box 8057
Gaithersburg, MD 20898-8057
301/496-1752

National Osteoporosis Foundation
2100 M Street N.W.
Washington, DC 20037
202/223-3336

CHAPTER 11—ALZHEIMER'S DISEASE:
THE ENDLESS NIGHT

Books

Gruetzner, H. *Alzheimer's: A Caregiver's Guide and Sourcebook.* New York: Wiley, 1992.

Mace, N., and P. Rabins. *The 36-Hour Day. A Family Guide to Caring for Persons with Alzheimer's Disease, Related Dementing Illnesses and Memory Loss in Later Life.* Baltimore: Johns Hopkins, 1991.

McGowin, D. F. *Living in the Labyrinth. A Personal Journey Through the Maze of Alzheimer's.* New York: Delacorte Press, 1993.

U.S. Congress. Office of Technology Assessment. *Confused Minds, Burdened Families: Finding Help for People with Alzheimer's and Other Dementias.* Washington D.C.: U.S. Government Printing Office, 1990.

U.S. Department of Health and Human Services. National Institutes of Health. 1993. *Advisory Panel on Alzheimer's Disease. Fourth Report to the Advisory Panel on Alzheimer's Disease.* NIH Publication no. 93-3520.

Articles

Bennett, D. A., and D. A. Evans. Alzheimer's disease. *Disease-a-Month* 38(1): 1–64 (Jan. 1992).

Breitner, J. C., B. A. Gau, K. A. Welsh, and others. Inverse association of anti-inflammatory treatments and Alzheimer's disease: Initial results of a co-twin control study. *Neurology* 44(2): 227–232 (Feb. 1994).

Caralis, P. V. Ethical and legal issues in the care of Alzheimer's patients. *Medical Clinics of North America* 78(4): 877–893 (Jul. 1994).

Collins, C. E., B. A. Given, and C. W. Given. Interventions with family caregivers of persons with Alzheimer's disease. *Nursing Clinics of North America* 29(1): 195–207 (Mar. 1994).

Katzman, R. Education and the prevalence of dementia and Alzheimer's disease. *Neurology* 43(1): 13–20 (Jan. 1993).

Murphy, M. The molecular pathogenesis of Alzheimer's disease: Clinical prospects. *Lancet* 340(8834–8835): 1512–1515 (Dec. 19–26, 1992).

Perls, T. T. The oldest old. *Scientific American* 272(1): 70–75 (Jan. 1995).

Rocca, W. A. Frequency, distribution, and risk factors for Alzheimer's disease. *Nursing Clinics of North America* 29(1): 101–111 (Mar. 1994).

Rosenberg, R. N. A causal role for amyloid in Alzheimer's disease: The end of the beginning. *Neurology* 43(5): 851–856 (May 1993).

Roth, M. E. Advances in Alzheimer's disease. A review for the family physician. *Journal of Family Practice* 37(6): 593–607 (Dec. 1993).

Schneider, L. S. and P. N. Tariot. Emerging drugs for Alzheimer's disease: Mechanisms of action and prospects for cognitive enhancing medications. *Medical Clinics of North America* 78(4): 911–934 (Jul. 1994).

Suhr, S. T., and F. H. Gage. Gene therapy for neurologic disease. *Archives of Neurology* 50(11): 1252–1268 (Nov. 1993).

Van Dijk, P. T., D. W. Dippel, and J. D. Habbema. Survival of patients with dementia. *Journal of the American Geriatrics Society* 39(6): 603–610 (Jun. 1991).

Vellas, B. J., J. L. Albarede, and P. J. Garry. Diseases and aging: Patterns of morbidity with age; relationship between aging and age-associated diseases. *American Journal of Clinical Nutrition* 55(6 Suppl): 1225S–1230S (Jun. 1992).

Vitiello, M. V., D. L. Bliwise, and P. N. Prinz. Sleep in Alzheimer's disease and the sundown syndrome. *Neurology* 42(7 Suppl 6): 83–93; discussion 93–94 (Jul. 1992).

Yi, E. S., I. L. Abraham, and S. Holroyd. Alzheimer's disease and nursing. New scientific and clinical insights. *Nursing Clinics of North America* 29(1): 85–99 (Mar. 1994).

Sources

Alzheimer's Association
919 N. Michigan Avenue, Suite 1000
Chicago, IL 60611
800/272-3900

Alzheimer's Disease Education and Referral Center
P.O. Box 8250
Silver Spring, MD 20907
301/495-3311

American Association of Retired Persons (AARP)
601 E Street N.W.
Washington, DC 20049
202/434-2277

National Institutes of Health
National Institute on Aging
9000 Rockville Pike
Bethesda, MD 20892
800/222-2225 (Information Center)

National Institutes of Health
National Institute of Neurological Disorders and Stroke
Bldg. 31, Room 8A06
9000 Rockville Pike
Bethesda, MD 20892
800/352-9424

INDEX